COMBINATION THERAPY FOR ASTHMA AND CHRONIC OBSTRUCTIVE PULMONARY DISEASE

LUNG BIOLOGY IN HEALTH AND DISEASE

Executive Editor

Claude Lenfant
Director, National Heart, Lung and Blood Institute
National Institutes of Health
Bethesda, Maryland

COMBINATION THERAPY FOR ASTHMA AND CHRONIC OBSTRUCTIVE PULMONARY DISEASE

Edited by

Richard J. Martin
Monica Kraft

National Jewish Medical and Research Center
Denver, Colorado

MARCEL DEKKER, INC.   NEW YORK · BASEL

BS

ISBN: 0-8247-0371-5

This book is printed on acid-free paper.

Headquarters
Marcel Dekker, Inc.
270 Madison Avenue, New York, NY 10016
tel: 212-696-9000; fax: 212-685-4540

Eastern Hemisphere Distribution
Marcel Dekker AG
Hutgasse 4, Postfach 812, CH-4001 Basel, Switzerland
tel: 41-61-261-8482; fax: 41-61-261-8896

World Wide Web
http://www.dekker.com

The publisher offers discounts on this book when ordered in bulk quantities. For more information, write to Special Sales/Professional Marketing at the headquarters address above.

Current printing (last digit):
10 9 8 7 6 5 4 3 2 1

PRINTED IN THE UNITED STATES OF AMERICA

07-01-02

INTRODUCTION

Asthma is a very "old" disease. Although many credit Moses Maimonides' (1135–1204) famous *Treatise on Asthma* with its first description, Hippocrates (460–375 B.C.) actually appears to have described it first in his *Corpus Hippocraticum*. The reason for this "error" is that at first asthma (or asma, as it was then called) was viewed as a symptom (panting or shortness of breath) rather than a disease.

In contrast, chronic obstructive pulmonary disease (COPD) is a much more recent disease entity. The anatomical features of emphysema—a close cousin of COPD—were first described by Matthew Baillie in 1793 (in *The Morbid Anatomy of Some of the Most Important Parts of the Human Body*). The first use of the term COPD, however, appears to have been by William A. Briscoe in 1965 (1), who used it to describe a condition characterized by chronic cough and expectoration associated with reduced airflow as measured by the forced expiratory volume during a fixed time period (i.e., 1 second). Since then, the definition of COPD has been extensively discussed, modified, and refined. Nonetheless, it appears that universal agreement on what precisely defines this condition has yet to be achieved. This is important because it bears on the best treatment options for COPD.

During the past two decades, many advances have been made in the treatment of patients with asthma and COPD. With regard to the former, the recognition that asthma is essentially an inflammatory disease led to many new and systematic therapeutic approaches that have provided significant improvements in patient care. These progressive advances have been reported in many volumes of the Lung Biology in Health and Disease series.

Similarly, since its inception, this series has published a number of volumes on COPD. The first (Vol. 9), *Chronic Obstructive Lung Disease,* edited by Thomas L. Petty and published in 1978, contains a chapter entitled "Respiratory and Pharmacologic Therapy in COPD." It demonstrates strikingly the commonality of some pharmacological agents used in the treatment of asthma and COPD; indeed, bronchodilators (such as theophylline) and anti-inflammatory drugs (such as cromolyn sodium and steroids) are part of the armamentarium used in both diseases. That, however, was in 1978! Today we know much more about the use and effectiveness of these and other agents, either alone or in combination, in asthma and in COPD. However, because there are more therapeutic options, there may be more uncertainty, if not confusion, about what modifications to prescribe and when to prescribe them.

This volume addresses these questions. The editors, Drs. Richard Martin and Monica Kraft, both from the National Jewish Medical and Research Center in Denver, Colorado, have assembled well-recognized experts in the specific pharmacological agents that are discussed. I believe the theme of this volume is novel and unique, and it is a most valuable addition to the Lung Biology in Health and Disease series. There is no doubt that, as the editors state in their Preface, this volume "will assist clinicians in making the best treatment choices for their patients, which ultimately will improve their quality of life."

Claude Lenfant, M.D.
Bethesda, Maryland

Reference

1.   Briscoe WA, Nash ES. The slow space in chronic obstructive pulmonary disease. Ann NY Acad Sci 1965; 121:706–722.

PREFACE

Understanding of the pathophysiology of asthma and chronic obstructive pulmonary disease (COPD) has greatly increased over the past decade. Because of this explosion of knowledge, treatment strategies have also changed. It is now known that inflammation is a significant component of both disease processes, especially asthma. Therefore, use of anti-inflammatory agents has become the mainstay of therapy for asthma and some cases of COPD. However, we have also learned that these medications are not without significant side effects, particularly after long-term use. This information has led us to the use of combination therapy for both disease processes. We now know that, in asthma, the combination of inhaled corticosteroids and long-acting β_2-agonists, theophylline, and leukotriene modifiers can result in a "steroid-sparing" effect—decreased corticosteroid requirement and side effects for the same efficacy.

Recently, knowledge has been acquired about the use of anticholinergic medications (a class of medications typically reserved for patients with COPD) in acute asthma. The treatment of COPD has also expanded to include the combination of inhaled β_2-agonists plus anticholinergics with or without theophylline and corticosteroids. Leukotriene modifiers may also benefit this population, but the literature is still sparse in this area.

The objective of this book is to examine the therapies used in the treatment of asthma and COPD separately, in combination, and in regard to dose timing. In addition to mechanistic information, chapters shed light on the efficacy of using several therapeutic agents, describing the literature in these areas. We hope that this information will assist clinicians in making the best treatment choices for their patients, which ultimately will improve their quality of life.

Richard J. Martin
Monica Kraft

CONTRIBUTORS

Gilbert E. D'Alonzo, D.O.   Professor, Department of Medicine, Temple University School of Medicine, Philadelphia, Pennsylvania

Gordon Dent, Ph.D.   Division of Respiratory Cell and Molecular Biology, University of Southampton School of Medicine, Southampton, England

Jeffrey M. Drazen, M.D.   Division of Pulmonary and Critical Care, Department of Medicine, Brigham and Women's Hospital and Harvard Medical School, Boston, Massachusetts

Monica Kraft, M.D.   Department of Medicine, National Jewish Medical and Research Center, Denver, Colorado

Alan R. Leff, M.D.   Professor and Chief, Section of Critical Care Medicine, Department of Medicine, The University of Chicago, Chicago, Illinois

Richard J. Martin, M.D. Department of Medicine, National Jewish Medical and Research Center, Denver, Colorado

Klaus F. Rabe, M.D. Chairman and Head, Department of Pulmonology, Leiden University Medical Center, Leiden, The Netherlands

Alain E. Reinberg, M.D., Ph.D. Unité de Chronobiologie et Chronopharmacologie, Fondation Adolph de Rothschild, Paris, France

Stephen I. Rennard, M.D. Pulmonary Division, Department of Internal Medicine, University of Nebraska Medical Center, Omaha, Nebraska

Michael H. Smolensky, Ph.D. Professor, School of Public Health, University of Texas Health Science Center, Houston, Texas

Joseph D. Spahn, M.D. Divisions of Clinical Pharmacology and Allergy–Clinical Immunology, Department of Pediatrics, National Jewish Medical and Research Center, Denver, Colorado

Mary E. Strek, M.D. Assistant Professor, Department of Medicine, The University of Chicago, Chicago, Illinois

E. Rand Sutherland, M.D. Department of Medicine, National Jewish Medical and Research Center, Denver, Colorado

Stanley J. Szefler, M.D. Divisions of Clinical Pharmacology and Allergy–Clinical Immunology, Department of Pediatrics, National Jewish Medical and Research Center, Denver, Colorado

Michael E. Wechsler, M.D. Division of Pulmonary and Critical Care, Department of Medicine, Brigham and Women's Hospital and Harvard Medical School, Boston, Massachusetts

CONTENTS

Contents *xi*

1

Inhaled Glucocorticoids

JOSEPH D. SPAHN and STANLEY J. SZEFLER

National Jewish Medical and Research Center
Denver, Colorado

I. Introduction

Glucocorticoids (GC) are among the most potent and effective class of medications available for use in both the acute and chronic manifestations of asthma (1,2). As outlined below, they have been used in the treatment of asthma for nearly 50 years, long before a rationale was developed to explain their actions (3–5). Much of the early enthusiasm regarding oral GC therapy in asthma was dampened with the realization that long-term use resulted in a number of debilitating adverse effects. Therefore, research was directed toward reducing the side-effect profile by delivering GC directly into the airway. Within 20 years, potent GCs delivered via effective metered-dose inhalers (MDIs) were developed and have revolutionized the way we care for asthmatics. No other asthma medication available today can improve asthma symptoms, decrease morbidity, improve baseline pulmonary function, and reduce BHR to the same extent as inhaled GC therapy can. In addition, by virtue of the fact that small quantities of GC are delivered topically, the incidence of adverse effects is greatly diminished compared to chronically administered oral GC therapy. This chapter provides a brief history of the development of inhaled GC, the mechanisms of inhaled glucocorticoid action, an overview of their clinical efficacy, followed by a discussion of their potential for adverse effects.

II. History

The first attempt to administer GC by the inhaled route came in 1951, when Gelfand reported improvement in four of five asthmatics treated with aerosolized cortisone suspended in saline (6) (Fig. 1). The effect was likely due to systemic absorption of the drug, in that very large doses (50 mg) were used. In contrast, a subsequent double-blind placebo-controlled study evaluating aerosolized hydrocortisone hemisuccinate at a much lower dose (15 mg/day) failed to show significant improvement in asthma symptoms compared to placebo (7). Other studies evaluating hydrocortisone and prednisolone in the late 1950s and early 1960s showed variable effects, but the general consensus was that these drugs were not effective, either because of insufficient potency of the GC used, inefficient delivery of the drug to the lower airway, or rapid clearance of the GC from the bronchial tree (8).

The decade of the 1960s heralded the development of both the "modern" pressurized MDI, which effectively delivered GCs to the lower airway, and the development of dexamethasone, a potent GC. Shortly after its release, several studies demonstrated that dexamethasone delivered topically via a pMDI (Decadron Respihaler®) resulted in improved asthma control and significant oral GC dose reduction in those with steroid-dependent asthma (9–12). Unfortunately, not all patients demonstrated improvement in asthma con-

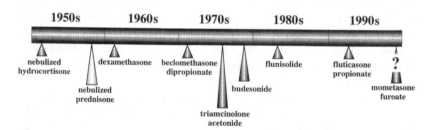

Figure 1 Time line of glucocorticoid development in the treatment of asthma. Note that mometasone furoate is currently undergoing Phase III clinical trials and may be approved for use before the millennium.

trol and/or oral GC dose reduction. Children and adolescents appeared to respond more favorably than adults, as did those with a recent diagnosis of asthma.

The recognition that inhaled dexamethasone therapy resulted in significant adverse effects came soon after its introduction. In fact, many of the initial studies demonstrating dexamethasone's efficacy found it to significantly suppress the hypothalamic-pituitary-adrenal (HPA) axis. Dennis and Itkin (12) made the important observation that despite significant oral GC dose reduction, many steroid-dependent asthmatics continue to display cushingoid stigmata while they are on inhaled dexamethasone. Of interest, these investigators were also the first to describe oral and laryngeal candidiasis as complications of inhaled GC therapy. In retrospect, these findings are not surprising, given that the amount of inhaled dexamethasone required for clinical efficacy was similar in magnitude to the dexamethasone equivalent dose of the oral GC that many of these patients were on. Thus, although effective, inhaled dexamethasone did not offer significant advantages over oral GC in terms of providing superior topical to systemic potency (13).

The first inhaled steroid to offer superior topical to systemic potency was beclomethasone dipropionate (BDP). BDP was initially developed as a topical GC for use in atopic dermatitis, but by the early 1970s a pressurized MDI delivering BDP at a dose of 50 µg per actuation was developed. In 1972, two open-label studies found inhaled BDP to have potent oral GC–sparing effects in patients with steroid-dependent asthma (14,15). Associated with significant reductions in oral GC dose were improvements in pulmonary function, decreased diurnal variability in peak expiratory flow rates, and less need for supplemental bronchodilator use. Of importance, BDP therapy did not result in suppression of the HPA axis. Furthermore, many steroid-dependent asthmatics treated with BDP developed steroid withdrawal syndrome as their oral steroid dose was tapered and eventually discontinued. Patients also reported exacerbations of their eczema and/or allergic rhinitis as their oral steroid dose was discontinued; in some cases, the patient's cushingoid stigmata disappeared. These observations strengthened the concept that BDP's efficacy came from its topical effects.

Controlled studies soon followed that confirmed the above findings (16–19). In a classic study from the Medical Research Council published in 1974 (16), BDP (400 and 800 µg/day) was found to be superior to placebo in terms of oral GC reduction and asthma symptoms in a large number of steroid-dependent asthmatics. This study was among the first to demonstrate dose-dependent effects of inhaled GC therapy, both in terms of clinical efficacy and adverse effects, with a greater percentage of patients tapered off oral GC therapy and a greater incidence of oral candidiasis in those treated with high-dose BDP compared to those treated with low-dose BDP. Another large double-blind, placebo-controlled study evaluated the long-term effects of inhaled BDP, betamethasone valerate, or orally administered prednisone (17). The investigators found the inhaled GCs to be as effective as prednisone in the management of severe asthma. In addition, a daily dose of 400 µg/day of BDP was found to be equivalent to 7.5 mg/day of prednisone, but without the adverse effects.

These studies laid the foundation for the acceptability and widespread use of inhaled GC therapy for chronic asthma. Over the ensuing 20–25 years, several other potent topical steroids—such as flunisolide, triamcinolone acetonide, budesonide (BUD), and fluticasone propionate—have become available for use in asthma. The concomitant use of spacer devices has further contributed to the optimization of topical effects while minimizing systemic effects. We now have a good understanding of the clinical efficacy and the potential for adverse effects associated with inhaled GC therapy in asthma. Great strides have also been made in our understanding of the mechanism(s) of GC action both at the molecular and cellular levels. The following sections briefly discuss the progress made regarding each of these areas.

III. Mechanisms of Action

A. Effects at the Molecular Level

Given their lipid composition, GCs are readily absorbed, diffusing easily across the cell membrane. Once inside the cytoplasm, they bind with high affinity to a specific intracytoplasmic receptor termed the *glucocorticoid receptor* (GCR). Upon binding, the GC-GCR complex is translocated into the nucleus (20), where it dimerizes (21), followed by binding to specific DNA sites, termed *glucocorticoid response elements* (GRE), upstream from the promoter regions of steroid-responsive genes (22). GC-GCR binding to the GRE results in either up- or downregulation of gene products (23–25). There are between 10 and 100 genes with GRE sites that can be directly influenced by GCs (26).

Of importance, many of the genes encoding for proinflammatory cytokines lack GREs. Thus, alternative avenues for GC action in suppressing inflammation must be employed. The major alternative pathway comes from the ability of GC to interfere with the ability of nuclear transcription factors such as AP-1 and NF-κB to upregulate the immune response. Nuclear transcription factors play an important role in amplifying the inflammatory cascade by upregulating the transcription of proinflammatory cytokine genes (27–29). Thus, by interfering with their ability to enhance proinflammatory cytokine production, GCs can effectively inhibit the expression of cytokines that do not have GREs. Glucocorticoids can also interfere with transcription-factor binding by stimulating the induction of proteins such as IκBα, which can neutralize specific transcription factors (30,31). Last, GCs can also influence posttranscriptional events such as RNA translation, protein synthesis, and protein secretion. In particular, GCs have been shown to decrease the stability of interferon-γ mRNA by activation of a ribonuclease that degrades the AU-rich sequences in the untranslated region of this gene (32).

B. Effects at the Cellular Level

The mucosal inflammatory response seen in asthma is associated with the production of cytokines, the upregulation of adhesion molecules on both leukocytes and vascular endothelium, the influx of inflammatory cells into the airway, and the production of mediators of inflammation, including histamine, leukotrienes, prostaglandins, PAF, and the eosinophil-derived basic proteins (33). GCs have profound inhibitory effects on nearly every aspect of the above inflammatory response. Although incompletely understood, the anti-inflammatory effects of GCs are thought to come primarily from their ability to inhibit the transcription of cytokines. By inhibiting the production of essentially all of the cytokines involved in allergic inflammation, the inflammatory response can be significantly suppressed. Specifically, in vitro GC exposure results in the inhibition of production of interleukin-1 (IL-1) (34), IL-2 (35), IL-3 (36), IL-4 (37,38), IL-5 (39,40), IL-6, (41), IL-13, granulocyte-macrophage colony stimulating factor (GM-CSF) (42,43), and tumor necrosis factor alpha (TNF-α) (43). Many, if not all, of these cytokines are thought to be directly or indirectly involved in airway inflammation.

Studies evaluating the effect of inhaled GC therapy on allergic inflammation in asthmatics have only recently been accomplished. These studies have employed bronchoscopy with bronchoalveolar lavage (BAL) and/or endobronchial biopsy before and following a course of inhaled GC therapy. One of the first controlled studies evaluated the effect of BUD (1200 μg/day) or terbutaline for 3 months on airway inflammation in 14 adult asthmatics (44). BUD was associated with an increase in the number of intact ciliated epithelial cells lining the airway epithelium and a reduction in the number of eosinophils within the airway epithelium. Reductions in the number of eosinophils and activated T lymphocytes (CD25-positive) obtained from BAL fluid of asthmatics treated with high-dose BDP have also been noted (45). A recent study from Trigg et al. (46) evaluated the effect of high-dose BDP therapy (1000 μg/day) or placebo for 4 months in a group of 25 mild asthmatics. In contrast to the above studies, this study failed to find reductions in T-helper and activated T cells following BDP therapy, while significant reductions in tissue eosinophils and activated eosinophils (EG2-positive) were found. Of significance, BDP was associated with diminished epithelial expression of GM-CSF and a reduction in the thickness of the lamina reticularis compared to placebo.

Fluticasone propionate (FP) has also been shown to result in significant reductions in airway inflammatory cells and mediators of inflammation from both BAL fluid and airway tissue of adults with asthma (47,48). Of interest, even short-term (3-week) low-dose FP (500 μg/day) therapy resulted in reduced airway inflammation (48). Associated with the decrease in airway inflammation was a reduction in the thickness of the lamina propria, suggesting that FP can also modulate the intensity of airway remodeling. This is the second study published to date suggesting that inhaled GC can attenuate airway remodeling. In this case, a lower dose of FP given over a shorter period was associated with similar results as those seen with the Trigg study (46).

Exhaled nitric oxide (NO) can be elevated in asthmatics and may serve as a noninvasive marker of allergic inflammation. A recent study evaluated the effect of BUD (1600 μg/day) on exhaled NO levels (49). Following 3 weeks of BUD therapy, exhaled NO levels fell from 203 to 120 ppb compared to no change following placebo administration. Last, inhaled GC therapy has also been demonstrated to downregulate T-lymphocyte activation in the peripheral blood of asthmatics (50).

Although inhaled GC therapy has been shown to suppress inflammation, it does not completely abolish airway inflammation. This point was demonstrated by Sont et al. (51), who performed bronchoscopy with bronchial biopsies on 26 adults with mild to moderate asthma receiving chronic inhaled GC therapy (BDP or BUD, mean dose of 654 μg/day). Despite a moderately high dose of inhaled GC therapy, the investigators found significant numbers of eosinophils, T lymphocytes, and mast cells within the lamina propria. Of interest, significant correlations were noted between the inflammatory cells and bronchial hyperresponsiveness but not with symptom scores, pulmonary function measures, or supplemental β-agonist use.

In summary, inhaled GC therapy results in reductions in inflammatory cell infiltration into bronchoalveolar lavage fluid, the epithelium, and within the lamina propria. In addition, there are preliminary data suggesting that inhaled GCs can reduce the thickness of the lamina reticularis. These data support the hypothesis that inhaled GCs act topically by suppressing allergic inflammation. Of importance, inhaled GCs may also attenuate airway remodeling.

IV. Efficacy of Inhaled GCs in Asthma

Asthma is a chronic respiratory disease characterized by reversible airflow limitation and airway hyperresponsiveness to a variety of stimuli in which airway inflammation plays a significant role. Given that inflammation is involved in the pathogenesis of asthma, drugs that interfere with the inflammatory response should be effective in the treatment of this disease. Thus, it is not surprising that, by virtue of their anti-inflammatory properties, GCs have become the cornerstone of asthma therapy. With that said, a vast body of literature has accumulated over the past 25 years supporting the clinical efficacy of inhaled GC therapy in children and adults with asthma. This section provides a general overview of clinical efficacy, highlighting important articles that demonstrate the effectiveness of inhaled GC therapy (see Table 1 for a summary of the beneficial effects of inhaled GC therapy).

A. Effect on Bronchial Hyperresponsiveness and Lung Function

Increased airway responsiveness, or bronchial hyperresponsiveness (BHR), is a sentinel feature of asthma that has been shown to correlate with disease severity, frequency of symptoms, and need for treatment (52). Although the precise relationship remains elusive, airway inflammation may contribute to bronchial hyperresponsiveness (53,54); however, the two conditions are not necessarily directly linked (55). Studies evaluating the effect of inhaled GC therapy in asthma have consistently demonstrated a favorable effect on BHR in both adults and children with asthma (56–66). Decreases in BHR from two- to sevenfold have been reported within 6 weeks of instituting inhaled GC therapy, with a plateau effect usually reached by 8 weeks of therapy. Although inadequately studied, inhaled GC therapy appears to be as effective or more effective than oral GC therapy in reducing BHR (67).

Van Essen-Zandvliet et al. (65), in one of the largest published studies evaluating inhaled GC therapy in children, studied 116 children with moderate asthma who were randomly assigned to either salbutamol and BUD (600 μg/day) or salbutamol only over a 22-month period. The children on BUD had

Table 1 Effects of Inhaled Glucocorticoids

A. Anti-inflammatory effects
   1. Reduction in inflammatory cell infiltrate
   2. Reduction in cytokine expression
   3. Possible reduction in airway remodeling
B. Clinical effects
   1. Reduction in symptoms (nocturnal awakening, cough)
   2. Reduction in supplemental β-agonist use
   3. Reduction in need for oral GCs during exacerbations
   4. Oral GC–sparing effects (FP and BUD)
   5. Reduction in need for hospitalization with acute asthma
   6. Possible reduction in asthma morbidity/mortality
   7. Possible sustained remission in a minority of patients
C. Effects on lung function
   1. Improved morning and evening PEF rates
   2. Reduction in diurnal variation of PEF rates
   3. Improved baseline FEV_1 values
   4. Reduction in lung volumes (TLC, RV) toward the normal range
   5. Reduction in BHR

Key: GC, glucocorticoid; FP, fluticasone propionate; BUD, budesonide; BHR, bronchial hyperresponsiveness.

a 1.4-doubling-dose decrease in BHR at 4 months of therapy, and this decrease continued throughout the study. In fact, a plateau effect had not been reached even after 22 months of BUD therapy. Associated with the decrease in BHR were significant improvements in lung function and asthma symptoms. The children randomized to BUD had an 11% improvement in their prebronchodilator FEV_1 compared to the children on placebo. This improvement in baseline prebronchodilator FEV_1 was maintained throughout the study. The children on placebo therapy fared poorly, with over 40% requiring withdrawal from the study secondary to poor asthma control and nearly 50% requiring at least one oral GC burst secondary to an asthma exacerbation. In marked contrast, only 14% of patients on BUD required supplemental courses of prednisone. Finally, the three children requiring hospitalization during the study were all in the placebo-treated group.

    Similar results have been noted in adult asthmatics. Haahtela et al. (64), studied the effect of BUD (1200 μg/day) or terbutaline in 103 newly diagnosed adult asthmatics over a 96-week period and found a 1-doubling-dose reduction in BHR in the group treated with BUD. Unlike the case in the pediatric study, a plateau effect was reached at 8 weeks, which was sustained throughout the study. Associated with the reduction in BHR were significant improvements in symptom scores and PEF rates and a decreased need for supplemental β_2-agonist use. A greater number of patients randomized to the placebo group ($n = 10$) were withdrawn from the study secondary to poor asthma control compared to those randomized to BUD ($n = 1$).

In addition to improving PEFR and FEV_1 values, GC therapy has also been shown to reduce lung hyperinflation in children with moderate to severe asthma (68,69). Last, BUD has been shown to protect against unlimited airway narrowing to methacholine in adults with moderate to severe asthma (70). When given increasing doses of methacholine, most asthmatics will reach a point in that no further loss of lung function will occur despite these increasing concentrations. In other words, a plateau effect to increasing methacholine occurs. A subset of patients with moderate to severe asthma exists in whom a plateau effect never occurs; rather, they develop unlimited and progressive airway narrowing. This phenomenon has significant clinical ramifications in that these patients are thought to be at increased risk for developing near fatal or fatal asthma exacerbations. In this study, the investigators first identified asthmatics who failed to develop a plateau effect to methacholine. These patients then received BUD (1600 µg/day) or placebo for 12 weeks. Of no surprise, those on BUD displayed a significantly improved BHR. More importantly, approximately two-thirds of the subjects developed a maximal-response plateau to methacholine after 12 weeks of BUD therapy. This study suggested that inhaled GCs have the ability to restore the normal limitation to broncho-constriction and, by doing so, have the potential to prevent the development of life-threatening airflow obstruction during an acute asthma exacerbation.

B. Protective Effect on Asthma Morbidity/Mortality

The above studies suggested that inhaled GC therapy would be associated with less asthma morbidity. Given the relatively rare occurrence of asthma hospitalizations and life-threatening events, epidemiological studies have been required to address whether inhaled GC therapy is indeed associated with reduced asthma morbidity. Ernst et al. (71), using a nested case-control analysis of a historical cohort of over 12,000 asthmatics from Canada, found subjects on chronic BDP therapy (defined as using ≥ 1 canister a month of BDP) to be one-tenth as likely to die or have a near-fatal asthma exacerbation compared to asthmatics not on inhaled GCs. Of note, this was the second study published by this group of investigators using this cohort of asthmatics (72). Their other study, which received a significant amount of attention, found an association between regular β-agonist use and fatal and near-fatal asthma. Thus, while β-agonist use may be associated with increased risk of asthma morbidity, inhaled GC use was associated with a significant protective effect.

During 1997–1998, two epidemiological studies were published demonstrating a protective effect of inhaled GCs on hospitalization for acute asthma (73,74). Donahue et al. (73) found asthmatics on inhaled GCs to be 50% less likely to be hospitalized with acute asthma than those not on inhaled GCs. Employing β-agonist use as a surrogate marker of disease severity, they found GCs to confer even greater protective effects, with a 70% reduction noted. The study by Blais et al. (74) sought to evaluate the effectiveness of inhaled GCs in preventing readmission to the hospital in those who were placed on inhaled GCs following an initial hospitalization. Inhaled GC therapy was associated with a 40% reduction in the rate of rehospitalization from day 15 to 6 months. This protective effect was lost after 6 months of therapy. The authors attributed the loss of protective effect after 6 months to confounding by severity.

C. Oral GC–Sparing Effect of the "Second-Generation" Inhaled GCs

The newly released second-generation inhaled GCs appear to display significant oral steroid–sparing effects. Second-generation GCs such as FP and to a lesser extent BUD display greater topical to systemic potencies, with the end result being a better therapeutic index. Because FP binds to the glucocorticoid receptor with high affinity (75) and possesses a prolonged GC receptor binding time (76), it displays the greatest topical anti-inflammatory effects. In addition, it undergoes extensive first-pass hepatic metabolism, rendering >98% of the swallowed portion inactive (77,78). With that said, systemic bioavailability is dependent on both oral bioavailability (drug absorbed from the gastrointestinal tract) and pulmonary bioavailability (drug absorbed from the lung). At present, all of the inhaled GC preparations display pulmonary bioavailability, as all drug delivered to the lung eventually enters the systemic circulation. In the case of FP, lung absorption is the sole source of systemic bioavailability (79). These two features, high topical anti-inflammatory effects and extensive first-pass metabolism, give this compound a high topical to systemic potency ratio and is the basis for its enhanced clinical efficacy. In a recently published randomized, placebo-controlled, multicenter study, over 80% of the patients randomized to receive high-dose FP therapy (2000 µg/day) were completely tapered off their oral GCs (80). In addition, those on high-dose FP had a significant improvement in their lung function despite the significant oral steroid dose reduction. Similar but less striking results were reported with BUD in a study by Nelson et al. (81). The ability of FP and BUD to result in significant oral steroid-sparing effects appears to be unique to these compounds in that similar effects have not been noted with the other available inhaled GCs (82).

D. Inhaled GCs as First-Line Therapy

Inhaled GC were initially reserved for use in patients with moderate to severe asthma (83), but as our understanding of this disease has advanced, inhaled GCs are now recommended for individuals with mild persistent asthma (84). The newly updated National Heart, Lung and Blood Institute (NHLBI) guidelines now recommend low-dose inhaled GC therapy (or cromolyn/nedocromil for children) as first-line therapy for mild persistent asthma (84). Inhaled GCs are also recommended in increasing doses for those with moderate and severe asthma. Whether inhaled GC therapy should be first-line therapy in children with mild asthma remains a topic of debate (85). Those that favor the use of inhaled GC therapy in mild asthma argue that since this medication reduces airway inflammation, BHR and need for supplemental β-agonist therapy, it should be used in all patients with persistent asthma of mild or greater severity. Given that inhaled GC therapy is not without the potential for adverse effects and that adequate long-term studies evaluating bone demineralization and growth delay have yet to be completed, others argue that its use should be reserved for those with more frequent symptoms—i.e., those with moderate to severe persistent asthma.

Two recent studies, one in children the other in adults, evaluated the efficacy and adverse effects of long-term BUD therapy in mild asthma (86,87). Of no surprise, both found BUD to be an effective asthma therapy with few adverse effects noted. Of significance, both made the intriguing observation that the longer an individual had asthma prior to the institution of inhaled GC therapy, the less improvement in pulmonary function was noted following institution of BUD therapy (Fig. 2). A third, uncontrolled study of 105 adult asthmatics treated with BUD over a 2-year period also found a significant negative correlation between duration of asthma symptoms and maximum increases in both PEF rates and FEV_1 (88). Of note, the correlations remained significant even after correcting for differences in baseline airway function. The results from these studies suggest that the longer the time from the initiation of symptoms and subsequent treatment with inhaled GCs, the less effective this form of therapy may be.

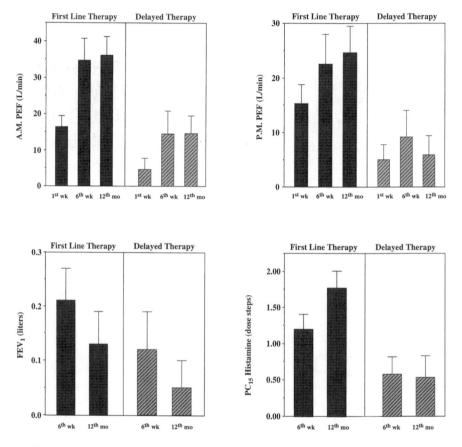

Figure 2 Comparison of improvements in patients treated with budesonide (BUD) as first-line therapy within 1 year of the diagnosis of asthma and patients treated with BUD more than 2 years after diagnosis. As noted in the figure, those who received BUD shortly after the diagnosis of asthma was made responded to a much greater extent than those who were placed on BUD 2 years later. (Data from Ref. 87.)

E. Inhaled GCs and Asthma Remission

Over the past couple of years, increased attention has been placed on whether chronic inhaled GC therapy can induce asthma remissions. Several of the properties of this class of medications—such as their ability to suppress airway inflammation, decrease BHR, and possibly their ability to prevent airway remodeling—support this concept. The recent observation that early institution of inhaled GCs results in the greatest potential for restoration of normal lung function further supports the concept that inhaled GC therapy can be a disease-modifying agent. Juniper et al. (89) were among the first to suggest that long-term therapy with an inhaled GC could result in sustained improvement after reducing or discontinuing therapy. After 1 year treatment with BUD, 14 subjects had their BUD dose halved ($n = 6$) or discontinued ($n = 8$), while 14 subjects were randomized to continue BUD at the same dose. Lung function, measurement of BHR, bronchodilator requirements, and asthma symptoms were quantitated after 6 weeks and again after 3 months. After 3 months, those whose dose had been tapered or discontinued had no change in BHR and did not require greater bronchodilator use than those who remained on the original dose of BUD. There was a small reduction in FEV_1 and symptoms at 3 months in those whose dose had been decreased. Of note, approximately 50% of the patients whose doses had been discontinued had a decrease in spirometry and an increase in BHR. Most likely to deteriorate were those with the greatest degree of BHR to start the study and who demonstrated less than a twofold improvement in BHR during the study. Nonetheless, the authors speculated that long-term treatment with BUD could potentially result in a permanent resolution of BHR and asthma. The major weakness of this study comes from the small number of patients (eight) who actually had their BUD discontinued and the short washout period (3 months).

Similar results were reported by Haahtela et al. (87). In this study, 37 newly diagnosed adult asthmatics who had received high-dose BUD (1200 µg/day) therapy for 2 years were randomized to receive either placebo or one-third the original dose of BUD (400 µg/day) for 1 year. The majority (74%) of patients randomized to the low-dose BUD group continued to maintain the improvements in lung function and BHR they had gained while on high-dose BUD. In contrast, only one-third of the subjects in the placebo group displayed sustained improvement. At the end of the year, significant declines in FEV_1, PEF rates, and BHR were noted in the placebo group compared to the BUD group. Of note, although the mean histamine provocative concentration resulting in a 15% decline in FEV_1 (PC_{15}) had worsened, it remained better than the baseline level at the start of the three year study. Thus, approximately one-third of the subjects who had been treated with long-term BUD appeared to sustain a prolonged remission with the remainder developing increasing disease activity in terms of worsening BHR.

Not all studies have demonstrated long-lasting or disease-modifying effects once inhaled GC therapy was discontinued. Osterman et al. (90) sought to investigate whether treatment with low-dose BUD (400 µg/day) in newly diagnosed asthma could influence the course of the disease. Seventy-five recent-onset (diagnosis made within 1 year) mild asthmatics (baseline FEV_1, 91%) were randomized to receive BUD 400 µg/day or placebo for 1 year with a follow-up period of 6 months off inhaled GCs. While on low-dose BUD, the subjects displayed significant improvements in morning PEF rates and BHR. During the 6-month washout, those gains had been lost to a large degree. The authors concluded that the improvements noted with low-dose BUD are short-lived without continued treatment.

Two important follow-up studies from the original Van Essen-Zandvliet (65) study on BUD therapy in childhood asthma sought to address the issue of remission in children with moderate asthma. In the first study (91), the investigators sought to determine whether long-term BUD therapy would result in remission of clinical asthma during therapy. Of the 53 children originally randomized to receive BUD (600 µg/day), 60% achieved an 8-month clinical remission at some point during the 3-year study. However, only one-third were in clinical remission upon completion of the study, and only 15% of the patients had a normal FEV_1 ($\geq$90%) and a normal PC_{20} value ($>$150 µg). Also of note, although long-term BUD therapy resulted in significant improvements in lung function and BHR, both parameters remained abnormal. The authors concluded that although long-term BUD therapy improved asthma symptoms and objective measures of asthma, it did not cure the disease. This point was strengthened in their second follow-up study (92). In this case, 28 children from the original cohort who had been stable on BUD for 2–3 years were randomized to continue their current BUD dose (8 patients; 600 µg/day) or to be completely tapered off BUD over 2 months (20 patients). All patients were followed over a 6-month period. Of the 20 patients in the placebo group, 8 had to be withdrawn during the 6-month follow-up and 5 required prednisone for poor asthma control, compared to none in the BUD group. In addition, much of the gain in lung function and reduction in BHR that these children displayed while on 2–3 years of BUD were lost by the end of the 6-month placebo period. Thus, long-term BUD treatment effectively suppressed the underlying mechanisms of asthma but, again, it did not cure the disease.

In summary, it appears as if inhaled GCs can induce a short-lived clinical remission during therapy. In addition, a couple of studies have suggested that a subset of mild adult asthmatics will undergo sustained remissions following at least a 1-year period of inhaled GC therapy. Unfortunately, there are no reliable predictors for who will undergo sustained remission. Last, some studies suggest that although the degree of BHR worsens off inhaled GC therapy, that BHR remains less than that noted before the institution of therapy. These data would suggest that long-term therapy with inhaled GCs might lead to mild modification of disease. It should be stressed that this issue of inhaled GCs inducing asthma remissions remains controversial and one that has been investigated neither adequately nor thoroughly. All of the studies published to date have employed very small numbers of patients. In every case, less than 50 subjects were studied. In addition, none of the studies were performed in young children, and no investigators studied the effect of inhaled GC administered for more than 3 years. Research in this area is greatly needed. Large, prospective, and long-term studies in both children and adults need to be performed before any evidence-based conclusions can be made.

F. Efficacy of Inhaled GCs in Asthma—Summary

In summary, studies evaluating inhaled steroid therapy have consistently reported significant reductions in BHR, fewer asthma symptoms, improved pulmonary function (PEF and FEV_1), less need for supplemental β-agonist use, and fewer exacerbations requiring courses of oral GCs (Table 1). In addition, epidemiological studies have demonstrated that inhaled GCs display protective effects against life-threatening and fatal asthma and protection against hospitalization and rehospitalization for acute asthma. Because inhaled GC therapy appears to be most effective if administered soon after the onset of the disease, there has been a trend toward earlier use of these medications. In fact, the newly revised NHLBI guidelines have now recommended inhaled GCs as first-line agents in all but patients with the mildest asthma. This recommendation has been met with some controversy, especially as it pertains to childhood asthma, given the propensity of these compounds to display systemic effects, as outlined below.

V. Inhaled GCs in COPD

A. Current Concepts of COPD

Chronic obstructive pulmonary disease (COPD) is a heterogeneous group of disorders—including chronic bronchitis, emphysema, and small airways disease—that lead to progressive, largely irreversible airflow obstruction which may be accompanied by airway hyperresponsiveness (93,94). COPD is characterized by cough, sputum production, and breathlessness associated with airflow obstruction. Patients generally have a progressive deterioration in lung function, which leads to substantial problems in their general health and quality of life, and eventual respiratory failure, and early death (95). COPD is one of the leading causes of death worldwide, with an increasing prevalence and mortality rate (96).

COPD occurs mostly in the elderly and is characterized by airflow obstruction that is not relieved completely with therapy (96). There are three distinct pathological processes, which may occur separately or, in many patients, concurrently: (1) destruction of alveolar walls, causing emphysema; (2) chronic bronchitis with hypersecretion of mucus; and (3) chronic asthma. Several pathological features of COPD distinguish it from asthma: (1) predominance of CD8 cells, (2) an increase in the number of neutrophils, (3) no thickening of the basement membrane, (4) no evidence of destruction of the airway epithelium, and (5) an increase in squamous metaplasia (97,98).

B. Pharmacotherapy of COPD

The aims of drug treatment for COPD are to cause bronchodilatation, reduce the work of breathing, reduce airway inflammation and tissue damage, and diminish hypersecretion of mucus or facilitate expectoration (99). Patients are seeking to reduce breathlessness, principally exercise-related, and productive cough. By definition, patients with COPD have a limited response to bronchodilator therapy. Nevertheless, the small responses may be accompanied by a subjective reduction in dyspnea and increased exercise tolerance. Guidelines for COPD pharmacotherapy have been developed by the American Thoracic Society and are summarized in Table 2 (100). Anticholinergics with a longer duration of action, such as oxitropium, require less frequent use and may facilitate patient compliance with regular therapy. A recent placebo-controlled study found that twice-daily salmeterol reduced symptom scores and raised morning PEF rates in patients with stable COPD 65 years of age and above (101). There have been different responses to trials of corticosteroids, presumably reflecting, in part, differences in type of patient. In perhaps 10% of stable COPD patients, FEV_1 improves in response to treatment with corticosteroids, but long-term use is limited by side effects. There is some evidence that inhaled corticosteroids can limit or prevent the accelerated decline in lung function associated with COPD.

Table 2 American Thoracic Society Guidelines for Drug
Treatment in Chronic Obstructive Pulmonary Disease

Step 1	Mild, variable symptoms
	β_2-agonist as needed
Step 2	Mild-to-moderate continuing symptoms
	Ipratropium 96–8 h
	β_2-agonist as needed, or regularly
Step 3	Step 2 unsatisfactory or increased symptoms
	Add sustained-release theophylline
	Consider sustained-release β_2-agonist
Step 4	Control of symptoms suboptimal
	Consider course of oral steroids
	Possible inhaled steroids (if oral steroids appear to help)
Step 5	Severe exacerbation
	Increase β_2-agonist dosage
	Increase ipratropium dosage
	Theophylline i.v.
	Steroids i.v.
	Antibiotics if indicated

Source: From Ref. 100.

C. Efficacy of Oral Steroid in COPD

There is some evidence that systemic corticosteroids have a role to play in the treatment of acute exacerbations of COPD (99). The evidence that they can modify the rate of progression of stable disease is more contradictory. Retrospective analysis of Dutch data has assessed the effectiveness of systemic corticosteroids on the rate of decline in FEV_1 in patients with COPD (102). The study included 139 patients with moderately severe COPD (mean $FEV_1 = 1.2$ L) who were referred to the clinic between 1964 and 1972 and who fulfilled the entry criteria. Until 1968, patients without specific contraindications were treated with oral prednisolone. After this date, increasing awareness of the adverse effects of corticosteroids and the advent of inhaled preparations led to a gradual change to the latter route of administration. Patients treated with ≥ 10 mg prednisolone daily appeared to exhibit a slower rate of decline in FEV_1 than patients on smaller doses or no corticosteroids.

D. Efficacy of Inhaled Corticosteroids in COPD

The evidence that inhaled corticosteroids are of benefit in COPD, either clinically or pathophysiologically, is scanty, yet these agents are widely used in the management of this disorder (97,103). This discrepancy is partly due to the inevitable diagnostic confusion between asthma in the elderly and COPD. Another reason is that, faced with a patient for whom few other treatments are of clear-cut benefit, physicians will try a treatment they judge to be safe, even if the likelihood of benefit is low. Another reason is that during acute exacerbations of COPD, systemic steroids may speed recovery—an effect that is taken as evidence that steroids will be of help in that individual in the long term.

It is commonly thought that the 15% of patients who respond to steroids represent a group with a substantial chronic asthmatic component. This view is supported by a study that showed that among patients with a clinical diagnosis of COPD, those with biopsy features of asthma (high number of eosinophils and thickening of the basement membrane) were the ones who improved with high-dose prednisolone over 2 weeks (104). The limited number of studies of the effect of steroids on airways inflammation of COPD have shown little evidence of an acute anti-inflammatory effect (105), although there may be some effect on airway protein leakage (106).

Recent guidelines (100,107) on the management of COPD indicate that inhaled corticosteroids are recommended only for those patients who show a clear objective response to a formal trial of either oral or high-dose inhaled steroids. For an unselected group of patients with COPD, a positive trial of steroids is defined as a 15% increase in baseline FEV_1, with an absolute increase of greater than 200 mL. A change of this magnitude is seen in 10–15% of patients with COPD. It is not clear how to manage the remaining 80–90% of patients who do not respond to steroids. Therefore, other outcome measures must be considered.

E. Measures of Efficacy of Inhaled Steroids

Short-term inhaled corticosteroids in COPD have had little effect on airway hyper-responsiveness or FEV_1 at doses that improve asthma (108–111). Keatings et al. (105) investigated the effect of inhaled BUD 800 μg twice daily for 2 weeks in 13 patients with severe COPD (predicted mean FEV_1, 35%). They found no clinical improvement in lung function or symptom scores and no significant change in inflammatory markers.

Longer-term treatment has shown some benefit on lung function, but studies generally have not distinguished between COPD and asthma (112,113). Three studies, of at least 2 years duration, showed an improvement in FEV_1 after the addition of inhaled corticosteroids to bronchodilator therapy (112–114). Dompeling et al. (112) in a 4-year prospective study showed that addition of beclomethasone dipropionate (BDP) 800 µg daily to bronchodilator therapy, given alone for the first 2 years of the study, among patients with obstructive lung disease significantly improved FEV_1. This improvement lasted for 6 months, after which FEV_1 declined, although the rate of decline was less than that seen before treatment with BDP. However, that study also involved asthmatic patients and did not have a placebo control group. The results are less impressive when postbronchodilator FEV_1 is evaluated (Fig. 3).

Kerstjens et al. (113), showed in a 2-year study that beclomethasone dipropionate 800 µg daily significantly improved FEV_1 in obstructive lung disease during the first 3 months of treatment compared with an inhaled anticholinergic agent or placebo. Again, however, no distinction was made between patients with COPD and asthma. Renkema et al. (114) studied the effects of BUD 1.6 mg or BUD 1.6 mg plus oral prednisolone compared with placebo for 2 years in 58 patients with COPD. The two active treatments significantly reduced pulmonary symptoms but had no significant effect on decline of lung function or the frequency or duration of exacerbations.

In addition, improvements in lung function were reported in several studies. Weiner et al. (115) showed that a significant improvement in FEV_1 with BUD was seen only in patients who had an increase in FEV_1 of more than 20% on β_2-agonists. Chanez et al. (104) reported that patients with larger numbers of eosinophils and thicker reticular basement membrane on bronchial biopsy (i.e., features of asthma) are more likely to respond to corticosteroids than are patients with COPD without these features.

Van Schayck et al. (116) investigated predictors of response to inhaled steroids in COPD patients. They found that bronchodilator reversibility and more substantial airways obstruction assessed by the ratio of FEV_1 to forced vital capacity resulted in a greater improvement in FEV_1 during treatment with inhaled steroids. These findings plus the study by Paggiaro et al. (93) related to duration of COPD suggest that patients with more severe airflow obstruction, especially with a long history of symptoms or any features consistent with asthma, are more likely to respond to treatment with inhaled steroids.

Paggiaro et al. (93) compared high-dose fluticasone propionate (FP), 500 µg twice daily, versus placebo in a study of 6 months duration. Patients

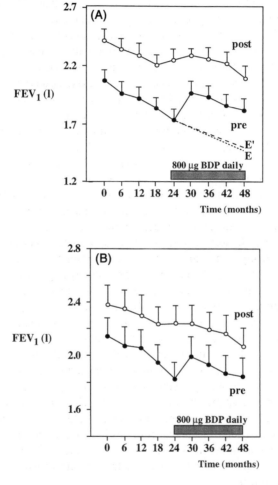

Figure 3 Forced expiratory volume in 1 second before and after bronchodilator therapy during the 4-year study period. (A) All patients ($n = 48$). (B) Patients with chronic obstructive pulmonary disease. BDP, beclomethasone dipropionate; E, the extrapolated endpoint if bronchodilator therapy alone had been continued during the third and fourth years of treatment; E', the extrapolated endpoint with a correction for regression to the mean. (From Ref. 112.)

had moderately impaired pulmonary function with less than 8% reversibility in FEV_1 after bronchodilator and no evidence of blood eosinophils. The primary outcome variable was exacerbation rate, and secondary outcome variables included symptoms, pulmonary function, 6-min walking distance, and breathlessness. Thirty-seven percent or 51 patients in the placebo group compared with 32% or 45 in the FP group had had at least one exacerbation by the end treatment ($p = 0.449$). Significantly more patients had moderate or severe exacerbations in the placebo group than in the FP group (86% vs. 60%, $p < 0.001$). Diary card and clinic morning peak expiratory flows improved significantly in the FP group ($p < 0.001$, $p = 0.048$, respectively), as did clinic FEV_1, ($p < 0.001$), forced vital capacity ($p < 0.001$), and midexpiratory flow ($p = 0.01$). Symptom scores for median daily cough and sputum volume were significantly lower with FP treatment than with placebo ($p = 0.004$ and $p = 0.016$, respectively). At the end of treatment, patients on FP had increased their 6-min walking distance significantly more than those on placebo ($p = 0.032$). FP was tolerated as well as placebo, with few adverse effects and without a clinically important effect on mean serum cortisol concentration.

Therefore, the key observations of the study by Paggioro et al. (93) were that (1) the overall rate of exacerbations was lower than predicted from pilot studies; (2) there was no significant difference between the groups in overall rates of exacerbation; (3) there was a shift in severity of exacerbations, with fewer patients in the active-treatment group having severe exacerbations; (4) there was a small but clinically and statistically significant improvement in peak expiratory flow rate of 15 L/min in the inhaled-steroid group and small improvements in spirometry, symptoms, and walking distance; and (5) the only predictor of response was a duration of COPD greater than 10 years. Earlier onset of symptoms among responders could be interpreted as being due to the contribution of a component of asthma to their airflow obstruction. In view of previous observations, this study raises questions on whether lower doses could be equally effective and whether the effect would be lost with long-term treatment.

Two large-scale studies are designed to determine whether inhaled corticosteroids slow the decline of FEV_1 in patients with COPD: (1) The European Respiratory Society Study on Chronic Obstructive Pulmonary Disease (EUROSCOP), which is being conducted in patients with mild COPD (117) and from which initial results suggest that any effect is small and transitory, and (2) The International Study of Obstructive Lung Disease ISOLDE study of more severe COPD (118).

F. Future Directions

In regard to the present management of COPD, the key observations to date regarding the role of inhaled steroids in COPD management include the following (97):

1. There should be no change in the recommendations in the COPD guidelines (107) that patients who show striking response to oral or inhaled corticosteroids should be treated with inhaled steroids.
2. A small absolute improvement in pulmonary function is associated with clinical benefit in terms of symptoms, exercise capacity, and possible severity of exacerbations.
3. If so, a reasonable approach would be to lower the threshold for concluding that a patient's illness has undergone a clinically important improvement with inhaled steroids.
4. If after several months of treatment with high-dose inhaled steroids, peak flow improves by 15 L/min or more and the severity and the number of exacerbations fall, the patient should continue on inhaled steroids.
5. If these variables do not improve, there is no compelling reason to continue with inhaled steroids.

Since it is difficult to demonstrate clinical predictors of response to inhaled steroids, an area that may justify further investigation is whether pathological appearances—especially eosinophils or thickened basement membrane—should be used to predict a response (97). Available studies imply that current treatment of COPD is unsatisfactory. Obviously, avoidance or cessation of smoking is the key to improving the outlook for patients with COPD. However, even if patients succeed in giving up smoking, there will still be many symptomatic patients for the foreseeable future.

It is important to understand the mechanisms of COPD. Present evidence suggests that the inflammation present in COPD is poorly responsive to steroids and that, unlike asthma, this inflammation of the airways is not the primary problem in the disease. New treatments for COPD are therefore needed (119). In designing clinical trials, short-term trials should look at outcomes measures such as (1) prevention of exacerbations of COPD (which are a common and important clinical problem); (2) exercise capacity; and (3) quality of life. Long-term studies should look at overall decline in pulmonary function, such as pre- and postbronchodilator FEV_1.

VI. Adverse Effects of Inhaled GC Therapy

Although the topical to systemic potency of inhaled GCs make the likelihood of GC-associated adverse effects much smaller than that of oral GCs, the potential for systemic absorption and hence systemic effects exists. In general, the development of adverse effects from inhaled GC therapy is dependent on the dose and the frequency with which the inhaled GC is given (120). High doses (1000 μg/day) administered frequently (four times daily) are most likely to result in an increase in both local and systemic adverse effects.

A. Local Adverse Effects

The most commonly encountered adverse effects from inhaled GC therapy are local and consist of oral candidiasis and dysphonia (Table 3). As is the case for systemic complications, these effects are dose-dependent and are most common in individuals on high-dose inhaled and oral GC therapy (121,122). Thrush is thought to occur as a result of local immunosuppression, while dysphonia occurs as a result of vocal cord muscle myopathy (123). The incidence of these local effects can be greatly minimized by using a spacer device, which reduces the oropharyngeal deposition of the drug (124,125). In addition, mouth rinsing using a "swish and spit" technique following inhaled GC inhalation

Table 3 Adverse Effects of Inhaled Glucocorticoid Therapy

A. Local effects
    1. Oral candidiasis (thrush)
    2. Dysphonia
B. Systemic effects
    1. Adrenal suppression
    2. Potential for growth suppression in children
    3. Potential for adverse effects on bone metabolism
    4. Other rare but reported adverse effects
        a. Opportunistic infection
        b. Development of cushingoid features
        c. Addisonian crisis
        d. Dermal thinning
        e. Psychosis
        f. Hypoglycemia

results in less drug left in the oropharynx and less chance of the drug being absorbed from the GI tract.

B. Systemic Adverse Effects

Although the risk for developing systemic adverse effects is much smaller for inhaled than for oral GC therapy, the potential for toxicity remains. The systemic effects of inhaled GCs are dependent on the dose delivered, the pharmacokinetic profile of the GC (i.e., degree of first-pass hepatic metabolism), the method of delivery of the GC, and individual differences in steroid sensitivity among patients (120). Several systemic effects have been reported, including suppression of the HPA axis, growth suppression, effects on bone metabolism, dermal thinning, cataracts/glaucoma, hypoglycemia, weight gain, psychosis, and opportunistic infection (Table 3).

Adrenal Suppression

Inhaled GC therapy can result in suppression of the HPA axis. The degree of suppression is largely dependent on the dose and frequency of the inhaled GC delivered, duration of treatment, route of administration, and time of day the drug is administered (125). There are two major methods of assessing HPA axis function (126). The first measures basal adrenal activity. Examples of this method include single morning cortisol determinations (the least sensitive method), serial serum cortisol concentrations over a fixed period of time (very sensitive), or 24-h urinary cortisol excretion (also very sensitive). The other method measures response to stimulation (ACTH or metyrapone) or stress (insulin-induced hypoglycemia). There have been a large number of studies evaluating HPA function in asthmatics; most have measured basal cortisol activity with single morning serum cortisol determinations (127–129) or 24-h urinary cortisol excretion (130–132), while others have measured response to stimulation (133,134). The preponderance of data would suggest doses of 400 µg/day or less are not associated with changes in the HPA axis, but that as the inhaled dose is increased to above 1000 µg/day, HPA axis suppression clearly occurs. High-dose FP therapy appears to have a much greater effect on HPA axis suppression than the other inhaled GCs, as discussed below (135,136).

Several studies, in both adults and children, have evaluated the effect of FP on HPA axis suppression. The majority have shown FP to have comparable systemic effects to either BDP or BUD, especially at the doses of FP recommended for the treatment of mild and moderate asthma (176–440 µg/day)

(137–140). The same cannot be said regarding high-dose FP therapy (i.e., dose $\geq$1000 µg/day). A number of studies have demonstrated significantly greater effects on HPA axis suppression than with equivalent doses of BUD (135,136,141,142). These studies found FP to have a greater likelihood to suppress plasma cortisol, urinary cortisol, and ACTH levels, with the greatest degree of suppression noted at doses of $\geq$1000 µg/day. Specifically, Clark et al. (135) studied 12 adult asthmatics in a double-blind, placebo-controlled crossover design comparing single doses of either inhaled BUD (400, 1000, 1600, or 2000 µg) or FP (500, 1000, 1500, or 2000 µg) administered at 2200 h and found FP to exhibit at least a twofold greater degree of adrenal suppression than BUD on a microgram-per-microgram basis. The interpretations from this study are limited by its design—i.e., a single-dose study with the drug administered at 2200 h (maximizing potential adrenal suppression).

A subsequent study from the same group (141) studied the effect of chronic dosing of either FP or BUD administered twice daily over 4 days and found FP to have a more profound suppressive effect on both morning cortisol levels and overnight urinary cortisol/creatine ratios compared to BUD, with a 3.5-fold difference in potency between the two drugs. Similar results were reported by Boorsma et al. (136), who compared the relative systemic potency of FP and BUD administered twice daily over 4 days in nonasthmatic adults. These investigators found fluticasone to have a 3.7- to 5.2-fold greater systemic potency ratio than BUD. Of note, high-dose FP (2000 µg/day) resulted in a reduction of over 80% in the average cortisol level and 89% suppression of the 8 morning level, compared to 27 and 11% suppression for 2000 µg/day of BUD respectively. Last, Donnelly et al. (142) studied high doses of BUD and FP (BUD 800, 1600, 3200 µg/day vs. FP 750, 1500, 2000 µg/day both delivered via pMDI) over a 5-day period in 28 healthy, nonasthmatic adults using suppression of plasma cortisol levels over a 24-h period on the fifth day of each treatment period. In addition, they evaluated for suppression of 8 A.M. cortisol values upon completion of each treatment period. Both drugs were found to result in a dose-dependent suppression of plasma cortisol levels at all time points through out the 24-h collection period. Both drugs also resulted in suppression of 8 A.M. cortisol values. As seen in the other studies, FP was found to be approximately three times more potent in suppressing plasma cortisol concentrations than BUD over a 24-h period.

From these studies, FP at doses of $\geq$1000 µg/day can be expected to result in clinically significant adrenal suppression. This is an important and possibly unique observation for FP. Thus, one should use high-dose FP only in patients with severe, poorly controlled asthma or in patients with steroid-dependent asthma. Once the patient's asthma is better controlled or the oral steroid dose has been significantly tapered, attempts should be made to titrate the FP dose downward. Whether or not modest reductions in the HPA axis are of clinical relevance remains to be determined. Even though it is extremely unlikely that an asthmatic on less than 1000 µg/day would develop an addisonian crisis due to adrenal suppression, the fact that measurable changes in the HPA axis are present indicates systemic absorption; thus HPA axis suppression could serve as a marker for other systemic effects.

Growth Suppression

Growth suppression is the steroid-associated adverse effect that causes the most concern for clinicians caring for children (143). Whether clinically significant growth suppression can occur with chronic inhaled GC therapy remains a controversial area, with some studies suggesting that doses as low as 400 µg/day of BDP can result in suppression of linear growth. Unfortunately, almost all of the studies that have attempted to determine the effect of inhaled GCs on growth have been limited. Many studies have evaluated growth over short periods using knemometry (144,145). Of significance, reductions in the growth rate of the lower leg noted in short-term knemometry studies cannot be used to predict an adverse effect on long-term statural growth (146). Other studies evaluating growth over longer periods have not been placebo-controlled, while some studies have included too heterogeneous a patient population in terms of scatter of ages of children enrolled. The following discussion attempts to summarize the data given the above limitations.

Before one can address the effect of inhaled GC therapy on growth, one must first take into account the observation that asthma, especially poorly controlled asthma, can affect growth adversely (147,148). Ninan and Russell, in one of the few studies that considered this variable, evaluated the growth of 58 children with asthma over a 5-year period (149). All children were prepubescent at entry (mean age 3.5 years for males, 4.4 years for females) and were followed for nearly 2 years before receiving inhaled GC therapy. In addition, each child's asthma was classified as being in good, moderate, or poor control according to asthma symptoms prior to beginning inhaled GC therapy. These investigators found that the study group as a whole had diminished growth velocity at the start of the study, with a mean height velocity standard deviation (HVSD) score of −0.51. The children whose asthma was in good control had the least evidence for growth suppression prior to the institution of inhaled GC therapy and continued to grow at the same rate while on therapy

(HVSD score -0.01 pre vs. -0.07 during iGC treatment). In contrast, the subjects whose asthma was poorly controlled grew poorly regardless of whether or not they were receiving inhaled GCs (HVSD score -1.50 pre vs. -1.55 during). Of interest, those with moderately controlled asthma actually demonstrated improved growth velocity while on inhaled GC therapy, with the HVSD score increasing from -0.83 to -0.49. These investigators concluded that poor asthma control, more than inhaled GC therapy, affected growth significantly.

There have now been four controlled studies demonstrating growth suppression using moderate doses of beclomethasone over a period of 7 to 12 months (150–153). In the first study, Tinkelman et al. (150) compared BDP 84 μg administered four times daily (336 μg/day) to theophylline in 195 children 6 to 16 years old with mild to moderate asthma over a 12-month period. Suppression of growth velocity was noted in the group treated with BPD, with the males being most affected. Doull et al. (151), studied the effect of 400 μg/day BDP or placebo in 94 children with mild asthma (7 to 9 years old) for 7 months, followed by a 4-month washout period. Following 7 months of either BDP or placebo, the children randomized to BDP had growth significantly less than the children on placebo (2.66 vs. 3.66 cm), with no significant catch-up growth noted during the 4-month washout period. Of note, the growth suppression occurred in the absence of HPA axis suppression, a finding also noted by Tinkelman et al. (150). The third study evaluated the effect of 1 year of therapy with BDP (400 μg/day) vs. salmeterol in 67 children (mean age 10.5 years, range 6–16 years) with mild to moderate asthma (152). BDP was found to be superior to salmeterol in terms of efficacy (improved pulmonary function, reduced BHR, and decreased need for oral GC use). However, the average annual growth was significantly reduced, with a reduction in linear growth of 1.4 cm resulting in -0.28 SDS (Fig. 4). A disturbing feature of this study was the indication of continuing effect throughout the period of BDP treatment. This is in contrast to the results obtained in the fourth study, as outlined below. In this study, by Simons et al. (153), 241 children were randomized to receive BDP 400 μg/day, salmeterol 100 μg/day, or placebo for 1 year. BDP was noted to be the most effective drug, with significant reductions in BHR, rescue albuterol use, and fewer withdrawals from the study due to poor asthma control. Evaluation of growth was also included, with those on BDP displaying some degree of growth suppression. Those on BDP grew 3.96 cm for the year, compared to 5.04 cm and 5.4 cm for the placebo and salmeterol groups respectively. Of potential significance, the growth-suppressive effect of BDP appeared to be greatest during the first 3 months of

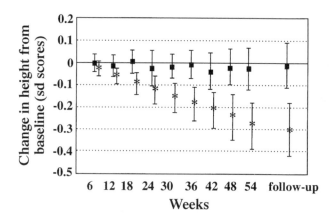

Figure 4 Change in height from baseline. Change in height as SDS (mean, 95% CI) during treatment with salmeterol (closed squares) or beclomethasone (asterisks). (From Ref. 152.)

therapy (Fig. 5). The growth curve for BDP appeared to parallel that of the other treatment groups from 3 months on.

Complicating the issue further is the observation that asthma can delay the onset of puberty (154,155). Studies using inhaled GC therapy in older children and in which a reduction in growth velocity is noted may actually be demonstrating an exaggerated decline in growth velocity seen immediately before the onset of puberty (156). A study by Merkus et al. (157) evaluated the long-term (22 months) effect of either BUD (600 µg/day) or placebo on growth rates of 40 asthmatic teenagers (mean age 12.8 years) compared to the growth rates of 80 age-matched, nonasthmatic controls (Fig. 6). Growth rates among the male asthmatics were found to be significantly decreased compared to those of age-matched nonasthmatic controls, but when the growth rates between the asthmatics treated with placebo vs. BUD were compared, those treated with BUD had better growth rates (−0.44 cm/year for BUD vs. −0.70 cm/year for placebo). Thus, the growth delay noted among the adolescent asthmatics was most likely due to a delay in puberty and not to the long-term BUD therapy.

Many of these studies have been criticized, as none of them had growth as their primary outcome variable. They also have methodological flaws in that they either fail to adequately assess pubertal status, lack baseline growth velocity data, display significant differences in baseline height or age between

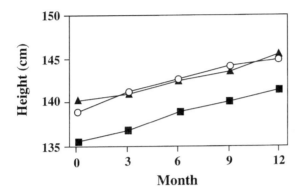

Figure 5 Mean height at baseline and after 3, 6, 9, and 12 months of treatment. Overall, during months 1 through 12, the mean increase in height was 3.96 cm in the beclomethasone dipropionate (BDP) group, 5.04 cm in the salmeterol group, and 5.04 in the placebo group. The effect of BDP on height appeared to be greatest during months 1 through 3. After this period, the slopes of the lines were parallel for the three treatment groups. The effect of BDP on growth differed significantly from the effect of placebo at 6 months ($p = 0.002$), 9 months ($p < 0.001$), and 12 months ($p < 0.001$) and differed from the effect of salmeterol at 9 and 12 months ($p < 0.001$ for both comparisons). The effect of salmeterol on growth did not differ significantly from that of placebo at any time. (From Ref. 153.)

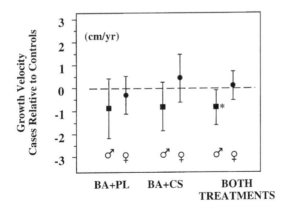

Figure 6 Differences in growth velocity according to sex and treatment in cases and controls. Treatments: BA + PL, albuterol + placebo; BA + CS, albuterol + BUD; *, $p < 0.04$ cases compared to controls (paired t-test). (From Ref. 157.)

the different treatment groups, or lack appropriate untreated control groups. In one of the few published studies that sought specifically to evaluate growth, Allen et al. (158) compared the growth of over 300 children randomized to receive FP 100 µg/day, FP 200 µg/day, or placebo for 1 year. After 1 year of FP therapy, no difference in height was noted between either dose of FP and placebo. It should be stressed that relatively low doses of FP were used in this study, which may therefore not be reflective of the growth pattern at higher doses, especially given the observation that significant adrenal suppression occurs at lower doses of FP compared to the other inhaled GCs. In fact, there has been a recent report of growth suppression in a small number of children treated with high-dose FP therapy (159). Six children with severe asthma who continued to be symptomatic despite being on high-dose BDP or BUD were subsequently placed on FP at doses ≥1000 µg/day. All of the children displayed improved asthma control while on the high-dose FP, but decreases in growth velocity were observed. Of no surprise, significant adrenal suppression was also noted. There are several limitations to this study in that it was neither prospective nor controlled, but it does make the important observation that high-dose FP therapy may be associated with adverse effects.

Although inhaled GC therapy can suppress short-term linear growth, long-term studies have not shown differences in growth (86) or attainment of adult height in GC patients compared to asthmatics not on inhaled GC and nonasthmatic controls (155,160). Unfortunately, these studies are limited by the fact that they were either retrospective or lacked adequate controls. In an intriguing follow-up to the Doull study outlined above (151), the investigators reanalyzed their previously published growth data that had demonstrated a loss of approximately 1 cm after 7 months of BDP therapy (161). Using a random-effects regression model on 50 children who had received BDP, they found the greatest loss of linear growth occurred during the first 6 weeks of therapy (Table 4). By week 19 and extending through week 30, there was no difference in linear growth compared to the growth before beginning BDP. These data and those of the Simons study (153) suggest that the growth-suppressive effects of inhaled GC therapy may be transient and short-lived. However, the results of these studies differ from those of the Verberne study (152).

A large 5-year randomized, multicenter study sponsored by the National Institutes of Health, the Childhood Asthma Management Program (CAMP), is an ongoing study designed to answer many of the questions regarding inhaled GC use in childhood asthma. This study, in which over 1000 children

Table 4 Comparison of Growth When Not Receiving Beclomethasone Dipropionate with Growth During Treatment, Segregated by 6-Week Divisions

Period	Growth (mm/week)	Difference between treatment and no treatment	95% Confidence interval	p Value
No treatment	0.140	—		
Weeks 0–6	0.073	−0.067	−0.120–−0.015	0.011
Weeks 7–12	0.094	−0.046	−0.098–−0.005	0.076
Weeks 13–18	0.093	−0.047	−0.100–−0.005	0.079
Weeks 19–24	0.138	−0.002	−0.054–0.051	0.935
Weeks 25–30	0.120	−0.02	−0.099–0.058	0.607

Source: From Ref. 151.

have been randomized to receive either placebo, nedocromil, or BUD, is designed to measure the natural history of childhood asthma. In addition, it will significantly enhance the field of our current knowledge in terms of both the efficacy and adverse effects of the two study medications. Of particular interest is whether 5 years of BUD therapy will adversely affect growth in addition to other potential adverse effects, including changes in bone metabolism or osteoporosis.

Osteoporosis

Osteoporosis, is the most predictable and debilitating GC-associated adverse effect in asthmatic patients dependent on chronic oral GC therapy. All patients who have been on >7.5 mg prednisone (or equivalent) daily for at least 6 months are at risk for developing osteoporosis (162). Despite the fact that osteoporosis can be a debilitating complication of GC therapy, there have been, until recently, a paucity of studies evaluating the effect of inhaled GC on bone metabolism and even fewer studies evaluating the effect of inhaled GC on bone mineral density. GCs exert negative effects on bone formation by inhibiting osteoblast function, in addition to increasing bone resorption. Several markers are available for use in analyzing the effects of GC on bone metabolism (163). The carboxypeptide of type I procollagen (PICP), osteocalcin, and alkaline phosphatase are serum markers of osteoblast function, while urinary hydroxyproline, and pyridinolone, and serum tartrate–resistant acid phosphatase (TRAP) and type I collagen carboxy-terminal propeptide (ICTP) are markers of bone resorption. Short-term studies have demonstrated dose-dependent suppression of serum osteocalcin levels with both BDP (164,165) and BUD (166). A study designed to assess the long-term effects of inhaled GCs on bone metabolism evaluated serum PICP and ICTP levels in 70 patients randomized to receive beclomethasone dipropionate (800 µg/day) compared to 85 patients randomized to receive bronchodilator therapy alone over a 2.5-year period (167). Of some surprise, although decreases in serum osteocalcin levels were noted shortly after treatment (4 weeks), there were no differences in markers of bone resorption or bone formation between the two groups upon completion of the 2.5-year study. The authors concluded that long-term changes in bone turnover during inhaled GC treatment should not be deduced from short-term studies with single serum parameters of bone function. They also stated that long-term studies utilizing bone densitometry need to be performed to adequately determine the potential for detrimental effects on bone metabolism.

To assess the clinical relevance of inhaled GC therapy on bone metabolism, studies utilizing bone densitometry should be performed. Bone densitometry is the most sensitive way to assess for the presence of osteoporosis (168,169). The detection and quantitation of the degree of osteoporosis is important; as the degree of osteoporosis increases, so too does the risk for fracture (170). There have been only a few studies using bone densitometry in asthmatics on inhaled GC therapy. Most have been cross-sectional, while a few have been prospective, controlled studies. Two recently published cross-sectional studies highlight the discrepancies in results that characterize many of the studies evaluating adverse effects with inhaled GC therapy. Hanania et al. (171) studied 36 asthmatics, 18 treated with BDP (mean dose, 1323 µg/day; median duration, 24 months) and 18 treated with bronchodilator alone. Biochemical markers of bone metabolism as well as bone mineral density were measured in all subjects. The investigators found significant reductions in osteocalcin levels in the group on BDP compared to those on bronchodilator therapy. In addition, those on BDP had significantly decreased bone mineral density of the femoral neck compared to age-matched controls. Of note, significant inverse correlations were found between bone mineral density and the dose duration (product of the average daily dose of inhaled GC in grams and the duration of therapy in months) of inhaled GC therapy.

Whereas Hanania et al. (171) found inhaled GC therapy to result in a dose-dependent reduction in bone density, Luengo et al. (172) found no difference in bone mineral density among 48 asthmatic patients on inhaled GC (BDP or BUD; mean dose 662 ± 278 µg/day for 10.6 years) compared to 48 age- and sex-matched nonasthmatic controls at baseline or after 2 years of observation. Similar results were noted by Konig et al. (173) in a cross-sectional study performed in children. Using biochemical markers of bone metabolism plus BMD, these investigators studied the effect of BDP (300–600 ng/day) in asthmatic children over a 2-year period with asthmatic children not on inhaled GSs and nonasthmatic children used as their control groups. BDP in doses up to 800 µg/day had no effect on osteocalcin levels or bone mineral density, but the asthmatics had lower osteocalcin levels than their age-matched, nonasthmatic peers.

A lingering and as yet inadequately addressed question is the effect of severe asthma on bone density. A recent study by Wisniewski et al. (174) sought to assess the magnitude of BMD reduction in relation to inhaled GC use after adjusting for confounding variables such as age, physical activity, past oral GC use, and asthma severity. A total of 81 subjects were recruited, 47 of whom were on inhaled GC (620 µg/day for 7.8) and 34 who had never received oral or inhaled GC. Overall, there was no difference in BMD between the group on inhaled GC therapy compared to the group not on inhaled GCs. There was, however, a statistically significant reduction in BMD in women with increasing dose of inhaled GC, equivalent to a 0.11-SD reduction in lumbar BMD for every year's use of inhaled GC at a dose of 1000 μg/day after correcting for confounding factors. In addition, the authors found no association between asthma severity and reduction in BMD. This is the second study that demonstrated a dose duration effect of inhaled GC on BMD (171). From this study, if BMD is lost in a linear fashion, the combination of dose plus duration of therapy must be considered, in that a 30-year course of 1000 μg/ day of inhaled GC would result in a BMD 3 SD below the mean. This conclusion must be tempered by the fact that it is unclear whether BMD loss occurs in a linear fashion.

Pauwels et al. (175) evaluated the efficacy and safety of FP and BDP in 340 adults with moderate to severe asthma in a 12-month double-blind crossover study. All subjects had been on 800 to 2000 μg/day of either BUD or BDP before randomization to receive FP (500, 750, or 1000 μg/day) or BDP (1000, 1500, or 2000 μg/day). At baseline, the mean morning cortisol levels in both treatment groups were within normal limits, with no change noted during the 12-month study. Despite normal cortisol levels, the BMD of the lumbar spine and femoral neck was significantly decreased compared with that of healthy control subjects, with Z-scores of -0.68 and 0.18, respectively. After 6 months of FP therapy, serum osteocalcin levels increased, as did the BMD of the lumbar spine and femoral Ward's triangle, while a decrease in BMD was found in the femoral neck following BDP therapy. This study also suggests that one can manifest evidence of systemic adverse effects without displaying adrenal suppression. Second, those with moderate to severe asthma may already have diminished BMD. Third, FP may have a better safety profile than BDP.

Given the discrepancy in results among the above studies, Toogood et al. performed bone density studies in 69 adult asthmatics in an attempt to differentiate between the effect of inhaled GC compared to the potential effect of other variables, such as past or current oral GC use, age, physical activity level, and postmenopausal state on bone density (176). They found inhaled GC therapy to result in a dose-dependent reduction of bone mineral density, with a decrease of approximately 0.5 SD for each increment of inhaled GC dose of 1 mg/day. Of some surprise, a larger lifetime exposure to inhaled GCs was associated with a more normal lumbar bone density. Toogood and colleagues speculated that this "protective effect" was due to reconstitution of bone mineral density following conversion from oral to inhaled GC therapy. Last, postmenopausal women on estrogen replacement therapy were likely to have normal bone density. In conclusion, it was found that the daily dose but not the duration of therapy adversely affects bone density and that estrogen therapy may offset inhaled GC effects on bone demineralization in postmenopausal women (176).

The issue of osteoporosis as it relates to inhaled GC use in childhood asthma has been inadequately studied. Complicating this issue is the lack of adequate healthy control reference ranges with which to compare values. In one of the largest studies published to date, Agertoft and Pedersen (177) performed total-body BMD determinations on a group of 157 asthmatic children treated with BUD at a mean dose of 500 µg/day for a mean duration of 4.5 years. For their control population, they performed BMD determinations on 111 age-matched asthmatics not on inhaled GC therapy. The authors found no differences between the two groups in any measure studied, including bone mineral density, total bone calcium, or bone mineral capacity. In summary, many factors appear to contribute to the development of osteoporosis, including dose, frequency of administration, and duration of use in addition to time of use above a "threshold" dose. Information is needed on how to manage steroid-induced osteoporosis, especially in cases where chronic high-dose inhaled GCs are indicated to manage severe persistent asthma.

Cataracts/Glaucoma

Cataracts and glaucoma are known ophthalmological complications of chronic systemic GC therapy (178–180). Two recent reports have suggested that chronic inhaled GC therapy is also associated with the development of these complications (181,182). Both studies have received substantial coverage in the lay press, and both are large epidemiological studies that found weak but statistically significant associations between inhaled GC therapy and either cataracts or glaucoma. It should be noted that in both studies elderly individuals were evaluated, with a mean age in the cataract study of 66 years, while only subjects 65 years old and over were evaluated in the glaucoma study. In addition, none of these studies provided any indication of clinical significance or visual impairment. In the study by Garbe et al. (182), individuals on high-dose inhaled GC therapy ($\geq$1500 µg/day) for prolonged periods of time ($\geq$3 months) were at greatest risk for the development of glaucoma, with an odds ratio of 1.44. Cummings et al. also found an increased risk for the development of subcapsular cataracts with higher cumulative lifetime doses of inhaled GC therapy, with the highest prevalence found in subjects whose lifetime dose was >2000 mg (181). Whether the results of these studies apply to inhaled GC use in children remains to be determined, although smaller short-term studies have not found associations between inhaled GC therapy and cataract formation (130,183). In the past year, Agertoft and Pedersen have published a large study suggesting that long-term BUD therapy in asthmatic children is not associated with the development of cataracts (184). Slit-lamp evaluations were performed on 157 asthmatic children on BUD an average of 4.5 years and in 111 age-matched asthmatic controls. Only one posterior subcapsular cataract was identified. This was in a child receiving BUD, but it was a known cataract with the diagnosis made 2 years before the child was placed on BUD therapy. The authors concluded that long-term treatment with BUD is unlikely to cause cataracts and that ophthamalogical surveillance is probably not warranted.

Other Adverse Effects

A number of other adverse effects have been associated with inhaled GC therapy, including hypoglycemia (185), the development of cushingoid features (186), opportunistic infections (187–189) dermal thinning (190,191), and psychosis (192). Most of these adverse effects have been reported as case reports, with few controlled studies performed to objectively evaluate the potential for and significance of these complications.

C. Inhaled GC Adverse Effects—Summary

In summary, while this area remains controversial, most would agree that high-dose (>1000 µg/day for children, 2000 µg/day for adults) therapy for extended periods of time is most likely to be associated with greatest risk for adverse effects. The adverse effects of greatest concern include HPA axis suppression, growth suppression, and the insidious development of osteoporosis (Table 3). At present many questions remain regarding the clinical significance of these adverse effects. Studies designed to address these concerns are in progress (e.g., the CAMP study); until a clear consensus emerges, it is prudent to use the lowest tolerated inhaled GC dose and to keep in mind that systemic effects can occur in those patients who require high-dose therapy for long periods of time for adequate asthma control.

VII. Combination Therapy for Asthma

Given that chronic inhaled GC therapy is not without risk for potential adverse effects and that some asthmatics remain symptomatic while on inhaled GC therapy, there has been a trend toward using combination therapy in patients with moderate and severe persistent asthma. Over the past 5 years, several studies have been published which in general show the combination of inhaled GCs plus a long-acting bronchodilator to be as effective or more effective than high-dose inhaled GC alone (193–196). Woolcock et al. (194), in 1996, published a study that sought to determine the most effective therapy in patients who were symptomatic despite being on BDP therapy. Subjects were randomized to receive either a double dose of BDP or a combination of BDP and the long-acting β-agonist salmeterol. Upon completion of the study, the combination of BDP plus salmeterol was found to as effective or more effective than high-dose BDP. In the ensuing 2 years, more studies have been published comparing low-dose inhaled GCs with a long-acting bronchodilator vs. high-dose inhaled GC therapy alone, with similar results reported. Pauwels et al. (195) enrolled over 850 asthmatics with moderate airflow obstruction (baseline FEV_1 75% of predicted) into a randomized, double-blind study where they received one of four treatments administered twice daily: (1) BUD 100 μg plus placebo; (2) BUD 100 μg plus formoterol 12 μg; (3) BUD 400 μg plus placebo; or (4) BUD 400 μg plus formoterol 12 μg for 1 year. The addition of formoterol to low-dose BUD resulted in a 29% reduction in severe asthma exacerbations, compared to a reduction of 49% with high-dose BUD, and a further reduction in exacerbations to 63% if formoterol was added to high-dose BUD. Asthma symptoms and lung function improved with the formoterol and the higher dose of BUD, with the greatest improvements noted with formoterol. The authors concluded that in patients with persistent symptoms despite treatment with inhaled GC, the addition of formoterol to BUD therapy or a higher dose of BUD may be beneficial. Evans et al. (196) studied the effect of low-dose BUD and sustained-release theophylline vs. high-dose BUD in a group of 62 patients with mild to moderate asthma and found both treatments to be equally effective in improving lung function. Of note, morning serum cortisol levels were significantly (but clinically insignificant) suppressed in the high-dose BUD but not in the low-dose group. Perhaps the most interesting aspect of this study came from the analysis of the monthly costs of various treatment modalities. Combination therapy with BUD and salmeterol was most expensive followed by high-dose BUD therapy alone, while the combination of low-dose BUD and theophylline was by far the least expensive.

Whether combination therapy with inhaled GCs and leukotriene-modifying agents will offer superior efficacy while minimizing the potential for adverse effects has yet to be determined. A recent study from Japan using pranlukast, a leukotriene receptor antagonist (not available in this country), found pranlukast to offer inhaled GC-sparing effects (197). Asthmatics who required high-dose BDP therapy (>1500 μg/day) to control their asthma were recruited. After a 2-week run-in period, the inhaled GC dose was reduced by 50% and the patients were randomized to receive either pranlukast or placebo for 6 weeks. Upon completion of the study, those randomized to receive placebo were symptomatic, had significant declines in their lung function, and had elevated levels of eosinophil cationic protein (ECP) and exhaled nitric oxide (eNO) compared to their baseline values. In contrast, those on pranlukast were able to maintain their lung function, had no worsening in symptoms, and had stable ECP and eNO values. Although this study was not designed to determine whether the combination of low-dose inhaled GC plus pranlukast was as effective as high-dose inhaled GC therapy, the results would suggest that combination therapy may offer significant advantages.

VIII. Summary

Inhaled GCs are among the most thoroughly studied and scrutinized medications used to treat asthma. They are now the preferred medication for control of persistent asthma. Inhaled GC therapy results in improvements in almost every efficacy parameter chosen and include reduction in symptoms, improvements in quality of life and airway caliber, and reductions in BHR, morbidity, and even mortality from asthma (Table 1). At the forefront are studies suggesting that early intervention and long-term therapy may offer the potential to affect long-term outcome. In other words, these drugs may display disease-modifying or remittive properties. On the other hand, there are some ominous features suggesting that long-term high-dose therapy may increase the potential for adverse effects such as growth suppression, bone mineral loss, and ocular disorders. This should be borne in mind as we move to treat at an early time of disease onset, which often occurs in young children (<2 years of age); develop higher potency inhaled GCs (e.g., FP); improve delivery systems to increase lung delivery, which may consequently increased systemic availability; and advocate long-term therapy. It will be important to define maximally safe and minimally effective doses of the available inhaled GCs and corresponding delivery systems. Physicians should use products that are well studied in the specific patient category they are managing. For example, there is extensive information on the dosing guidelines of BUD in children. We should also effectively incorporate nonsteroid asthma controllers to limit the use of inhaled GCs. We should also incorporate our new knowledge of GC mechanisms of action and limitations in activity, combined with increased understanding of the pathophysiology of asthma to develop new drugs.

Acknowledgments

This chapter is supported in part by National Institutes of Health grant number HL-36577 and General Clinical Research Center Grant 5 M01 RR00051.

References

1. Szefler SJ. Glucocorticoid therapy for asthma: clinical pharmacology. J Allergy Clin Immunol 1991; 88:147–164.
2. Spahn JD, Leung DYM. The role of glucocorticoids in the management of asthma. Allergy Asthma Proc 1996; 17:341–350.
3. Randolph TG, Rollins JP. The effect of cortisone on bronchial asthma. J Allergy 1950; 21:288–295.
4. Carryer HM, Koelsche GA, Prickman LE, Maytum CK, Lake C, Williams HL. The effect of cortisone on bronchial asthma and hay fever occurring in subjects sensitive to ragweed pollen. J Allergy 1950; 21:282–287.
5. Feinberg SM, Dannenberg TB, Malkiel S. ACTH and cortisone in allergic manifestations: therapeutic results and studies on immunological and tissue reactivity. J Allergy 1951; 22:195–210.
6. Gelfand ML. Administration of cortisone by the aerosol method in the treatment of bronchial asthma. N Engl J Med 1951; 245:293–294.
7. Brockbank W, Brebner H, Pengelly CDR. Chronic asthma treated with aerosol hydrocortisone. Lancet 1956; 2:807.
8. Reed CE. Aerosol glucocorticoid treatment of asthma: adults. Am Rev Respir Dis 1990; 141:S82–S88.
9. Crepea SB. Inhalation corticosteroid (dexamethasone PO₄) management of chronically asthmatic children. J Allergy 1963; 34:119–126.
10. Arbesman CE, Bonstein HS, Reisman RE. Dexamethasone aerosol therapy for bronchial asthma. J Allergy 1963; 34:354–361.

11. Snider GL, Frank MI, Aaronson AL, Radner DB, Kaplan MA, Mosko MM. The effect of dexamethasone aerosol on airway obstruction in bronchial asthma. Dis Chest 1963; 44:408–415.

12. Dennis M, Itkin IH. Effectiveness and complications of aerosol dexamethasone phosphate in severe asthma. J Allergy 1964; 35:70–76.

13. Toogood JH, Lefcoe NM. Dexamethasone aerosol for the treatment of ''steroid dependent'' chronic bronchial asthmatic patients. J Allergy 1965; 36:321–332.

14. Brown HM, Storey G, George WHS. Beclomethasone dipropionate: a new steroid aerosol for the treatment of allergic asthma. BMJ 1972; 1:585–590.

15. Clark TJH. Effect of beclomethasone dipropionate delivered by aerosol in patients with asthma. Lancet 1972; 1:1361–1364.

16. Brompton Hospital/Medical Research Council Collaborative Trial. Double-blind trial comparing two dosage schedules of beclomethasone dipropionate aerosol in the treatment of chronic asthma. Lancet 1974; 2:303–307.

17. British Thoracic and Tuberculosis Association. Inhaled corticosteroids compared with oral prednisone in patients starting long-term corticosteroid therapy for asthma. Lancet 1975; 2:469–473.

18. Godfrey S, Konig P. Beclomethasone aerosol in childhood asthma. Arch Dis Child 1973; 48:665–670.

19. British Thoracic and Tuberculosis Association. A controlled trial of corticosteroids in patients receiving prednisone tablets for asthma. Br J Dis Chest 1976; 70:95–103.

20. Picard D, Yamomoto KR. Two signals mediate hormone dependent nuclear localization of the glucocorticoid receptor. EMBO J 1987; 6:3333–3340.

21. Tsai SY, Carlstedt-Duke J, Weigel NL, Dahlman K, Gustafsson JA, Tsai MJ, O'Malley BW. Molecular interactions of steroid hormone receptor with its enhancer element: evidence for receptor dimer formation. Cell 1988; 55:361–369.

22. Luisi BF, Xu WX, Otwinowski Z, Freedman LP, Yamamoto KR, Siegler PB. Crystallographic analysis of the interaction of the glucocorticoid receptor with DNA. Nature 1991; 352:497–505.

23. Sakai DD, Helms S, Carlstedt-Duke J, Gustafsson JA, Rottman FM, Yamamoto KR. Hormone-mediated repression of transcription: a negative glucocorticoid response element from the bovine prolactin gene. Genes Dev 1988; 2:1144–1154.

24. Diamond MI, Miner JN, Yoshinaga SK, Yamamoto KR. Transcription factor interactions: selectors of positive or negative regulation from a single DNA element. Science 1990; 249:1266–1272.

25. Yang-Yen H-F, Chambard J-C, Sun Y-L, Smeal T, Schmidt TJ, Drouin J, Karin M. Transcriptional interference between c-Jun and the glucocorticoid receptor: mutual inhibition of DNA binding due to direct protein-protein interaction. Cell 1990; 62:1205–1215.

26. Barnes PJ, Greening AP, Crompton GK. Glucocorticoid resistance in asthma. Am J Respir Crit Care Med 1995; 152:S125–S142.

27. Schule R, Rangarajan P, Kliewer S, Ransone LJ, Bolado J, Yang N, Verma IM, Evans R. Functional antagonism between oncoprotein c-Jun and the glucocorticoid receptor. Cell 1990; 62:1217–1226.

28. Adcock IM, Brown CR, Gelder CM, Shirasaki H, Peters MJ, Barnes PJ. The effects of glucocorticoids on transcription factor activation in human peripheral blood mononuclear cells. Am J Physiol 1995; 37:C331–C338.

29. Ray A, Prefontaine KE. Physical association and functional antagonism between the p65 subunit of transcription factor NF-kappa B and the glucocorticoid receptor. Proc Natl Acad Sci USA 1994; 91:752–756.

30. Scheinman RI, Cogswell PC, Lofquist AK, Baldwin AS. Role of transcriptional activation of $I\kappa B\alpha$ in mediation of immunosuppression by glucocorticoids. Science 1995; 270:283–286.

31. Auphan N, DiDonato JA, Rosette C, Helmberg A, Karin M. Immunosuppression by glucocorticoids: inhibition of NF-κB activity through induction of IkB synthesis. Science 1995; 270:286–290.

32. Peppel K, Vinci JM, Baglioni C. The AU-rich sequences in the 3′ untranslated region mediate the increased turnover of interferon mRNA induced by glucocorticoids. J Exp Med 1991; 173:349–355.

33. Hegele RG, Hogg JC. The Pathology of Asthma: An Inflammatory Disorder. In Szefler SJ, Leung DYM, eds. Severe Asthma: Pathogenesis and Clinical Management. New York: Marcel Dekker, 1996:61–76.

34. Borish L, Mascali JJ, Dishuck J, Beam WR, Martin RJ, Rosenwasser LJ. Detection of alveolar macrophage-derived IL-1β in asthma: inhibition with corticosteroids. J Immunol 1992; 149:3078–3082.

35. Boumpas DT, Older SA, Anastassiou ED, Tsokos GC, Nelson D, Balow JE. Dexamethasone inhibits human IL-2 but not IL-2R gene expression in vitro at the level of nuclear transcription. J Clin Invest 1991; 87:1739–1747.

36. Culpepper JA, Lee F. Regulation of IL-3 expression by glucocorticoids in cloned murine T lymphocytes. J Immunol 1985; 135:3191–3197.

37. Wu CY, Fargeas C, Nakajima T, Delespesse G. Glucocorticoids suppress the production of interleukin 4 by human lymphocytes. Eur J Immunol 1991; 21:2645–2647.

38. Byron KA, Varigos G, Wooton A. Hydrocortisone inhibition of human interleukin-4. Immunology 1992; 77:624–626.

39. Rolfe FG, Hughes JM, Armour CL, Sewell WA. Inhibition of interleukin-5 gene expression by dexamethasone. Immunology 1992; 77:494–499.

40. Robinson D, Hamid Q, Ying S, Bentley A, Assoufi B, Durham S, Kay AB. Prednisolone treatment in asthma is associated with modulation of bronchoalveolar lavage cell interleukin-4, interleukin-5, and interferon-γ cytokine gene expression. Am Rev Respir Dis 1993; 148:401–406.

41. Tobler A, Meier R, Seitz M, Dewald B, Baggiolini M, Fey MF. Glucocorticoids downregulate gene expression of GM-CSF, NAP-1, IL-8, IL-6, but not M-CSF in human fibroblasts. Blood 1992; 79:45–51.

42. Kato M, Schleimer RP. Anti-inflammatory steroids inhibit granulocyte/macrophage colony stimulating factor production by human lung tissue. Lung 1994; 172:113–124.

43. Waage A, Bakke O. Glucocorticoids suppress the production of tumor necrosis factor by lipopolysaccharide-stimulated human monocytes. Immunology 1988; 63:299–302.

44. Laitinen LA, Laitinen A, Haahtela T. A comparative study of the effects of an inhaled corticosteroid, BUD, and a β2-agonist, terbutaline, on airway inflammation in newly diagnosed asthma. J Allergy Clin Immunol 1992; 90:32–42.

45. Wilson JW, Djukanovic R, Howarth PH, Holgate ST. Inhaled beclomethasone dipropionate downregulates airway lymphocyte activation in atopic asthma. Am J Respir Crit Care Med 1994; 149:86–90.

46. Trigg CJ, Manolitsas ND, Wang J, Calderon MA, McAulay A, Jordan SE, Herdman MJ, Jhalli N, Duddle JM, Hamilton SA, Devalia JL, Davies RJ. Placebo-controlled immunopathologic study of four months of inhaled corticosteroids in asthma. Am J Respir Crit Care Med 1994; 150:17–22.

47. Booth H, Richmond I, Ward C, Gardiner PV, Harkawat R, Walters EH. Effect of high dose inhaled fluticasone propionate on airway inflammation in asthma. Am J Respir Crit Care Med 1995; 152:45–52.

48. Olivieri D, Chetta A, Del Donno M, Bertorelli G, Casalini A, Pesci A, Testi R, Foresi A. Effect of short-term treatment with low-dose inhaled fluticasone propionate on airway inflammation and remodeling in mild asthma: a placebo-controlled study. Am J Respir Crit Care Med 1997; 155:1864–1871.

49. Kharitonov SA, Yates DH, Barnes PJ. Inhaled glucocorticoids decrease nitric oxide in exhaled air of asthmatic patients. Am J Respir Crit Care Med 1996; 153:454–457.

50. Majori M, Piccoli LM, Bertacco S, Cuomp A, Cantini L, Pesci A. Inhaled beclomethasone dipropionate downregulates CD4 and CD8 T-lymphocyte activation in peripheral blood of patients with asthma. J Allergy Clin Immunol 1997; 100: 379–382.

51. Sont JK, Van Krieken JHJM, Evertse CE, Hooijer R, Willems LNA, Sterk PJ. Relationship between the inflammatory infiltrate in bronchial biopsy specimens and clinical severity of asthma in patients treated with inhaled steroids. Thorax 1996; 51:496–502.

52. Hargreave FE, Ryan G, Thomson NC, Ryan G, Thomson NC, O'Byrne PM, Latimer K, Juniper EF, Dolovich J. Bronchial responsiveness to histamine or methacholine in asthma: measurement and clinical significance. J Allergy Clin Immunol 1981; 68:347–355.

53. Barnes PJ. New concepts in the pathogenesis of bronchial hyperresponsiveness and asthma. J Allergy Clin Immunol 1989; 83:1013–1026.

54. Chung KF. Role played by inflammation in the hyperreactivity of the airways in asthma. Thorax 1986; 41:657–662.

55. Power C, Sreenan S, Hurson B, Burke C, Poulter LW. Distribution of immuno-

competent cells in the bronchial wall of clinically healthy subjects showing bronchial hyperresponsiveness. Thorax 1993; 48:1125–1129.

56. Kraan J, Koeter GH, VD Mark TW, Sluiter HJ, De Vries K. Changes in bronchial hyperreactivity induced by 4 weeks of treatment with antiasthmatic drugs in patients with allergic asthma: a comparison between BUD and terbutaline. J Allergy Clin Immunol 1985; 76:628–636.

57. Ryan G, Latimer KM, Juniper EF, Roberts RS, Tech M, Hargreave FE. Effect of beclomethasone dipropionate on bronchial hyperresponsiveness to histamine in controlled non-steroid dependent asthma. J Allergy Clin Immunol 1985; 75: 25–30.

58. Dutoit JI, Salome CM, Woolcock AJ. Inhaled corticosteroids reduce the severity of bronchial hyperresponsiveness in asthma but oral theophylline does not. Am Rev Respir Dis 1987; 136:1174–1178.

59. Svendsen UG, Frolund L, Madsen F, Nielson NH, Holstein-Rathlou N-H, Weeke B. A comparison of the effects of sodium cromylglycate and beclomethasone dipropionate on pulmonary function and bronchial hyperreactivity in subjects with asthma. J Allergy Clin Immunol 1987; 80:68–74.

60. Kerrebijn KF, Van Essen-Zandvliet EEM, Neijens HJ. Effect of long-term treatment with inhaled corticosteroids and beta-agonists on the bronchial hyperresponsiveness in children with asthma. J Allergy Clin Immunol 1987; 79:653–659.

61. Kraan J, Koeter GH, Van Der Mark TW, Boorsma MM, Kukler J, Sluiter HJ, De Vries K. Dosage and time effects of inhaled BUD on bronchial hyperreactivity. Am J Respir Dis 1988; 137:44–48.

62. Juniper EF, Kline PA, Vanzieleghem MA, Ramsdale EH, O'Byrne PM, Hargreave FE. Effect of long-term treatment with an inhaled corticosteroid (BUD) on airway hyperresponsiveness and clinical asthma in non-steroid-dependent asthmatics. Am Rev Respir Dis 1990; 142:832–836.

63. Waalkens HJ, Gerristen J, Koeter GH, Krouwels FH, Van Aalderen WMC, Knol K. BUD and terbutaline or terbutaline alone in children with mild asthma: effects on bronchial hyperresponsiveness and diurnal variation in peak flow. Thorax 1991; 46:499–503.

64. Haahtela T, Jarvinen M, Kava T, Kiviranta K, Koskinen S, Lehtonen K, Nikander K, Persson T, Reinikainen K, Selroos O, Sovijarvi A, Stenius-Aarniala B, Svahn T, Tammivaara R, Laitinen LA. Comparison of a β2-agonist, terbutaline, with an inhaled corticosteroid, BUD, in newly diagnosed asthma. N Engl J Med 1991; 325:388–392.

65. Van Essen-Zandvliet EE, Hughes MD, Waalkens HJ, Duiverman EJ, Pocock SJ, Kerrebijn KF. Effects of 22 months of treatment with inhaled corticosteroids and/or beta-2-agonists on lung function, airway responsiveness, and symptoms in children with asthma. Am J Respir Dis 1992; 146:547–554.

66. Djukanovic R, Wilson JW, Britten KM, Wilson SJ, Walls AF, Roche WR, Howarth PH, Holgate ST. Effect of an inhaled corticosteroid on airway

inflammation and symptoms in asthma. Am Rev Respir Dis 1992; 145:669–674.

67. Jenkins CR, Woolcock AJ. Effect of prednisone and beclomethasone dipropionate on airway responsiveness in asthma: a comparative study. Thorax 1988; 43:378–384.

68. Nikolaizik WH, Preece MA, Warner JO. One year follow-up study of endocrine and lung function of asthmatic children on inhaled BUD. Eur Respir J 1997; 10:2596–2601.

69. Sekerel BE, Tuncer A, Saraclar Y, Adalioglu G. Inhaled BUD reduces lung hyperinflation in children with asthma. Acta Pediatr 1997; 86:932–936.

70. Booms P, Cheung D, Timmers MC. Protective effect of inhaled BUD against unlimited airway narrowing to methacholine in atopic patients with asthma. J Allergy Clin Immunol 1997; 99:330–337.

71. Ernst P, Spitzer WO, Suissa S, Cockroft D, Habbick B, Horwitz RI, Boivin J-F, McNutt M, Buist AS. Risk of fatal and near fatal asthma in relation to inhaled corticosteroid use. JAMA 1992; 268:3462–3464.

72. Spitzer WO, Suissa S, Ernst P, Horwitz RI, Habrick B, Cockroft D, Boivin J-F, McNutt M, Buist AS, Reebuck AS. The use of beta-agonists and the risk of death and near death from asthma. N Engl J Med 1992; 326:501–506.

73. Donahue JG, Weiss ST, Livingston JM, Goestch MA, Greineder DK, Platt R. Inhaled steroids and the risk of hospitalization for asthma. JAMA 1997; 277:887–891.

74. Blais L, Ernst P, Boivin J-F, Suissa S. Inhaled corticosteroids and the prevention of readmission to hospital for asthma. Am J Respir Crit Care Med 1998; 158:126–132.

75. English AF, Neate MS, Quint DJ, Sareen M. Biological activities of some corticosteroids used in asthma. Am J Respir Crit Care Med 1994; 149 (suppl):A212.

76. Hogger P, Rohdewald P. Binding kinetics of fluticasone propionate to the human glucocorticoid receptor. Steroids 1994; 59:597–602.

77. Phillips GH. Structure-activity relationships of topically active steroids: the selection of fluticasone propionate. Respir Med 1990; 84(suppl A): 19–23.

78. Harding SM. The human pharmacology of fluticasone propionate. Respir Med 1990; 84(suppl A):25–29.

79. Lipworth BJ. New perspectives on inhaled drug delivery and systemic bioactivity. Thorax 1995; 50:105–110.

80. Noonan M, Chervinsky P, Busse WW, Weisberg SC, Pinnas J, DeBoisblanc BP, Boltomsky H, Pearlman D, Repsher L, Kellerman D. Fluticasone propionate reduces oral prednisone use while it improves asthma control and quality of life. Am J Respir Crit Care Med 1995; 152:1467–1473.

81. Nelson HS, Bernstein IL, Fink J, Edwards TB, Spector SL, Storms WW, Tashkin DP. Oral glucocorticosteroid-sparing effect of BUD administered by Turbuhaler: a double blind, placebo-controlled study in adults with moderate to severe chronic asthma. Chest 1998; 113:1264–1271.

82. Hummel S, Lehtonen L. Comparison of oral-steroid sparing by high-dose and low-dose inhaled steroid in maintenance treatment of severe asthma. Lancet 1992; 340:1483–1487.

83. Expert Panel Report. Guidelines for the Diagnosis and Management of Asthma. NIH publication No. 91-3042. Bethesda, MD: National Institutes of Health, National Heart, Lung and Blood Institute, 1991.

84. Expert Panel Report 2: Guidelines for the Diagnosis and Management of Asthma. NIH publication No. 97-4051. Bethesda, MD: National Institutes of Health, National Heart, Lung and Blood Institute, 1997.

85. Drazen JM, Israel E. Treating mild asthma—when are inhaled steroids indicated (editorial)? N Engl J Med 1994; 331:737–739.

86. Agertoft L, Pedersen S. Effects of long-term treatment with an inhaled corticosteroid on growth and pulmonary function in asthmatic children. Respir Med 1994; 88:373–381.

87. Haahtela T, Jarvinen M, Kava T, Kiviranta K, Koskinen S, Lehtonen K, Nikander K, Persson T, Selroos O, Sovijarvi A, Stenius-Aarniala B, Svahn T, Tammivaara R, Laitinen LA. Effects of reducing or discontinuing inhaled BUD in patients with mild asthma. N Engl J Med 1994; 331:700–705.

88. Selroos O, Pietinalho A, Lofroos A-B, Riska H. Effect of early vs. late intervention with inhaled corticosteroids in asthma. Chest 1995; 108:1228–1234.

89. Juniper EF, Kline PA, Vanzieleghem MA, Hargreave FE. Reduction of BUD after a year of increased use: a randomized controlled trial to evaluate whether improvements in airway responsiveness and clinical asthma are maintained. J Allergy Clin Immunol 1991; 87:483–489.

90. Osterman K, Carlholm M, Ekelund J, Kiviloog J, Nikander K, Nilholm L, Salomonsson P, Strand V, Venge P. Zetterstrom O. Effect of 1 year daily treatment with 400 mcg BUD (Pulmicort Turbuhaler) in newly diagnosed asthmatics. Eur Respir J 1997; 10:2210–2215.

91. Van Essen-Zandvliet EE, Hughes MD, Waalkens HJ, Duiverman EJ, Kerrebijn KF. Remission of childhood asthma after long-term treatment with an inhaled corticosteroid (BUD): can it be achieved? Eur Respir J 1994; 7:63–68.

92. Waalkens HJ, Van Essen-Zandvliet EE, Hughes MD, Gerritsen J, Duiverman EJ, Knol K, Kerrebijn KF. Cessation of long-term treatment with inhaled corticosteroid (BUD) in children with asthma results in deterioration. Am Rev Respir Dis 1993; 148:1252–1257.

93. Paggiaro PL, Dahle R, Bakran I, Frith L, Hollingworth K, Efthimiou J, on behalf of the International COPD study group. Multicentre randomised placebo-controlled trial of inhaled fluticasone propionate in patients with chronic obstructive pulmonary disease. Lancet 1998; 351:773–780.

94. Fletcher CM, Pride NM. Definitions of emphysema, bronchitis, asthma, and airflow obstruction: 25 years on from the Ciba symposium. Thorax 1984; 39:81–85.

95. Fletcher CM, Peto R. The natural history of chronic airflow obstruction. BMJ 1978; 1:1645–1648.

96. Thom TJ. International comparisons in COPD mortality. Am Rev Respir Dis 1989; 140:27–34.
97. Barnes NC. Inhaled steroids and COPD. Lancet 1998; 351:766–767.
98. Humbert M. Airways inflammation in asthma and chronic bronchitis. Clin Exp Allergy 1996; 25:735–737.
99. Greening A. Pharmacotherapy in COPD. Eur Respir Rev 1997; 7:45, 243–248.
100. American Thoracic Society. Standards for the diagnosis and care of patients with chronic obstructive pulmonary disease (COPD). Am J Respir Crit Care Med 1995; 152:S77–S120.
101. Ulrik CS. Efficacy of inhaled salmeterol in the management of smokers with chronic obstructive pulmonary disease: a single centre randomised, double-blind, placebo-controlled, crossover study. Thorax 1995; 50:750–754.
102. Postma DS, Peters I, Sluiter HJ. Moderately severe chronic airflow obstruction: can corticosteroids slow down obstruction? Eur Respir J 1988; 1:22–26.
103. Siafakas NM, Vermiere P, Pride NB, Paoletti P, Gibson J, Howard P, Vernault JC, Decromer M, Higenbottom T, Postma DS, Rees J. Optimal assessment and management of chronic obstructive pulmonary disease (COPD): European Respiratory Society consensus statement. Eur Respir J 1995; 8:1398–1420.
104. Chanez P, Vignola AM, O'Shaughnessy T, Enander I, Dechun LI, Jeffery PK, Bousquet J. Corticosteroid reversibility in COPD is related to features of asthma. Am J Respir Crit Care Med 1997; 155:1529–1534.
105. Keatings VM, Jatakanon A, Worsdell YM, Barnes PJ. Effects of inhaled and oral glucocorticoids in inflammatory indices in asthma and COPD. Am J Respir Crit Care Med 1997; 155:542–548.
106. Llewellyn-Jones CG, Harris TAJ, Stockley RA. The effect of fluticaone propionate on sputum of patients with chronic bronchitis and emphysema. Am J Respir Crit Care Med 1996; 153:616–621.
107. British Thoracic Society guidelines for the management of chronic obstructive pulmonary disease. Review and position statement. Thorax 1997; 52 (suppl 1).
108. Engel T, Heining JH, Madson O, Hanson M, Weeks ER. A trial of inhaled BUD on airways responsiveness in smokers with chronic bronchitis. Eur Respir J 1989; 2:935–939.
109. Auffarth B, Postma DS, DeMonchy JGR, Van der Mark TW, Boorsma M, Koeter GH. Effects of inhaled BUD on spirometry, reversibility, airway responsiveness and cough thresholdin smokers with COPD. Thorax 1991; 46:327.
110. Weir DC, Gove RI, Robertson AJ, Burge SP. Corticosteroid trials in non-asthmatic chronic airflow obstruction. Thorax 1990; 45:112–117.
111. Pride NB, Taylor RG, Lins H, Joyce H, Watson A. Bronchial hyper-responsiveness as a risk factor for progressive airflow obstruction in smokers. Bull Eur Physiopathol Respir 1987; 23:369–375.
112. Dompeling E, van Schayck CP, van Grunsven PM, Van Herwaarden CLA, Akkermans R, Molema J, Folgering H, Van Weel C. Slowing the deterioration

of asthma and chronic obstructive pulmonary disease observed during bronchodilator therapy by adding inhaled corticosteroids: a 4-year prospective study. Ann Intern Med 1993; 118:770–778.

113. Kerstjens HAM, Brand PLP, Hughes MD, Robinson NJ, Postma DS, Sluiter HJ, Bleecker ER, Dekhuijzen PNR, DeJong PM, Mengelers HJJ, Overbeek SE, Schoonbrood DFME. A comparison of bronchodilator therapy with or without inhaled corticosteroid therapy for obstructive airways disease. N Engl J Med 1992; 327:1413–1419.

114. Renkema TEJ, Schouten JP, Koeter GH, Postma DS. Effects of long-term treatment with corticosteroids in COPD. Chest 1996; 109:1156–1162.

115. Weiner P, Weiner M, Azgad Y, Zamir D. Inhaled BUD therapy for patients with stable COPD. Chest 1995; 108:1568–1571.

116. Van Schayck CP, van Grusven PM, Dekhuijzen PNR. Do patients with COPD benefit from treatment with inhaled corticosteroids? Eur Respir J 1996; 9:1969–1972.

117. Pauwels RA, Lofdahl CG, Pride NB, Postma DS, Laitinen LA, Ohlsson SV. European Respiratory Society study on chronic obstructive pulmonary disease (EUROSCOP): hypothesis and design. Eur Respir J 1992; 51:1254–1261.

118. Burge PS, Calvenley PMA, Daniels JME. The acute effects of oral prednisolone in patients with COPD in the ISOLDE trial: responders and non-responders. Am J Respir Crit Care Med 1996; 153(suppl 4):A126.

119. Barnes PJ. New therapies for chronic obstructive pulmonary disease. Thorax 1998; 53:137–147.

120. Toogood JH. Complications of topical steroid therapy for asthma. Am Rev Respir Dis 1990; 141:S89–S96.

121. Toogood JH. High-dose inhaled steroid therapy for asthma. J Allergy Clin Immunol 1989; 83:528–536.

122. Williams AJ, Baghat MS, Stableforth DE, Cayton RM, Shenoi PM, Skinner C. Dysphonia caused by inhaled steroids: recognition of a characteristic laryngeal abnormality. Thorax 1983; 38:813–821.

123. Toogood JH, Baskerville J, Jennings B, Lefcoe NM, Johansson S-A. Use of spacers to facilitate inhaled corticosteroid treatment of asthma. Am Rev Respir Dis 1984; 129:723–729.

124. Toogood JH, Jennings B, Baskerville J, Lefcoe N, Newhouse M. Assessment of a device for reducing oropharyngeal complications during beclomethasone treatment of asthma. Am Rev Respir Dis 1981; 123:113.

125. Meltzer EO, Kemp JP, Welch MJ, Orgel HA. Effect of dosing schedule on efficacy of beclomethasone dipropionate aerosol in chronic asthma. Am Rev Respir Dis 1985; 131:732–736.

126. Pedersen SE. Efficacy and safety of inhaled corticosteroids in children. In: Schleimer RP, Busse WW, O'Byrne PM, eds. Inhaled Glucocorticoids in Asthma. New York: Marcel Dekker, 1997:551–606.

127. Johansson SA, Andersson KE, Brattsand R. Topical and systemic potencies of

BUD, beclomethasone dipropionate, and prednisone in man. Eur J Respir Dis 1982; 63 (suppl 122):74–84.

128. Ebden P, Jenkins A, Houston G. Comparison of two high dose corticosteroid aerosol treatments, beclomethasone dipropionate (1500 µg/d), and BUD (1600 µg/d) for chronic asthma. Thorax 1986; 41:869–874.

129. Springer C, Avital A, Maayan CH. Comparison of BUD and beclomethasone dipropionate for treatment of asthma. Arch Dis Child 1987; 62:815–819.

130. Warner J, Nikolaizik W, Marchant J. The systemic effects of inhaled corticosteroids. J Allergy Clin Immunol 1989; 83:220–225.

131. Brown PH, Blundell G, Greening AP, Crompton GK. Hypothalamo-pituitary-adrenal axis suppression in asthmatics inhaling high dose corticosteroids. Respir Med 1991; 85:501–510.

132. Pedersen S, Fuglsang G. Urinary cortisol excretion in children treated with high doses of inhaled corticosteroids: a comparison of BUD and beclomethasone. Eur Respir J 1988; 1:433–435.

133. Baran D. A comparison of inhaled BUD and beclomethasone dipropionate in childhood asthma. Br J Dis Chest 1987; 81:170–175.

134. Prahl P, Jenson T, Bjorregaard-Anderson H. Adrenocortical function in children on high dose aerosol therapy. Allergy 1987; 42:541–544.

135. Clark DJ, Grove A, Cargill RI, Lipworth BJ. Comparative adrenal suppression with inhaled BUD and fluticasone propionate in adult asthmatic patients. Thorax 1996; 51:262–266.

136. Boorsma M, Andersson N, Larsson P, Ullman A. Assessment of relative systemic potency of inhaled fluticasone and BUD. Eur Respir J 1996; 9:1427–1432.

137. Dahl R, Lundback B, Malo JL, Mazza JA, Nieminen MM, Saarelainen P, Barnacle H. A dose-ranging study of fluticasone propionate in adult patients with moderate asthma. Chest 1993; 104:1352–1358.

138. Gustafsson P, Tsanakas J, Gold M, Primhak R, Radford M, Gillies. Comparison of the efficacy and safety of inhaled fluticasone propionate 200 µg/day with inhaled beclomethasone dipropionate 400 µg/day in mild and moderate asthma. Arch Dis Child 1993; 69:206–211.

139. Lipworth BJ, Clark DJ, McFarlane LC. Adrenocortical activity with repeated twice daily dosing of fluticasone propionate and BUD given via a large volume spacer to asthmatic children. Thorax 1997; 52:686–689.

140. Hoekx JCM, Hedlin G, Pedersen W, Sorva R, Hollingworth K, Efthimiou J. Fluticasone propionate compared with BUD: a double blind trial in asthmatic children using powder devices at a dosage of 400 µg/day. Eur Respir J 1996; 9:2263–2272.

141. Clark DJ, Lipworth BJ. Adrenal suppression with chronic dosing of fluticasone propionate compared with BUD in adult asthmatic patients. Thorax 1997; 52:55–58.

142. Donnelly R, Williams KM, Baker AB, Badcock CA, Day RO, Seale JP. Effects

of BUD and fluticasone on 24-hour plasma cortisol: a dose response study. Am J Respir Crit Care Med 1997; 156:1746–1751.

143. Ellis EF. Adverse effects of corticosteroid therapy (editorial). J Allergy Clin Immunol 1987; 80:515–517.

144. Wolthers OD, Pedersen S. Controlled study of linear growth in children during treatment with inhaled glucocorticosteroids. Pediatrics 1992; 89:839–842.

145. Wolthers OD, Pedersen S. Growth of asthmatic children during treatment with BUD: a double blind trial. BMJ 1991; 303:163–165.

146. Pedersen S, Agertoft L. Relationship between short-term lower leg growth and long-term statural growth in asthmatic children treated with BUD. Am J Respir Crit Care Med 1995; 56:13.

147. Reimer LG, Morris HG, Ellis EF. Growth of asthmatic children during treatment with alternate-day steroids. J Allergy Clin Immunol 1975; 55:224–231.

148. Russell G. Asthma and growth. Arch Dis Child 1993; 69:695–698.

149. Ninan TK, Russell G. Asthma, inhaled corticosteroid treatment, and growth. Arch Dis Child 1992; 67:703–705.

150. Tinkelman DG, Reed CE, Nelson HS, Offord KP. Aerosol beclomethasone dipropionate compared with theophylline as primary treatment of chronic, mild to moderately severe asthma in children. Pediatrics 1993; 92:64–77.

151. Doull IJM, Freezer NJ, Holgate ST. Growth of prepubertal children with mild asthma treated with inhaled beclomethasone dipropionate. Am J Respir Crit Care Med 1995; 151:1715–1719.

152. Verberne AAPH, Frost C, Jan Roorda RJ, Van Der Laag H, Kerrebijn KJ. One year treatment with salmeterol compared with beclomethasone in children with asthma. Am J Respir Crit Care Med 1997; 156:688–695.

153. Simons FER, and the Canadian Beclomethasone Dipropionate-Salmeterol Xinafoate Study Group. A comparison of beclomethasone dipropionate, salmeterol, and placebo in children with asthma. N Engl J Med 1997; 337:1659–1665.

154. Martin AJ, Landau LI, Phelan PD. The effect on growth of childhood asthma. Acta Pediatr Scand 1981; 70:683–688.

155. Balfour-Lynn L. Childhood asthma and puberty. Arch Dis Child 1985; 60:231–235.

156. Lemanske RF, Allen DB. Choosing a long-term controller medication in childhood asthma: the proverbial two-edged sword (editorial). Am J Respir Crit Care Med 1997; 156:685–687.

157. Merkus PJFM, Van Essen-Zandvliet EEM, Duiverman EJ, Van Houwelingen HC, Kerrebijn KF, Quanjer PH. Long-term effect of inhaled corticosteroids on growth rate in adolescents with asthma. Pediatrics 1993; 91:1121–1126.

158. Allen DB, Bronsky EA, LaForce CF, Nathan RA, Tinkelman DG, Vandewalker ML, Konig P, and the Fluticasone Propionate Asthma Study Group. Growth in asthmatic children treated with fluticasone propionate. J Pediatr 1998; 132:472–477.

159. Todd G, Dunlop K, McNaboe J, Ryan MF, Carson D, Shields MD. Growth and adrenal suppression in asthmatic children treated with high-dose fluticasone propionate. Lancet 1996; 348:27–29.

160. Silverstein MD, Yunginger JW, Reed, CE, Petterson T, Zimmerman D, Li JCL, O'Fallon WM. Attained adult height after childhood asthma: effect of glucocorticoid therapy. J Allergy Clin Immunol 1997; 99:466–474.

161. Doull IJM, Campbell MJ, Holgate ST. Duration of growth suppressive effects of regular inhaled corticosteroids Arch Dis Child 1998; 78:172–173.

162. Lukert BP, Raisz LG. Glucocorticoid-induced osteoporosis: pathogenesis and management. Ann Intern Med 1990; 112:352–364.

163. Toogood JH. Effects of inhaled steroid therapy for asthma on skeletal metabolism. In: Schleimer RP, Busse WW, O'Byrne PM, eds. Inhaled Glucocorticoids in Asthma. New York: Marcel Dekker, 1997:607–626.

164. Teelucksingh S, Padfield PL, Tibi L, Gough KJ, Holt PR. Inhaled corticosteroids, bone formation, and osteocalcin. Lancet 1991; 338:60–61.

165. Pouw EM, Prummel MF, Oosting H, Roos CM, Endert E. Beclomethasone inhalation decreases serum osteocalcin concentrations. BMJ 1991; 302:627–628.

166. Wolthers OD, Riis BJ, Pedersen S. Bone turnover in asthmatic children treated with oral prednisone or inhaled BUD. Pediatr Pulmonol 1993; 16:341–346.

167. Kerstjens HAM, Postma DS, Van Doormaal JJ, Van Zanten AK, Brand PLP, Dekhuijzen PNR, Koeter GH. Effects of short term and long term treatment with inhaled corticosteroids on bone metabolism in patients with airways obstruction. Thorax 1994; 49:652–656.

168. Johnston CC, Slemenda CW, Melton LJ. Clinical use of bone densitometry. N Engl J Med 1991; 324:1105–1109.

169. Seeman E, Wagner HW, Offord KP, Kumar R, Johnson WJ, Riggs BL. Differential effects of endocrine dysfunction on the axial and appendicular skeleton. J Clin Invest 1982; 69:1302–1309.

170. Cummings SR, Black DM, Nevitt M, Browner W, Cauley J, Ensrud K, Genant HK, Palermo L, Scott J. Bone density at various sites for prediction of hip fracture. Lancet 1993; 341:72–75.

171. Hanania NA, Chapman KR, Sturtridge WC, Szalai JP, Kestin S. Dose-related decreases in bone density among asthmatic patients treated with inhaled corticosteroids. J Allergy Clin Immunol 1995; 96:571–579.

172. Luengo M, Del Rio L, Pons F, Picado C. Bone mineral density in asthmatic patients treated with inhaled corticosteroids: a case control study. Eur Respir J 1997; 10:2110–2113.

173. Konig P, Hillman L, Cervantes C, Levine C, Maloney C, Douglas B, Johnson L, Allen S. Bone metabolism in children with asthma treated with inhaled beclomethasone dipropionate. J Pediatr 1993; 122:219–226.

174. Wisniewski AF, Lewis SA, Green DJ, Maslanka W, Burrell H, Tattersfield AE. Cross sectional investigation of the effects of inhaled corticosteroids on bone

density and bone metabolism in patients with asthma. Thorax 1997; 52:853–860.
175. Pauwels RA, Yernault JC, Demedts MG, Geusens P. Safety and efficacy of fluticasone and beclomethasone in moderate to severe asthma. Am J Respir Crit Care Med 1998; 157:827–832.
176. Toogood JH, Baskerville JC, Markov AE, Hodsmon AB, Fraher LJ, Jennings B, Haddad RG, Drost D. Bone mineral density and the risk of fracture in patients receiving long-term inhaled steroid therapy for asthma. J Allergy Clin Immunol 1995; 96:157–166.
177. Agertoft L, Pedersen S. Bone mineral density in children with asthma receiving long-term treatment with inhaled BUD. Am J Respir Crit Care Med 1998; 157: 178–183.
178. Rooklin AR, Lampert SI, Jaeger EA, McGeady SJ, Mansmann HC. Posterior subcapsular cataracts in steroid-requiring asthmatic children. J Allergy Clin Immunol 1979; 63:383–386.
179. Toogood JH, Markov AE, Baskerville J, Dyson C. Association of ocular cataracts with inhaled and oral steroid therapy during long-term treatment of asthma. J Allergy Clin Immunol 1993; 91:571–579.
180. Skuta GL, Morgan RK. Corticosteroid-induced glaucoma. In: Ritch R, Shields MB, Krupin T, eds. The Glaucomas. St Louis: Mosby-Year Book, 1996:1177–1188.
181. Cumming RG, Mitchell P, Leeder SR. Use of inhaled corticosteroids and the risk of cataracts. N Engl J Med 1997; 337:8–14.
182. Garbe E, LeLorier J, Boivin J-F, Suissa S. Inhaled and nasal glucocorticoids and the risks of ocular hypertension or open-angle glaucoma. JAMA 1997; 277: 722–727.
183. Simons FER, Persaud MP, Gillespie CA, Cheang M, Shuckett EP. Absence of posterior subcapsular cataracts in young patients treated with inhaled glucocorticoids. Lancet 1993; 342:776–778.
184. Agertoft L, Larsen FE, Pedersen S. Posterior subcapsular cataracts, bruises and hoarseness in children with asthma. Eur Respir J 1998; 12:130–135.
185. Carrel AL, Somers S, Lemanske RF, Allen DB. Hypoglycemia and cortisol deficiency with low-dose corticosteroid therapy for asthma. Pediatrics 1996; 97:921–924.
186. Hollman GA, Allen DB. Overt glucocorticoid excess due to inhaled corticosteroid therapy. Pediatrics 1988; 81:452–455.
187. Shaikh WA. Pulmonary tuberculosis in patients treated with inhaled beclomethasone. Allergy 1992; 47:327–330.
188. Abzug MJ, Cotton MF. Severe chickenpox after intranasal use of corticosteroids. J Pediatr 1993; 123:577–579.
189. Sy MLT, Chin TW, Nussbaum E. Pneumocystis carinii pneumonia associated with inhaled corticosteroids in an immunocompetent child with asthma. J Pediatr 1995; 127:1000–1002.
190. Capewell S, Reynolds S, Shuttleworth D, Edwards C, Finlay AY. Purpura and

dermal thinning associated with high dose inhaled corticosteroids. BMJ 1990; 300:1548–1551.

191. Autio P, Karjalainen Risteli L, Risteli J, Kiistala U, Oikarinen A. Effects of an inhaled steroid (BUD) on skin collagen synthesis of asthma patients in vivo. Am J Respir Crit Care Med 1996; 153:1172–1175.

192. Lewis LD, Cochrane GM. Psychosis in a child inhaling BUD. Lancet 1983; 2: 634.

193. Greening AP, Ind PW, Northfield M, Shaw G and the Allen & Hanburys Limited UK Study Group. Added salmeterol versus higher-dose corticosteroid in asthma patients with symptoms on existing inhaled corticosteroid. Lancet 1994; 344:219–224.

194. Woolcock A, Lundback B, Ringdal N, Jacques LA. Comparison of addition of salmeterol to inhaled steroids with doubling of the dose of inhaled steroids. Am J Respir Crit Care Med 1996; 153:1481–1488.

195. Pauwels RA, Lofdahl CG, Postma DS, Tattersfield AE, O'Byrne P, Barnes PJ, Ullman A. Effect of inhaled formoterol and BUD on exacerbations of asthma. N Engl J Med 1997; 337:1405–1411.

196. Evans DJ, Taylor DA, Zetterstrom O, Chung KF, O'Connor BJ, Barnes PJ. A comparison of low-dose inhaled BUD plus theophylline and high-dose inhaled BUD for moderate asthma. N Engl J Med 1997; 337:1412–1418.

197. Tamaoki J, Kondo M, Sakai N, Nakata J, Takemura H, Nagai A, Takizawa T, Konno K. Leukotriene antagonist prevents exacerbation of asthma during reduction of high-dose inhaled corticosteroid. Am J Respir Crit Care Med 1997; 155:1235–1240.

2

β₂-Adrenergic Agonists

MARY E. STREK and ALAN R. LEFF

The University of Chicago
Chicago, Illinois

I. Historical Perspective

Airflow obstruction in asthma and chronic obstructive pulmonary disease (COPD) historically has been treated with virtually the same drugs despite very different pathogenetic mechanisms. The physiological limitation imposed by both conditions derives from increased work of breathing (caused by increase airway resistance and/or decreased lung elastance) and ventilation/perfusion mismatch, causing hypoxemia (1,2). Nonetheless, asthma has been defined physiologically as reversible airway obstruction (more recently, obstruction resulting directly from inflammation) (3), while obstruction in COPD has been defined anatomically either as distal airway disease of the emphysematous type or as chronic bronchitis (4).

The pathogenesis of asthma and COPD may have some common derivatives. Many patients with intractable asthma resemble clinically those with COPD, and many patients with COPD have substantially reversible airflow obstruction. This suggests that the distinction between COPD and asthma may to some extent be definitional. It now is clear that multiple phenotypes exist for asthma (5) and that COPD cannot be categorized properly according to classic phenotypes of emphysema or chronic bronchitis. Thus, it is not surprising that some patients with asthma are relatively refractory to β-adrenoceptor drugs, while some patients with COPD respond reasonably well to these medications.

It has been presumed that the mechanism of action of β-adrenoceptor drugs in both asthma and COPD is the relaxation of airway smooth muscle. In COPD, the affected site is largely the distal (<2 mm) airways of the lungs, whereas in asthma, the cartilagenous airways (larger-diameter airways) are generally those most affected. The inflammatory process in asthma is fundamentally dissimilar to that of COPD. Inflammation in COPD is fundamentally neutrophilic and nonimmunologically driven. With rare exception, patients with COPD acquire the disease through cigarette smoking. Asthma is a disease of idiopathic inflammation in which eosinophils are likely to play a greater role than neutrophils (6,7). The "remodeling" of airways in both processes is vastly different. Mucous obstruction and obliteration of terminal airways and alveoli characterizes the architectural changes of COPD (8). By contrast, asthma is characterized by smooth muscle hypertrophy not found in COPD, remarkable—and still unexplained—hypersensitivity to β-adrenoceptor blockade, epithelial shedding, mucous gland hyperplasia (also characteristic of COPD), and airway hyperresponsiveness to immunological (and nonspecific) stimuli (9,10). Histological sections of patients who have died of asthma reveal severely constricted airways, much in contrast to what is seen in COPD. Thus, it is somewhat surprising that β-adrenoceptor agonists are the most widely used compounds in the treatment of *both* COPD and asthma. In fact, in the United States, β-adrenoceptor drugs are used about twice as frequently as ipratropium, which has a specific indication from the Food and Drug Administration for treatment of COPD.

The therapeutic rationale for the use of β-adrenoceptor agonists in asthma probably derives from the historical conception at the turn of the century that asthma was a disease of autonomic imbalance (11). The notion that a physiologically antagonistic sympathetic–parasympathetic innervation of the autonomic nervous system existed abnormally in autonomic imbalance, favoring parasympathetic constriction, has persisted until recently (12). There is evidence that maximal parasympathetic activation is capable of overriding maximal sympathetic stimulation (13). However, there is no proprioceptor of airway caliber in humans, and there are no sympathetic nerves in human airway smooth muscle (14). Hence, sympathetic output is not increased in bronchoconstricting normal or asthmatic individuals in a homeostatic fashion (14). Thus, the use of β-adrenoceptor agonists to effect bronchodilation in human asthmatics derives from a fortuitous historical misconception of the pathogenesis of asthma. The scientific rationale for the use of β-adrenergic agonists in COPD is probably less clear. If the disease resides in small airways of the lung, which are destroyed ultimately by the inflammatory process, how might drugs that relax airway smooth muscle improve flow? Indeed, the expected level of improvement is modest, and one presumes that therapeutic benefit derives from relaxation of normal bronchomotor tone in airways that still remain patent and functional.

II. Pharmacological Mechanisms

A. Short-Acting Agents

The development of therapeutically acceptable β-adrenoceptor agonists for the treatment of asthma required pharmacological alteration of the molecular structure of naturally occurring catecholamines. Endogenously synthesized catecholamines include epinephrine (synthesized only in the adrenal medulla), norepinephrine (the transmitter at the myoneural junction for sympathetic transmission), and dopamine. Dopamine has no effect on airway smooth muscle (15), and norepinephrine has no substantial bronchodilating effect because it lacks significant β_2-adrenoceptor activity. The presence of one additional methyl group at the amino-terminal end of the catecholamine molecule on epinephrine (vs. norepinephrine) confers substantial β_2-adrenergeric activity to epinephrine, which is an efficacious bronchodilator. However, whether it is administered parenterally or by inhaler, its duration of action is quite short (around 15–20 min), as the drug is readily inactivated by the ubiquitous enzyme catechol-O-methyl transferase (COMT) (16). Epinephrine also contains significant α_1-, α_2-, and β_1- as well as β_2-adrenergic activity (17). This is less of a limitation in the treatment of acute asthmatic emergencies as it is for maintenance therapy for chronic asthma or COPD.

B. Agents with Improved Specificity

The first pharmacological breakthrough in the use of β-adrenoceptor agents for regular therapy in the treatment of asthma came with the development of isoproterenol. The addition of three terminal methyl groups (vs. 1 for epinephrine, Fig. 1) confers virtually complete β-adrenergic specificity to the molecule, although pharmacological activity is equivalent for both β_1- and β_2-adrenoceptor subtypes. Although this agent has been given in elixir form by oral administration, side effects, especially cardiovascular effects, are minimized by inhaled administration of the drug. The efficacy of isoproterenol is the greatest of any of the β-adrenoceptor drugs, but its short duration of action (still only about 15–30 min) and lack of β_2-receptor specificity detract significantly for the desirability of this drug as an agent for the regular treatment of asthma or COPD.

C. Agents with Medium Duration of Action

The development of β-adrenergic agonists of medium duration of action [3–4 h by metered-dose inhaler (MDI)] introduced a new concept in therapy with β-adrenoceptor drugs—i.e., their use as continuous maintenance therapy in patients with chronic asthma or COPD. The pharmacological imperative was to develop a compound that maintained β_2-adrenoceptor specificity but which could not be readily inactivated by COMT. This strategy was used in the development of metaproterenol (Figs. 1 and 2), in which the −OH groups were moved from the 3,4 position on the skeletal catecholamine benzene ring, where they occur in nature, to the 3,5 position. This achieved the goal of increasing duration of activity to 3–4 h when given by MDI and >6 h when administered orally. However, metaproterenol still lacked absolute specificity for the β_2-adrenoceptor, which was achieved in cogeners that followed—e.g., terbutaline and albuterol. For many years, terbutaline was used only as an orally administered β_2-specific adrenergic agent; administered in this way, it had a duration of action of 6–8 h. In sustained-action preparations, albuterol could be administered orally only twice daily. Albuterol achieved its longer duration of action by the substitution of a hydroxymethyl-group at the 3-position on the catecholamine ring, rather than by 3,5 −OH substitution (Fig. 1). Both approaches were equally effective for administration by MDI and oral

---

Figure 1 Evolution of compounds for treating asthma. Epinephrine, a naturally occurring cathecholamine, is rapidly metabolized and lacks β-adrenergic specificity. The addition of multiple CH_3 groups increases β_2-adrenergic specificity but decreased intrinsic activity for bronchodilation. Addition of longer *N*-side chains increases lipid solubility and increases β_2-adrenergic specificity even further (see Table 1). Duration of action also is increased substantially for formoterol and salmeterol.

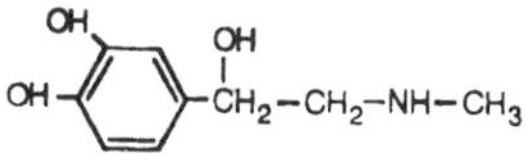

Epinephrine

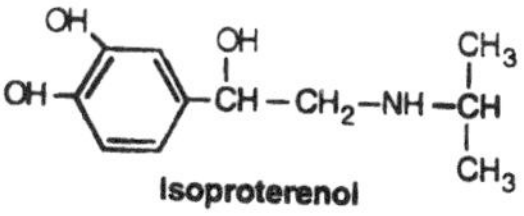

Isoproterenol

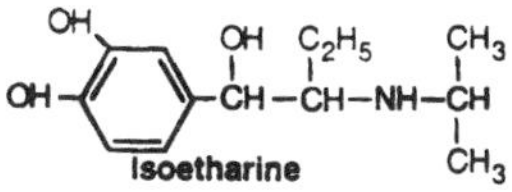

Isoetharine

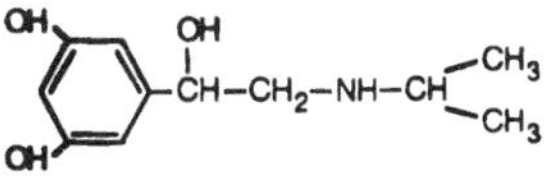

Metaproterenol

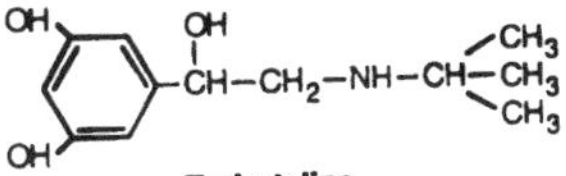

Terbutaline

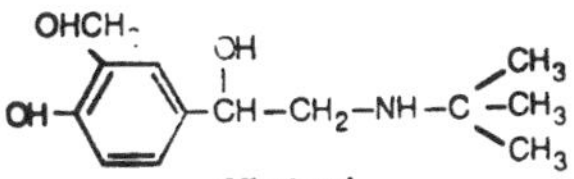

Albuterol

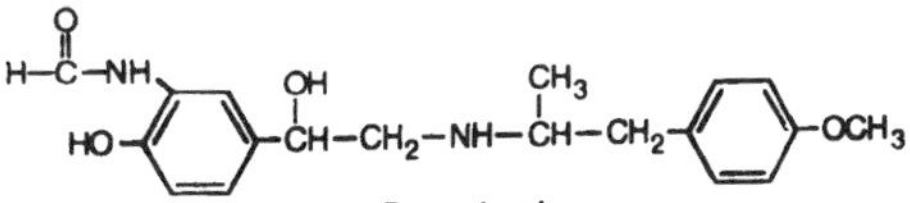

Formoterol

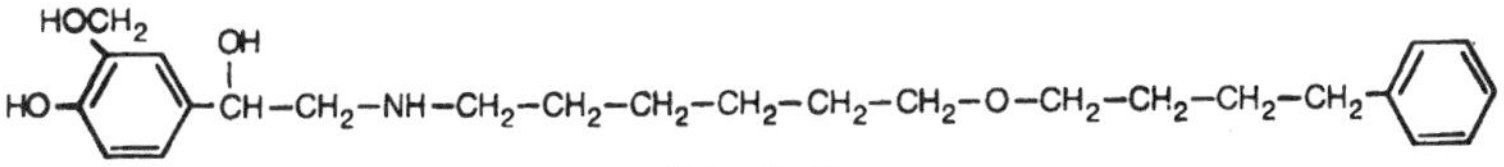

Salmeterol

Alternate Site:
Short ──▶ medium duration of activity

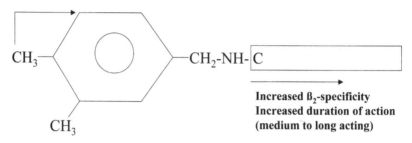

Figure 2 Pharmacological developmental strategies for sympathomimetic drugs. Duration of action is prolonged from short- to intermediate-acting drugs by moving the methyl groups on the benzene ring from the 3,4 to the 3,5 position or by substituting a hydroxymethyl group in the 3-position. This prevents degradation by catechol-*O*-methyltransferase. Additions to the terminal *N*-end of the molecule increase both β_2-adrenergic specificity of the compound and lipid solubility. Increased solubility and binding to the exocyte greatly increase duration of action.

administration, and the addition of a $-CH(CH_3)_3$ to the *N*-terminal end of the catecholamine skeleton now conferred near absolute β_2-adrenergic specificity to these compounds.

The development of compounds with near absolute β_2-receptor specificity offered the therapeutic promise of saturation kinetics of this receptor subtype, which has a special predilection for airway (and uterine) smooth muscle. However, several paradoxes remain. Asthmatic patients who are under relatively good control generally respond well to β_2-adrenergic agents but during exacerbations become refractory even to massive doses. The mechanism is presumed to result from exacerbation of the underlying inflammatory state, but this description lacks a defined mechanism. It may be that refractoriness to the activity of β_2-adrenergic agonists during acute asthmatic exacerbations relates more to the inability of airway smooth muscle to relax than to the augmentation of contraction caused by inflammation. Prior investigations have shown that normal airway smooth muscle in dogs relaxes less well to contraction caused by multiple agonists than to contraction caused by a single strong contractile agents (18,19). Similarly, the ''propranolol paradox'' remains unexplained. Why do some asthmatics (on some occasions) develop life-threatening bronchoconstriction to trivial amounts of β-adrenergic blocking agents while nonasthmatic humans tolerate massive quantities of these β-adrenoceptor blocking drugs (i.e., presumed total β-adrenoceptor blockade) with no detectable change in lung function? Failure of β-adrenergic agonists to work in acute asthma exacerbations may also result from airway edema, which on the mucosal side confers a mechanical contractile advantage to airways with an edematously narrowed lumen by LaPlace's law and on the serosal side may cause loss of airway tethering forces (lung interdependence forces).

The controversies surrounding the risk:benefit aspects of maintenance therapy with β-adrenergic agonists are discussed below. Used alone, medium-acting β-adrenergic agonists are now the standard of practice for mild intermittent asthma, and these drugs are indicated by the National Asthma Expert Panel (NAEP) of the National Heart, Lung and Blood Institute as well as by the World Health Organization as "reliever medications" for patients who require transient therapeutic augmentation (3). Despite the β₂ specificity of albuterol, terbutaline, and other sympathomimetic cogeners, systemic absorption can cause hypotension (there are β₂-adrenoceptors in vascular smooth muscle) and substantial tremulousness in skeletal muscle (see discussion below).

Fenoterol is a medium- to long-acting β-adrenoceptor agonist having a novel and complex side chain, which prolongs its activity in the airway. However, this drug is less β₂-specific than albuterol and terbutaline, and it may prolong the QTc interval in cardiac conduction. Unlike other β-adrenergic agonists, fenoterol has been associated specifically with increased cardiac toxicity when administered by MDI. Details of these concerns follow in the discussion below.

Concerns about toxicity and the necessary frequency of administration for optimal therapeutic effects have complicated the use of medium-acting β-adrenergic agonists in the treatment of asthma. Administration of these drugs four to six times per day, while effective, is at best inconvenient. The lack of an anti-inflammatory effect of β₂-adrenergic agents provides no control of the cellular infiltration and inflammation of chronic asthma. Thus, β-adrenoceptor agonists do not treat the underlying process. The situation in COPD is in some sense less complicated. Patients with highly compromised lung function who are continuously symptomatic are less reluctant to use these drugs more frequently. Furthermore, the evidence that corticosteroids are either efficacious or capable of modifying the inflammatory process in COPD is much less compelling than in asthma. Even so, medium-duration β-adrenergic agonists have a rapid decay time after administration. In asthmatic patients, the bronchodilator response declines immediately after administration and returns to near

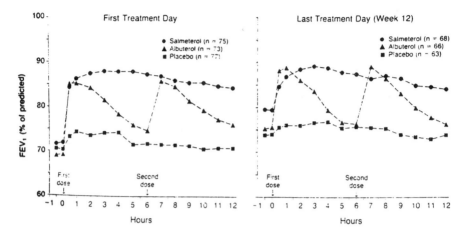

Figure 3 Relative duration of action of salmeterol and albuterol. The "sawtooth" effect of albuterol, which is more rapidly metabolized, is mitigated by steady-state bronchodilation over the 12-h period with salmeterol, which is sequestered within the membrane by binding to the exocyte of the β_2-adrenoceptor. (From Ref. 26.)

baseline after 3 h. In this context, maintenance therapy could also be described as "rescue" therapy for patients who are treated with β-adrenergic agonists (Fig. 3).

D. Long-Duration Preparations

The description of the optimal β_2-adrenoceptor drug would be as follows: (1) long duration of action; (2) stable steady-state duration of bronchodilation between administration of doses; (3) exceptional β_2:β_1 specificity; (4) minimal systemic side effects; and (5) improvement in quality-of-life measures. To a significant degree, these characteristics have been approximated by new generation β_2-adrenoceptor drugs.

Salmeterol is the only long-acting β-adrenoceptor agent available in the United States. It has a novel structure with a long side chain attached to the amino-terminal side of the molecule (Fig. 4); the long side chain terminates with a benzene ring. The molecule is extremely lipophilic. Intuitively, one might expect that a molecule of this size would lose most of its biological activity and bind only weakly to the β_2-receptor. However, the salmeterol molecule binds with considerable affinity and extreme specificity to the β_2-receptor ($85,000{:}1$ β_2:β_1) (Table 1). The mechanism of action is extremely novel. The

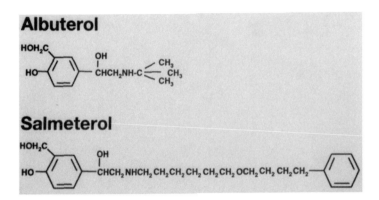

Figure 4 Chemical structures of albuterol and salmeterol. Salmeterol has a long side chain attached to the *N*-terminal side of the molecule. The long side chain ends with a benzene ring. Salmeterol is a highly lipid-soluble molecule, which greatly increases its duration of action compared to albuterol.

portion of the molecule that is homologous to albuterol binds reversibly to the β₂-adrenoceptor, and the ability of propranolol to block the relaxing effect of salmeterol in contracted human airway smooth muscle in vitro has been demonstrated (20,21). However, the relaxing effect persists when the same tissues are washed free of propranolol in vitro, suggesting that a portion of the molecule binds irreversibly to an inactive exocyte. This exocyte has now been characterized and is demonstrated schematically in Fig. 5, which illustrates the dual irreversible and reversible binding characteristics of the drug.

Table 1 Relative Specificity of Sympathomimetic Drugs for the β₂-Receptor

β-Agonist	Potency at β-receptor (isoprenaline = 1.0)		
	β₂ trachea (airways smooth muscle)	β₁ atria (cardiac tissue)	Selective ratio
Isoprenaline	1.00	1.0000	1
Fenoterol	0.60	0.0050	120
Formoterol	20.00	0.0500	400
Albuterol	0.55	0.0004	1375
Salmeterol	8.50	0.0001	85,000

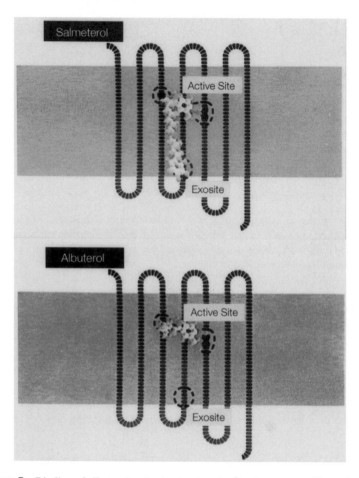

Figure 5 Binding of albuterol and salmeterol to the β_2-adrenoceptor. The active site links transmembrane domains. This binding is competitive. Binding to the exocyte by salmeterol distal to the active site is noncompetitive and greatly increases the drug's duration of action.

Because of its extreme lipophilicity and irreversible membrane-binding characteristics, both the catecholamine ring and the amino terminal side chain are "buried" within the membrane; thus the molecule resists enzymatic degradation. The prolonged half-life of salmeterol permits steady-state dosing (Fig. 3), in comparison with the "sawtooth" effects of the moderate-duration β-

adrenoceptor drugs, and twice-daily administration produces steady-state bronchodilation.

Formoterol is another lipophilic β_2-selective agonist (Fig. 1) with a physiological half-life identical to that of salmeterol. Its structure resembles that of fenoterol more, but to date there have been no suggestions of any unusual cardiovascular toxicity associated with this compound. The compound is not yet available for use in the United States, but its extensive use in Europe suggests that it will be virtually identical to salmeterol. A study of the functional and binding characteristics of these two long-acting β_2-adrenoceptor agonists showed that they are equipotent in relaxing maximally contracted guinea pig spirals, 10 times more potent than L-isoproterenol and fenoterol, and 100 times more potent than albuterol (22). Formoterol is more efficacious ($86 \pm 5\%$) than salmeterol ($62 \pm 3\%$) in inducing relaxation (percentage of maximal aminophylline relaxation). Both formoterol and salmeterol are highly selective for the β_2- versus β_1-receptor subtype. One study has suggested that both formoterol and salmeterol increase FEV_1 and significantly protect against methacholine-induced bronchoconstriction for up to 24 h (23).

E. Enantiomers of β₂-Selective Drugs

At least two enantiomeric forms of each β-adrenoceptor drug exist. Recent investigations have explored the potentially improved efficacy and diminished toxicity of the R form of albuterol known as levalbuterol, which has just been approved for use via nebulization in the United States. Some preliminary studies suggest that pure R albuterol might have a superior efficacy-to-toxicity ratio than that of the racemic mixtures now available for clinical use (24). Peer-reviewed clinical evidence for the superiority of pure R albuterol still is scant. No advantage of R albuterol over racemic albuterol was observed in the inhibition of stimulated secretion of eosinophil peroxidase from the peripheral blood eosinophils of either atopic or nonatopic asthmatic subjects (25). The potential advantages of selective enantiomers of salmeterol are of particular interest, since there are four separate enantiomers, but no data are yet available on the therapeutic benefits of specific enantiomers of these other β_2-adenoceptor drugs.

F. Tachyphylaxis and Additive Effects

The issue of tachyphylaxis to β-adrenergic agonists remains a subject of controversy. The bronchodilating effects of salmeterol persist without attenuation (Fig. 3) (26). However, some studies have shown that patients treated with β-adrenoceptor agonists develop some tolerance to the drugs—i.e., lesser effects are produced by the same dose of agonist (27). Chronic treatment with both medium- and long-duration β-adrenergic agonists has been noted to cause a decrease in protection after bronchoprovocation with exercise, methacholine, or allergen (28–30). Tolerance has also been noted with the long-acting β_2-adrenoceptor agonist formoterol. After 2 weeks of regular treatment with formoterol, mean FEV_1 at 12 h after the final dose of formoterol was not as great as 12 h after the initial dose 2 weeks earlier (31). As for many other receptors, repetitive stimulation may cause downregulation of receptor number, but this also does not imply necessarily diminished therapeutic efficacy. While the bronchoprotective effect of β-adrenoceptor agonists may decrease with time, numerous studies have demonstrated that it remains much greater than that of placebo. Other studies have demonstrated that tolerance to the bronchodilator effects does not occur with chronic use of these compounds (32,33). A fair conclusion would be that, if tolerance does develop, it is not clinically relevant (34,35).

In patients with persistent asthma, selection of the controller medication(s) as defined by NAEPP guidelines (3) is a matter of considerable discussion at present. Recent studies have demonstrated that patients failing to respond optimally to inhaled corticosteroids respond substantially better to the addition of inhaled β_2-adrenoceptor agonists than to a doubling of the dose of inhaled corticosteroid (36,37). Long-acting β_2-agonists also have been shown to improve quality of life in patients with asthma (38). Long-acting β-adrenoceptor agents are now being evaluated extensively for treatment of COPD. As efficacy measures are more difficult to achieve, improvement in quality of life will probably be an important determinant of the value of these drugs in the treatment of COPD.

III. Clinical Efficacy

A. Asthma

In most countries, inhaled β-adrenergic agonists are the most widely prescribed medications in the treatment of asthma (39). They are the treatment of choice as rescue medication for the acute relief of asthma symptoms, prevent exercise-induced bronchoconstriction, and provide lifesaving bronchodilation during acute asthma exacerbations. As discussed above, medium-duration β_2-adrenergic agonists are considered the standard of care for mild intermittent asthma, and these drugs are recommended by the NAEPP of the National

Heart, Lung and Blood Institute as well as the World Health Organization for use as "reliever medications" for asthmatic patients of all levels of severity when symptomatic relief is desired (3). Long-acting β$_2$-adrenergic agonists are currently recommended as "controller medication" for those patients already on inhaled corticosteroids who are still not optimally controlled (3). See Table 2 for a list of currently available medium- and long-acting inhaled β$_2$-adrenergic agonists.

β-adrenergic agonists are the most potent bronchodilating medications currently available for the treatment of asthma. In a study of the effects of bronchodilators and corticosteroids on airflow obstruction and airway hyper-responsiveness, Wempe et al. demonstrated that when administered as doubling doses until a plateau in FEV$_1$ was achieved, salbutamol caused greater bronchodilation than ipratropium (26.2 vs. 14.7% predicted FEV$_1$) and greater protection against histamine challenge (3.95 vs. 1.12 doubling concentrations) (40). This is twice the bronchodilation achieved with chronic treatment with either corticosteroids (inhaled budesonide 1.6 mg daily for 3 weeks or prednisone 40 mg daily for 8 days) or oral leukotriene-modifying agents (40,41). Wempe also found that the combination of nebulized salbutamol and ipratropium administered at a concentration 50% of that administered individually did not result in greater bronchodilation than salbutamol alone (40).

Studies have demonstrated that both medium- and long-acting inhaled β-adrenergic agonists provide clinically significant protection against acute bronchoconstriction provoked by exercise (28,42); cold, dry air (28,43); or allergen (44,45). A number of studies have demonstrated that a single dose of salmeterol provides clinically significant protection against exercise-induced

Table 2 β$_2$-Receptor Agonists Used to Treat Asthma and Chronic Obstructive Pulmonary Disease

Generic name	Trade name	Duration of action
Albuterol	Ventolin, Proventil	Medium (3–6 h)
Bitolterol	Tornalate	Medium
Metaproterenol	Alupent	Medium
Pirbuterol	Maxair	Medium
Terbutaline	Brethaire	Medium
Fenoterol	Not available in the United States	Medium
Salmeterol	Serevent	Long (12 h)
Formoterol	Not approved in the United States	Long

bronchospasm in adults for 12 h (46,47). A recent study of the effect of long-term therapy with salmeterol in subjects with exercise-induced asthma showed that the morning dose of salmeterol significantly decreased the degree of bronchospasm provoked by exercise throughout the month-long study (days 1, 14, and 29) (28). Inhaled β-adrenergic agonists are known to inhibit the early asthmatic response to allergen, presumably by direct bronchodilation and functional antagonism of bronchoconstriction. In an interesting study by Twentyman et al., nebulized albuterol was shown to decrease not only the early but also the late asthmatic reaction caused by inhaled allergen challenge and to attenuate the subsequent increase in airway responsiveness to histamine at a time when albuterol was no longer active (7.5 h after nebulization), suggesting that albuterol also acts by mechanisms not accounted for by direct relaxation of airway smooth muscle (44).

There is additional evidence that β-adrenergic agonists may have beneficial effects apart from their action on airway smooth muscle; however, conclusive evidence for a true anti-inflammatory effect is lacking. In a study of the nonbronchodilator effects of inhaled β-adrenergic agonists, O'Connor et al. compared the protective effects of inhaled terbutaline on the bronchoconstrictor responses to methacholine, which contracts airway smooth muscle directly, and adenosine 5′-monophosphate, which acts indirectly by mast-cell activation (48). Terbutaline caused a significantly greater inhibition of the response to adenosine 5′-monophosphate, suggesting an additional non-smooth-muscle effect, perhaps related to an action on airway mast cells. A study of inflammatory indices in patients with asthma as assessed by bronchoalveolar lavage failed to show any improvement after 8 weeks of therapy with salmeterol (49).

Long-acting β_2-adrenergic agonists have a clear role in the treatment of nocturnal asthma (50–52). In a study of the efficacy of inhaled salmeterol versus the combination of slow-release theophylline and ketotifen in patients with nocturnal asthma, salmeterol was much more effective in improving nocturnal symptoms (50). In addition, side effects were five times less frequent with salmeterol as compared with the theophylline-ketotifen combination therapy. In a study comparing sleep quality in patients with stable nocturnal asthma, salmeterol was superior to theophylline with fewer nocturnal arousals as assessed by polysomnography and improved daytime cognition as assessed by visual vigilance (51). In this study there was no patient preference for either therapy.

Numerous studies have also demonstrated the benefit of long-acting β_2-adrenergic agonists over an increased dose of inhaled corticosteroid in patients with moderate persistent asthma who require additional therapy (36,37,53). Woolcock et al. compared the efficacy and safety of adding one of two doses of salmeterol versus high-dose beclomethasone (1000 μg twice daily) in asthma patients with persistent symptoms on beclomethasone 500 μg twice daily. The addition of salmeterol at either dose resulted in greater improvement in lung function as assessed by peak expiratory flow rate and increased percentage of symptom-free days and nights; it also decreased the use of rescue albuterol when compared with doubling the dose of beclomethasone (37). There was no additional benefit to adding salmeterol 100 μg twice daily compared to 50 μg twice daily. A subsequent study by Pauwels et al. evaluated the effect of adding formoterol to lower and higher doses of the inhaled corticosteroid budesonide (53). The addition of formoterol to the lower dose of budesonide (100 μg twice daily) decreased rates of severe and mild asthma exacerbations by 26 and 40%, respectively, over the 1-year study period. Exacerbation rate decreased further with high-dose budesonide (400 μg twice daily) alone, but the greatest reduction in exacerbation rate was noted in the group of patients receiving both high-dose budesonide and formoterol. Lung function as assessed by both FEV_1 and peak expiratory flow rates was improved most in the groups that received formoterol as compared with those receiving budesonide alone.

There is evidence that with regular administration, tolerance or subsensitivity to β-adrenergic agonists may occur and that diminution in the protective effect against bronchoconstrictor stimuli may develop. A study by Sears et al. showed that regular use of fenoterol was associated with decreased asthma control compared with as-needed β-adrenergic agonist use (54). Regular treatment with albuterol 200 μg three times a day for 3 weeks was associated with an increase in the variability of the peak expiratory flow rate (55). A decrease in FEV_1 and increase in bronchial hyperreactivity to histamine was noted after therapy with regularly scheduled albuterol was discontinued. Recent studies suggest that this also results with chronic use of long-acting β-adrenergic agonists (28–31). When used long term, salmeterol continued to provide protection against exercise-induced asthma; however, the length of time the medication was active after a single dose decreased over time (28). As discussed above, the clinical relevance of these observations remains unclear at present. A recent, rigorously performed prospective evaluation of regularly scheduled versus as needed use of β₂-adrenergic agonists concluded that in patients with mild asthma, regular use of the β₂-adrenergic agonist albuterol was not harmful (56). There was no significant difference in peak expiratory flow variability, FEV_1, rescue albuterol use, asthma symptoms, asthma quality-of-life score, or airway responsiveness to methacholine between patients randomized to receive albuterol on a regular schedule or as needed. This study, however, also demonstrated that there was no clinical advantage to regularly scheduled use of β-adrenergic agonists. Long-acting β-adrenergic agonists are by design recommended for regularly scheduled use, and studies showing that long-term use of these agents is safe in patients already receiving inhaled corticosteroids fit with currect guidelines for their use (37,53). The addition of salmeterol to a regimen of inhaled budesonide resulted in improved asthma control, as discussed above, without causing an increase in bronchial hyperresponsiveness as assessed by histamine or an increase in exacerbation rates (37).

In summary, current treatment guidelines for asthma recommend that all patients receive a medium-duration β_2-adrenergic agonist to use on an as-needed basis (Table 2). Patients with moderate persistent asthma on inhaled corticosteroids who require additional therapy should in addition receive a long-acting β_2-adrenergic agonist. Either a medium- or long-acting β_2-adrenergic agonist is effective for patients with exercise-induced bronchoconstriction.

While β-adrenergic agonists may be given orally or by subcutaneous or intravenous injection, the preferred route of administration is by inhalation. This results in fewer side effects for a given degree of bronchodilation (57). Inhalation has replaced parenteral administration in the treatment of acute asthma exacerbations in the emergency room. Many studies have shown that an MDI, when properly used, can be as effective as a nebulizer in both adults and children with acute asthma (57).

B. COPD

Inhaled β-adrenergic agonists are also effective in the treatment of COPD; however, they produce less bronchodilation in patients with COPD than in those with asthma (58). In addition, unlike the case in patients with asthma, improvement in symptoms may occur without any significant improvement in airflow obstruction as measured by spirometry. This may occur in part because of a decrease in dynamic hyperinflation as measured by a decreased functional residual capacity, allowing patients with moderate to severe COPD to breathe more comfortably at a lower lung volume (59). This is one of the many reasons why reversibility of airflow obstruction with a single dose of inhaled β-adrenergic agonist should not be used as a criterion for predicting response to long-term bronchodilator therapy. In a recent study of reversibility in patients with COPD, it was noted that early bronchodilator response as assessed by FEV_1 15 min after inhalation of 200 μg of salbutamol imperfectly predicted maximum response to either salbutamol or salmeterol, which often occurred 1–2 h after salbutamol administration (60). Patients who failed to demonstrate an acute improvement in FEV_1 after salbutamol often had a significant response to salmeterol when assessed 2–4 h later.

Most treatment paradigms for COPD recommend the use of β_2-adrenergic agonists as second-line therapy for patients who do not have complete improvement with inhaled ipratropium (61). While this is the current recommendation, practice patterns indicate that inhaled β-adrenergic agonists remain the most widely prescribed medications for symptomatic relief in COPD. A recent long-term study of inhaled corticosteroids and bronchodilators in patients with COPD provides some evidence for this practice (62). The addition of the inhaled anticholinergic ipratropium to a regimen of inhaled terbutaline 500 μg four times a day conferred no additional benefit in terms of FEV_1, airway responsiveness to histamine, or symptom-free days as compared with placebo.

Long-acting β_2-adrenergic agonists have been shown to be of benefit in some patients with COPD. Lipworth et al. noted a small improvement in spirometric values 1 and 6 h after a single dose of salmeterol that was maintained after chronic dosing (63). In this same study, there was no improvement in lung volumes or exercise capacity, but symptoms of dyspnea on exertion improved. Salmeterol has also been shown to result in improved symptoms and morning peak expiratory flow rates in patients with moderate to severe COPD (64). Despite a modest gain in lung function, a clinically significant improvement in health and well-being was noted following 16 weeks of treatment with salmeterol (65). Formoterol has also been shown to be of benefit in patients with reversible obstructive aiways disease (66). Over the 6-month study, there was no difference in morning predose peak expiratory flow rate, use of rescue medication, and symptoms between patients receiving formoterol versus salmeterol. Mean evening predose peak expiratory flow rate, however, was superior at 2, 3, and 4 months in the group receiving formoterol.

IV. Systemic Effects

A. Side Effects

Side effects from β-adrenergic agonists are dose-dependent. Acute side effects include an increase in systolic blood pressure, a decrease in diastolic blood pressure, palpitations from reflex tachycardia, skeletal muscle tremor, hypokalemia, and increases in free fatty acids, insulin, and glucose in serum (67).

In addition, nonselective β-adrenergic agonists cause tachycardia, increased cardiac output, and arrhythmias. Chronic use of β-adrenergic agonists results in a decrease in the intensity of tremor and palpitations over time. Inhaled β-adrenergic agonists cause a widened (A-a) difference for oxygen, presumably due to an increase in ventilation/perfusion mismatching (67). The resultant decrease in P_{O_2} is generally small, short-lived, and of minimal clinical significance. In patients with COPD, side effects may be less well tolerated, especially in the elderly. In particular, tachycardia and arrhythmias can be of concern in those with preexisting cardiac disease. Serious cardiac side effects rarely occur at conventional doses despite the large number of patients with coexisting COPD and cardiac disease (see below).

B. Excess Mortality

Whether inhaled β-adrenergic agonists contributed to excess asthma mortality has been the subject of ferocious debate. Isolated instances of increased asthma mortality associated with the use of "forte"-strength isoproterenol in the 1960s and fenoterol use in the 1970s appear to have been causally related to the use of these β-adrenergic agonists (68). Studies have shown that fenoterol causes a greater peak effect on heart rate and serum potassium than albuterol at equivalent doses, leading some investigators to postulate that fenoterol is less $β_2$-selective than albuterol (69). Subsequently, a retrospective matched case-control study correlated asthma mortality with β-adrenergic agonist use, especially that of fenoterol (70). Reanalysis of these data, however, showed that the association between the use of inhaled β-adrenergic agonists and asthma mortality was confined to use in excess of recommended limits (71). In addition, a large study of 25,000 patients in Great Britain treated with either salmeterol or salbutamol concluded that excess mortality related to asthma did not occur over the 16 weeks of the study (72). After careful review of these studies, many have concluded that excess β-adrenergic agonist use is a *marker* of asthma severity and risk for subsequent mortality and not a true cause of excess asthma deaths.

While $β_2$-adrenergic agonists are generally well tolerated by patients with COPD, there are reports of arrhythmias, angina, and myocardial infarction developing following nebulized albuterol at a dose of 5.0 mg or terbutaline at a dose of 4.0 mg (69). A subsequent study identified preexisting cardiac disease as a marker for excess asthma mortality associated with β-adrenergic agonist use when administered either orally or by nebulization but not by MDI (73). This has led to the conclusion that in patients with preexisting cardiac disease, β$_2$-adrenergic agonists are safest when given by MDI and that nebulization of doses of albuterol above 2.5 mg should be avoided.

References

1. Wagner PD, Dantzker DR, Dueck R. Ventilation-perfusion inequality in chronic obstructive pulmonary disease. J Clin Invest 1977; 59:203–216.
2. Wagner PD, Dantzker DR, Iasovoni VE, et al. Pattern and time-course of ventilation-perfusion inequality in exercise-induced asthma. Am Rev Respir Dis 1978; 118:511–524.
3. National Asthma Expert Panel. Guidelines for the Diagnosis and Management of Asthma. National Institutes of Health Publication No. 97-405. Bethesda, MD: NIH, April, 1997.
4. West JB. Obstructive disease. In: Pulmonary Pathophysiology—The Essentials. Baltimore: Williams & Wilkins, 1977:59–91.
5. Leff AR. Future directions in asthma—is a cure possible? Chest 1997; 11:615–685.
6. Rabe KF, Munoz NM, Vita AJ, Morton BE, Magnussen H, Leff AR. Contraction of human bronchial smooth muscle caused by activated human eosinophils. Am J Physiol Lung Cell Mol Physiol 1994; 267:L326–L334.
7. Munoz NM, Hamann KJ, Vita A, Cozzi P, Baranowski S, Solway J, Leff AR. Activation of tracheal smooth muscle responsiveness by fMLP-treated HL-60 cells and neutrophils. Am J Physiol Lung Cell Mol Physiol 1993; 264:L222–L228.
8. Spencer H. Emphysema. In: Pathology of the Lung. New York: Pergamon Press, 1977:505–542.
9. White SR, Leff AR. Epithelium as a target. In: Holgate JS, Busse WW, eds, Inflammatory Mechanisms in Asthma. New York: Marcel Dekker, 1998:497–536.
10. Hogg J and Hegele RG. Postmortem pathology. In: Barnes PJ, Grunstein MM, Leff AR, Woolcock AJ, eds. Asthma. New York: Lippincott Raven, 1997:201–208.
11. Salter HH. On Asthma, Its Pathology and Treatment. London: Churchill, 1860.
12. Leff AR. The role of the adrenergic nervous system in asthma. In: Kaliner M, Barnes P, eds. Asthma: Pathophysiology and Treatment. New York: Marcel Dekker, 1991:357–384.
13. Leff A, Munoz NM. Selective autonomic stimulation of canine trachealis with dimethylphenylpiperazinium. J Appl Physiol 1981; 51:528–537.
14. Sands M, Douglas F, Green J, Banner A, Robertson G, Leff AR. Homeostatic regulation of bronchomotor tone by sympathetic activation during bronchocon-

striction in normal and asthmatic humans. Am Rev Respir Dis 1985; 132:993–998.

15. Leff AR, Munoz NM. Unpublished observations.

16. Jenne JW. Pharmacology of beta-adrenergic agonists. In: Leff AR, ed. Pulmonary and Critical Care Pharmacology and Therapeutics. New York: McGraw-Hill, 1996:483–487.

17. Hoffman BB, Lefkowitz RJ. Catecholamines, sympathomimetic drugs, and adrenergic receptor agonists. In: Hardman JG, Limbird LE, eds. The Pharmacological Basis of Therapeutics. New York: McGraw-Hill, 1996:199–248.

18. Russell JA. Differential inhibitory effect of isoproterenol on contractions of canine airways. J Appl Physiol 1984; 57:801–807.

19. White SR, Popovich KJ. Mitchell RW, Koenig SM, Mack MM, Munoz NM, Leff AR. Antagonism of relaxation to isoproterenol caused by agonist interactions. J Appl Physiol 1988; 64:2501–2507.

20. Nials AT, Coleman RA, Johnson M, Magnussen H, Rabe KF, Varday CJ. Effects of beta-adrenoceptor agonists in human bronchial smooth muscle. Br J Pharmacol 1994; 113:687–692.

21. Johnson M. Approaches to the design of long acting agonists at β-adrenoceptors. In: Small R, Johnson M, eds. β-Adrenoceptor Agonists and the Airways. London: Royal Society of Medicine Press, 1995:13–26.

22. Roux FJ, Grandordy B, Douglas JS. Functional and binding characteristics of long-acting β_2 agonists in lung and heart. Am J Respir Crit Care Med 1996; 153: 1489–1495.

23. Rabe KF, Jorres R, Nowak D, Behr N, Magnussen H. Comparison of the effects of salmeterol and formoterol on airway tone and responsiveness over 24 hours in bronchial asthma. Am Rev Respir Dis 1993; 147:1436–1441.

24. Perrin-Fayolle M, Blum PS, Morley J, Grosclaude M, Chambe M-T. Differential enantiomers of albuterol. Clin Rev Allergy Immunol 1996; 14:139–146.

25. Leff AR, Herrnreiter A, Naclerio RM, Baroody FM, Handley DA, Munoz NM. Effect of enantiomeric forms of albuterol on stimulated secretion of granular protein from human eosinophils. Pulm Pharmacol Ther 1997; 10:1097–1104.

26. Pearlman DS, Chervinsky P, LaForce C, Seltzer JM, Southern DJ, Kemp JP, Dockhorn J, Grossman J, Liddle RF, Yancy W, Cocchetto DM, Alexander WJ, Van As A. A comparison of salmeterol with albuterol in the treatment of mild-to-moderate asthma. N Engl J Med 1992; 327:1420–1425.

27. Nelson HS, Raine D Jr, Donner C, Posey WC. Subsensitivity to the bronchodilator action of albuterol produced by chronic administration. Am Rev Respir Dis 1977; 116:871.

28. Nelson JA, Strauss L, Skowronski M, Ciufo R, Novak R, McFadden ER. Effect of long-term salmeterol treatment on exercise-induced asthma. N Engl J Med 1998; 339:141–146.

29. Cheung D, Timmers MC, Zwinderman AH, Bel EH, Dijkman JH, Sterk P. Long-

term effects of a long-acting β_2-adrenoceptor agonist, salmeterol, on airway hyperresponsiveness in patients with mild asthma. N Engl J Med 1992: 327:1198–1203.

30. O'Connor BJ, Aikman SL, Barnes PJ. Tolerance to the nonbronchodilator effects of inhaled β_2-agonists in asthma. N Engl J Med 1992: 327:1204–1208.

31. Yates DH, Sussman HS, Shaw MJ, Barnes PJ, Chung KF. Regular formoterol treatment in mild asthma. Am J Respir Crit Care Med 1995; 152:1170–1174.

32. Ullman A, Hedner J, Svedmyr N. Inhaled salmeterol and salbutamol in asthmatic patients. Am Rev Respir Dis 1990; 142:571–575.

33. Arvidsson P, Larsson S, Löfdahl C-GA, Melander B, Wählander L, Svedmyr N. Formoterol, a new long-acting bronchodilator for inhalation. Eur Respir J 1989; 2:325–330.

34. Svedmyr N, Löfdahl C-GA. Physiology and pharmacodynamics of β-adrenergic agonists. In: Jenne J, ed. Drug Therapy for Asthma. New York: Marcel Dekker, 1987:177–211.

35. Tuttersfield A. Tolerance to β-agonists. Bull Eur Physiopathol Respir. 1985; 21: 51–55.

36. Greening AP, Ind PW, Northfield M, Shaw G. Added salmeterol versus higher-dose corticosteroid in asthma patients with symptoms on existing inhaled corticosteroid. Lancet 1994; 344:219–224.

37. Woolcock A, Lundback B, Ringdal N, Jacques LA. Comparison of addition of salmeterol to inhaled steroids with doubling of the dose of inhaled steroids. Am J Respir Crit Care Med 1996; 153:1481–1488.

38. Juniper EF, Johnston PR, Borkhoff CM, Guyatt GH, Boulet L-P, Haukioja A. Quality of life in asthma clinical trials: comparison of salmeterol and salbutamol. Am J Respir Crit Care Med 1995; 151:66–70.

39. O'Byrne PM, Kerstjens HAM. Inhaled β_2-agonists in the treatment of asthma. N Engl J Med 1996; 335:886–888.

40. Wempe JB, Postma DS, Breederveld N, Alting-Hebing D, van der Mark TW, Koeter GH. Separate and combined effects of corticosteroids and bronchodilators on airflow obstruction and airway hyperresponsiveness in asthma. J Allergy Clin Immunol 1992; 89:679–687.

41. Israel E, Rubin P, Kemp JP, Grossman J, Pierson W, Siegel SC, Tinkelman D, Murray JJ, Busse W, Segal AT, Fish J, Kaiser HB, Ledford D, Wenzel S, Rosenthal R, Cohn J, Lanni C, Pearlman H, Karahalios, Drazen JM. The effect of inhibition of 5-lipoxygenase by zileuton in mild-to-moderate asthma. Ann Intern Med 1993; 119:1059–1066.

42. Anderson S, Seale JP, Ferris L, Schoeffel R, Lindsay DA. An evaluation of pharmacotherapy for exercise-induced asthma. J Allergy Clin Immunol 1979; 64: 612–624.

43. O'Byrne PM, Morris M, Roberts R, Hargreave FE. Inhibition of the bronchial response to respiratory heat exchange by increasing doses of terbutaline sulfate. Thorax 1982; 37:913–917.

44. Twentyman OP, Finnerty JP, Holgate ST. The inhibitory effects of nebulized albuterol on the early and late asthmatic reactions and increase in airway responsiveness provoked by inhaled allergen in asthma. Am Rev Respir Dis 1991; 144: 782–787.

45. Twentyman OP, Finnerty JP, Harris A, Palmer J, Holgate ST. Protection against allergen-induced asthma by salmeterol. Lancet 1990; 336:1338–1342.

46. Anderson SD, Rodwell LT, Du Toit J, Young IH. Duration of protection by inhaled salmeterol in exercise-induced asthma. Chest 1991; 100:1254–1260.

47. Kemp JP, Dockhorn RJ, Busse WW, Bleecker ER, Van As A. Prolonged effect of inhaled salmeterol against exercise-induced bronchospasm. Am J Respir Crit Care Med 1994; 150:1612–1615.

48. O'Connor BJ, Fuller RW, Barnes PJ. Nonbronchodilator effects of inhaled β_2 agonists. Am J Respir Crit Care Med 1994; 150:381–387.

49. Gardiner PV, Ward C, Booth H, Allison A, Hendrick DJ, Walters EH. Effect of eight weeks of treatment with salmeterol on bronchoalveolar lavage inflammatory indices in asthmatics. Am J Respir Crit Care Med 1994; 150:1006–1011.

50. Muir JF, Bertin L, Georges D. Salmeterol versus slow-release theophylline combined with ketotifen in nocturnal asthma. Eur Respir J 1992; 5:1197–1200.

51. Selby C, Engleman HM, Fitzpatrick MF, Sime PM, Mackay TW, Douglas NJ. Inhaled salmeterol or oral theophylline in nocturnal asthma. Am J Respir Crit Care Med 1997; 155:104–108.

52. Weersink EJM, Douma RR, Postma DS, Koeter GH. Fluticasone propionate, salmeterol xinafoate, and their combination in the treatment of nocturnal asthma. Am J Respir Crit Care Med 1997; 155:1241–1246.

53. Pauwels RA, Lofdahl C-G, Postma DS, Tatterfield AE, O'Byrne P, Barnes PJ, Ullman A. Effect of inhaled formoterol and budesonide on exacerbations of asthma. N Engl J Med 1997; 337:1405–1411.

54. Sears MR, Taylor DR, Print CG, Lake DC, Li Q, Flannery EM, Yates DM, Lucas MK, Herbison GP. Regular inhaled beta-agonist treatment in bronchial asthma. Lancet 1990; 336:1391–1396.

55. Wahedna I, Wong CS, Wisniewski AFZ, Pavord ID, Tattersfield AE. Asthma control during and after cessation of regular $beta_2$-agonist treatment. Am Rev Respir Dis 1993; 148:707–712.

56. Drazen JM, Israel E, Boushey HA, Chinchilli VM, Fahy JV, Fish JE, Lazarus SC, Lemanske RF, Martin RJ, Peters SP, Sorkness C, Selzer SJ. Comparison of regularly scheduled with as-needed use of albuterol in mild asthma. N Engl J Med 1996; 335:841–847.

57. Nelson HS. β-adrenergic bronchodilators. N Engl J Med 1995; 333:499–506.

58. ATS Statement. Standards for the diagnosis and care of patients with chronic obstructive pulmonary disease. 1995; 152:S78–S121.

59. Tantucci C, Duget A, Similowski T, Zelter M, Derenne J-P, Milic-Emil J. Effect of salbutamol on dynamic hyperinflation in chronic obstructive pulmonary disease patients. Eur Respir J 1998; 12:799–804.

60. Cazzola M, Vinciguerra A, Di Perna F, Matera MG. Early reversibility to salbutamol does not always predict bronchodilation after salmeterol in stable chronic obstructive pulmonary disease. Respir Med 1998; 92:1012–1016.

61. Ferguson GT, Cherniack RM. Management of chronic obstructive pulmonary disease. 1993; 328:1017–1022.

62. Rutten-Van Molken, MPMH, Van Doorslaer KA, Jansen MCC, Kerstjens HAM, Rutten FFH. Costs and effects of inhaled corticosteroids and bronchodilators in asthma and chronic obstructive pulmonary disease. Am J Respir Crit Care Med 1995; 151:975–982.

63. Grove GA, Lipworth BJ, Reid P, Smith RP, Ramage L, Ingram CG, Jenkins RJ, Winter JH, Dhillon DP. Effects of regular salmeterol on lung function and exercise capacity in patients with chronic obstructive airways disease. Thorax 1996; 51:689–693.

64. Ulrik CS. Efficacy of inhaled salmeterol in the management of smokers with chronic obstructive pulmonary disease: a single centre randomised, double blind, placebo controlled, crossover study. Thorax 1995; 50:750–754.

65. Jones PW, Bosh TK, in association with an international study group. Quality of life changes in COPD patients treated with salmeterol. Am J Respir Crit Care Med 1997; 155:1283–1289.

66. Vervloet D, Ekstrom T, Pela R, Duce Gracia F, Kopp C, Silvert BD, Quebe-Fehling E, Della Cioppa G, Di Benedetto G. A 6-month comparison between formoterol and salmeterol in patients with reversible obstructive airways disease. Respir Med 1998; 92:836–842.

67. Wanner A. Is the routine use of inhaled β-adrenergic agonists appropriate in asthma treatment? Am J Respir Crit Care Med 1995; 151:597–599.

68. Barrett TE, Strom BL. Inhaled beta-adrenergic receptor agonists in asthma: more harm than good? Am J Respir Crit Care Med 1995; 151:574–577.

69. Jenne JW. Adverse effects of beta-adrenergic agonists. In: Leff AR, ed. Pulmonary and Critical Care Pharmacology and Therapeutics. New York: McGraw-Hill, 1996:497–503.

70. Spitzer WO, Suissa S, Ernst P, Horwitz RI, Habbick B, Cockcroft D, Boivin J-F, McNutt M, Buist AS, Rebuck AS. The use of β-agonists and the risk of death and near death from asthma. N Engl J Med 1992; 326:501–506.

71. Suissa S, Ernst P, Boivin JF, Horwitz RI, Habbick B, Cockroft D, Blais L, McNutt M, Buist AS, Spitzer WO. A cohort analysis of excess mortality in asthma and the use of inhaled β-agonists. Am J Respir Crit Care Med 1994; 149: 604–610.

72. Castle W, Fuller R, Hall J, Palmer J. Serevent nationwide surveillance study: comparison of salmeterol with salbutamol in asthmatic patients who require regular bronchodilator treatment. BMJ 1993; 306:1034–1037.

73. Suissa S, Hemmelgarn B, Blais L, Ernst P. Bronchodilators and acute cardiac death. Am J Respir Crit Care Med 1996; 154:1598–1602.

3

Theophylline

GORDON DENT

University of Southampton School
of Medicine
Southampton, England

KLAUS F. RABE

Leiden University Medical Center
Leiden, The Netherlands

I. Introduction

Theophylline is used widely in the treatment of asthma today, more than 60 years after its introduction. In recent years theophylline has been relegated to second- or third-line treatment for patients whose asthma does not respond well to corticosteroids and β_2-adrenoceptor agonists, but its value is recognized and the drug undergoes periodic reappraisals in the light of new scientific evidence of its effects and efficacy. Traditionally regarded as a bronchodilator, theophylline has begun recently to be thought of as possessing additional immunomodulatory or anti-inflammatory actions that account for its usefulness in patients in whom bronchodilation alone is unlikely to account fully for the drug's effectiveness. Improvement in basal lung function remains the therapeutic target of theophylline therapy, but the relative contribution made to long-term improvement of asthma symptoms by bronchodilation and by other actions remains open to debate. The actions of theophylline and some related alkylxanthine drugs in the airways and on cells involved in airway inflammation are reviewed here and their relationship to the therapeutic use of theophylline is discussed.

II. Historical Perspective

A. Discovery and Development of Theophylline

Methylxanthines have been recognized as being of use in the treatment of asthma for more than a century, strong coffee having been recommended as a reliever of asthma symptoms by Henry Hyde Salter in 1859 (1). Theophylline was first isolated from tea in 1888 by Albrecht Kossel, who characterized the compound as a dimethylxanthine by identifying its methylation product as caffeine, a trimethylxanthine (2). In contrast to theobromine, a dimethylxanthine purified from cocoa, theophylline had both methyl groups attached to the six-membered ring of the molecule's purine core (Fig. 1) and was confirmed to be 1,3-dimethylxanthine. Kossel was awarded the Nobel Prize in medicine in 1910 in recognition of his work on purines. Emil Fischer and Lorenz Ach went on to synthesize theophylline in 1895 (3), and industrial production was begun at the turn of the century by C.F. Boehringer and Sons.

Following Salter's demonstration of the clinical benefits of caffeine in asthmatic patients, the relaxant action of theophylline in human airways was demonstrated by Samson Raphael Hirsch in 1922 (4). The identification of theophylline as a bronchodilator supplemented its two other recognized effects as a diuretic and a cardiotonic drug (5,6). It was not until the late 1930s, however, that theophylline began to be used in the treatment of obstructive airways disease, following the description by George Hermann et al. of its beneficial effects in severe asthma (7).

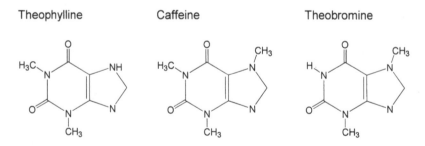

Figure 1   Chemical structure of methylxanthines: theophylline (1,3-dimethylxanthine), caffeine (1,3,7-trimethylxanthine), and theobromine (3,7-dimethylxanthine).

In the last quarter of the twentieth century, theophylline's use has become widespread, with the introduction of sustained-release formulations (8,9), improved availability of drug-monitoring techniques (10), and standardized dosing strategies (11,12) resulting in increased efficacy with clinically acceptable toxicity profiles. Theophylline is now one of the world's most prescribed therapies for asthma and chronic obstructive pulmonary disease (COPD) (13,14).

B. Chemistry of Theophylline

The plant alkaloids theophylline, caffeine, and theobromine are closely related in structure, belonging to the class of methylxanthines (Fig. 1). Xanthine itself is a derivative of purine, which forms the core of nucleosides and nucleotides, the purine bases. Purine nucleosides include adenosine, which is produced by many cells undergoing high metabolic activity; purine nucleotides include the 3':5'-cyclic monophosphates of adenosine (cyclic AMP) and guanosine (cyclic GMP), which are produced inside cells as "second messengers" in response to direct or receptor-mediated activation of adenylyl or guanylyl cyclase. This structural basis may underlie the two primary pharmacological actions of theophylline: antagonism of adenosine receptors and inhibition of cyclic nucleotide phosphodiesterases (PDE), the cyclic AMP/cyclic GMP–catabolizing enzymes.

Structure-activity studies of a series of xanthine derivatives have shown substitution at the 3- and 7-nitrogen atoms to influence the in vitro and in vivo bronchial relaxant activity of the compounds, while substitution at the 1-nitrogen and 8-carbon atoms affects the ability of the derivatives to act as antagonists at adenosine receptors (15). Thus, theophylline (1,3-dimethylxanthine) is effective as a bronchodilator and as an adenosine antagonist whilst enprofylline (3-propylxanthine) lacks a substituent at the N-1 position and is a poor antagonist at most classes of adenosine receptor but retains a bronchodilator potency greater than that of theophylline (16). Trisubstitution at the N-1, N-3, and N-9 positions leads to isomerization of the imidazyl ring of the purine group; the 8-9 double bond localizes to the 7-8 position, with consequent loss of pharmacological activity (17).

Synthetic xanthine derivatives have been studied as inhibitors of PDE. These include 3-isobutyl-1-methylxanthine (IBMX), enprofylline and a theobromine derivative, pentoxifylline [1-(5-oxohexyl)-3,7-dimethylxanthine]. These drugs are more potent than the plant alkaloids, both as PDE inhibitors and as relaxants of airways smooth muscle in vitro (18–20). Like theophylline

Table 1   Inhibition of PDE Isoenzymes by Theophylline and IBMX

Isoenzyme	Cell/Tissue	IC_{50}[a]	Reference
Theophylline			
1	Brain, bovine	280 μM[e]	(22)
2	Heart, rat	270 μM[b]	(22)
	Bronchus, human	55 μM[c]	(19)
3	Heart, rat	390 μM[b]	(22)
	Platelets, human	98 μM[b]	(22)
4	Trachea, dog	155 μM[b]	(22)
	Bronchus, human	150 μM[c]	(19)
	Eosinophils, human	290 μM[b]	(23)
5	Platelets, human	630 μM[e]	(22)
IBMX			
1	Heart, bovine	2.5 μM	(24)
	Brain, bovine	10 μM[e]	(25)
		8.9 μM[b]	(26)
	Trachea, bovine	5.0 μM	(27)
2	Heart, bovine	50 μM	(24)
	Heart, rat	6 μM[b]	(25)
		6.3 μM[b]	(26)
	Trachea, bovine	4 μM	(27)
3	Heart, bovine	2 μM	(24)
	Heart, rabbit	5 μM	(27)
	Heart, guinea pig	2 μM[b]	(28)
	Heart, rat	10 μM[b]	(26)
	Platelets, human	4 μM[b]	(25)
	Platelets, human	10 μM	(29)
4	Heart, bovine	15 μM	(24)
	Trachea, bovine	5 μM	(27)
	Trachea, dog	9 μM[b]	(28)
	Neutrophils, human	8 μMb	(25)
	Neutrophils, human	10 μM[b]	(30)
	Neutrophils, human	20 μM	(29)
	Eosinophils, human	14 μM[b]	(23)
5	Trachea, bovine	4.5 μM[d]	(27)
	Platelets, human	10 μM[e]	(25)
	Lung, human	1.8 μM[d]	(29)

[a] IC_{50} is the concentration causing 50% inhibition of enzyme activity.
The substrate was cyclic AMP 1 μM except for the following:
[b] Cyclic AMP 0.5 μM.
[c] Cyclic AMP 0.25 μM.
[d] Cyclic GMP 1 μM.
[e] Cyclic GMP 0.5 μM.
Source: Ref. 21.

(Table 1), IBMX and pentoxifylline inhibit all PDE isoenzyme families with approximately equal potency (19,31). Other xanthine derivatives exhibit selectivity for specific isoenzyme families; some are among the synthetic PDE inhibitors that have been investigated recently as potential antiasthma drugs (32–34).

III. Pharmacological Mechanisms

The widespread use of theophylline in the treatment of bronchial asthma prompted studies of the drug's biochemical actions in lung tissues to elucidate its mode of action. Theophylline is known to be both an inhibitor of PDE and an antagonist at adenosine receptors. Additionally, theophylline has been reported to increase extracellular concentrations of catecholamines through reuptake inhibition, but the relevance of this action to theophylline's clinical effects remains unclear (35,36).

While bronchodilation is theophylline's most widely recognized pharmacological action, alkylxanthines exhibit a range of actions on smooth muscle and inflammatory cells that may underlie theophylline's effectiveness in asthma and COPD. The relative contribution made to these actions by PDE inhibition and adenosine antagonism has been addressed in many cases.

A. Modes of Action of Theophylline

Phosphodiesterase Inhibition

Cyclic nucleotide phosphodiesterase (PDE; 3':5'-cyclic nucleotide 5'-nucleotidohydrolase, EC 3.1.4.17) comprises the group of enzymes that catalyse the hydrolysis of the 3'-ribose phosphate bond of cyclic AMP and cyclic GMP to form the 5'-nucleotide monophosphates, adenosine 5'-monophosphate (AMP) and guanosine 5'-monophosphate (GMP). Elevation of intracellular cyclic AMP levels is associated with smooth muscle relaxation (37), and the demonstration that theophylline inhibits PDE (38), thereby preventing breakdown of cyclic AMP, was assumed to explain theophylline's bronchodilator action.

PDE exists as several isoenzymes, forming at least eight "families" (39,40). While selective inhibitors have been developed to most of these families, many xanthine derivatives, including theophylline, act as nonselective PDE inhibitors, exhibiting similar inhibition of all isoenzymes (Table 1). As a consequence of this, theophylline elevates cyclic GMP as well as cyclic

AMP levels, leading to activation of both cyclic AMP- and cyclic GMP-dependent protein kinases (PKA and PKG). These protein kinases catalyze the phosphorylation of numerous proteins, especially ion channels and pumps, involved in the induction and maintenance of smooth muscle contraction (37,41–43). In fact, PKG has been suggested to be the predominant enzyme mediating the suppression of agonist-induced Ca^{2+} elevations in smooth muscle by cyclic AMP as well as mediating the actions of cyclic GMP produced in response to guanylyl cyclase activators such as nitric oxide (37,42). Thus, the nonselective profile of its PDE inhibition might endow theophylline with additional effectiveness.

The PDE-inhibitory potency of a range of natural and synthetic methylxanthines correlates closely with their ability to relax rat tracheal smooth muscle in vitro, although the relevance of this relationship to theophylline's clinical efficacy as a bronchodilator has been questioned in view of the slight inhibition of lung PDE activity achieved by concentrations of the drug within the conventional therapeutic range (15). However, the concentration dependencies of cyclic AMP PDE inhibition and bronchial smooth muscle relaxation in vitro by theophylline are similar (Fig. 2), and adenosine antagonism appears to be uninvolved in many aspects of bronchial smooth muscle relaxation (see Sec. III.B). Furthermore, a novel methylxanthine displaying negligible adenosine receptor antagonism—1,3-dimethyl-7-isobutylxanthine (isbufylline)—relaxes bronchial smooth muscle in vitro with 50 to 100 times higher potency than that with which it inhibits PDE, suggesting that only a small degree of PDE inhibition is required in the absence of adenosine antagonism to effect relaxation of airways smooth muscle (44). It should be noted, however, that isbufylline's potent in vivo bronchospasmolytic action was demonstrated against indirectly acting spasmogens such as antigen, arachidonic acid, platelet activating factor (PAF), and capsaicin, suggesting that the drug might owe much of its in vivo effectiveness to actions on inflammatory cells or sensory nerves rather than to direct relaxant actions on smooth muscle (45).

Theophylline is a weak bronchodilator in comparison to β-adrenoceptor agonists (14,46,47), and it is conceivable that the small degree of acute bronchodilation achieved at therapeutic concentrations of theophylline reflects the small degree of PDE inhibition. Studies with a range of synthetic 3-substituted alkylxanthines show strong correlation between potencies for cyclic AMP PDE inhibition and guinea pig tracheal smooth muscle relaxation, but correlation of relaxation with A_1 adenosine receptor antagonism was also observed for the same drugs (48). Drugs that were very weak PDE inhibitors were gener-

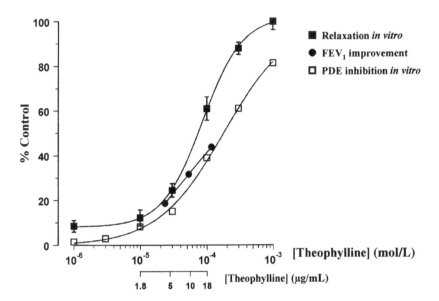

Figure 2 Concentration dependence of PDE inhibition in human bronchial homogenates (□) and relaxation of human bronchial rings in vitro (●) and bronchodilation in vivo (○). (From Refs. 58–60.)

ally also weak relaxants of airway smooth muscle but the most potent relaxants were those compounds with high potency both as PDE inhibitors and as adenosine antagonists. It remains unclear, therefore, whether PDE inhibition alone can account for the bronchodilator actions of alkylxanthines or if adenosine receptor antagonism also contributes.

Adenosine Receptor Antagonism

The purine nucleoside adenosine is produced throughout the body, particularly at sites of oxygen deprivation or increased ATP utilization (49). It is of particular interest as it causes bronchoconstriction in asthmatics but not in normal subjects (50) in addition to inducing contraction of asthmatic airways smooth muscle in vitro (51).

Theophylline is an antagonist at both the A_1 and A_2 classes of adenosine receptors (49) at concentrations within its therapeutic range, suggesting that this action might be more relevant than PDE inhibition to the clinical effects of theophylline. Structure-activity relationships, however, show the potency of xanthine derivatives in relaxing airways to be unrelated to their potency as adenosine antagonists (15). The contraction of isolated asthmatic bronchi in response to adenosine is abolished by a combination of a histamine H_1 receptor antagonist and a cysteinyl leukotriene receptor antagonist (51), indicating that an indirect action of adenosine, *via* released bronchoconstrictor mediators, may be more important than a direct action on airways smooth muscle, in which the contraction-promoting A_1 receptors are scarce (52).

Adenosine enhances allergic mediator release from lung mast cells, thus presenting a target for potential antiasthma drugs. In several species, the mast-cell degranulation response involves the A_3 receptor class, which is present in large quantities in the human lung and is only weakly antagonized by conventional xanthines such as theophylline (53,54). Evidence suggests, however, that theophylline inhibits both adenosine-dependent augmentation of mast-cell mediator release in vitro and adenosine-induced bronchoconstriction in vivo with greater potency than it exhibits against responses due to other stimuli (55–57). This suggests that adenosine receptor antagonism contributes to the pharmacological actions of theophylline, although it is assumed that many actions also involve PDE inhibition.

B. Pharmacological Actions of Theophylline

Bronchodilation

Theophylline relaxes human bronchial smooth muscle in vitro at concentrations similar to those that inhibit PDE-catalyzed cyclic AMP hydrolysis in tissue homogenates (Fig. 2) (58–60). Fifty percent maximal relaxation is achieved at a concentration of approximately 80 μM, corresponding roughly to 14 μg/mL (19). This relaxant activity is mimicked in large airways by selective inhibitors of the PDE3 isoenzyme family and by mixed PDE3/PDE4 inhibitors (20,61), but PDE3 inhibitors are largely ineffective in relaxing small airways (62), in contrast to theophylline, whose relaxant effect is independent of airway diameter (63).

The theophylline analogue 8-phenyltheophylline, which acts as an antagonist at adenosine receptors but has negligible PDE-inhibitory activity, has no effect on human bronchial smooth muscle tension (58). This suggests that adenosine antagonism is not involved in theophylline's bronchial relaxant properties in nonasthmatic airways in vitro. Low levels of endogenous adenosine production at resting tone in vitro may, however, account for the lack of effect of an adenosine antagonist; the situation in vivo is likely to be different and the role of adenosine antagonism cannot be predicted.

In vivo, theophylline causes measurable bronchodilation after oral or intravenous administration in patients with airway obstruction (see Sec. IV), while intravenous administration also improves lung function in normal subjects (47). This basal bronchospasmolytic action of the drug is less pronounced than its antibronchospastic effect: theophylline protects against the bronchoconstriction induced by histamine or muscarinic receptor agonists (e.g., methacholine, carbachol), with significant effects against histamine-induced bronchoconstriction occurring at serum theophylline concentrations below 5 μg/mL (64). It remains unclear whether this protective effect of theophylline involves actions in addition to bronchodilation.

Bronchoprotection

In addition to its acute bronchodilator action, theophylline has been demonstrated to exert significant protective effects against bronchoconstriction induced by recognized asthma triggers, including exercise and allergens, as well as experimental bronchoconstrictor agents such as histamine and methacholine. These experimental studies are useful in indicating the effectiveness of theophylline against particular types of bronchial reaction.

Histamine and Methacholine

Theophylline inhibits histamine- or methacholine-induced bronchoconstriction after oral or intravenous administration. A single oral dose of theophylline—producing a mean serum theophylline concentration of 13 μg/mL and a small bronchodilation (7.6% increase in FEV_1)—has been shown to protect asthmatic children against these reactions, with the provocation dose of inhaled constrictor required to reduce FEV_1 by 20% ($PD_{20}FEV_1$) increasing threefold for methacholine and twofold for histamine, although no correlation could be observed in these experiments between serum theophylline concentration and bronchoprotective effects (65). A 1.3-fold increase in $PD_{20}FEV_1$ to histamine has also been observed at a mean serum theophylline concentration of 13 μg/mL after several days' oral administration of a sustained-release theophylline preparation in adult asthmatics (66). In a study of asthmatic adults, in which histamine and methacholine reactivity were measured after each of three intravenous doses of aminophylline, a clear relationship could be observed between serum theophylline concentration and protection against both methacholine and histamine bronchial provocation, with a significant degree of protection against histamine-induced bronchoconstriction (measured as dose causing 100% increase in specific airways resistance, $PD_{100}sR_{aw}$)

occurring at serum theophylline concentrations as low as 3.2 μg/mL (64). In this study, theophylline protected more effectively against histamine- than against methacholine-induced bronchoconstriction, a finding that correlates intriguingly with in vitro data showing nonselective PDE inhibitors to relax histamine-contracted human bronchi more effectively than those contracted with methacholine, although there are insufficient data at present to propose a definite relation between these phenomena.

Exercise

Theophylline also exerts a concentration-dependent protective effect against exercise-induced bronchoconstriction in asthmatic subjects. Following administration of a single oral dose of theophylline to asthmatic children, a diminishing protection is observed over time, paralleling the decrease in mean serum theophylline concentration to 16, 13, and 10 μg/mL at 2, 4, and 6 h after administration, respectively (67). In mildly asthmatic adults treated with intravenous aminophylline (equivalent to 200 or 351 mg anhydrous theophylline), protection against exercise-induced bronchoconstriction (measured as decrease in FEV_1 or increase in sR_{aw}) is related to the dose and to serum concentration of theophylline, with significant protection observed after a dosage resulting in a mean serum concentration of 6.7 μg/mL and significantly greater protection after a dosage resulting in a mean concentration of 10 μg/mL (68). The degree of protection against exercise-induced bronchoconstriction by aminophylline does not correlate with the magnitude of acute bronchodilation, suggesting a difference in the mechanisms through which these actions are mediated (68).

Allergens

Intravenous infusion of theophylline (7.2 mg/kg loading dose followed by a maintenance infusion of 74 mg/h, leading to steady mean serum concentrations of approximately 10.5 μg/mL) or enprofylline (2.7 mg/kg followed by 71 mg/h, leading to steady serum concentrations of 2.7 μg/mL) causes a minor initial bronchodilation and a significant protection against both the immediate and late bronchoconstrictor responses (measured as decrease in FEV_1 and as decrease in specific airways conductance, sG_{aw}) to inhaled allergen (Fig. 3). Despite the fourfold lower serum concentration of enprofylline (associated with a slightly smaller initial bronchodilation), this drug exerted a greater protective effect against the late asthmatic reaction to inhaled allergen. Enprofylline's greater potency confirms the importance of PDE inhibition, relative to

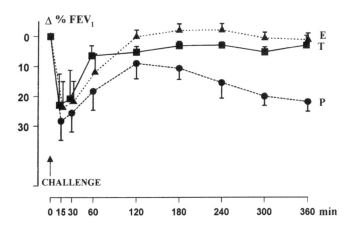

Figure 3 Effects of theophylline and enprofylline on early and late asthmatic reactions to allergen inhalation. The graph shows percentage change in FEV_1 following allergen inhalation in patients treated with placebo (P), theophylline (T), or enprofylline (E). (From Ref. 69.)

adenosine antagonism, in protection against bronchial reactions in an experimental asthmatic response.

Toluene diisocyanate (TDI), a common trigger of occupational asthma in subjects sensitized through chronic exposure to isocyanates in the workplace, induces a typical asthmatic dual reaction of immediate and delayed bronchoconstriction after inhalation. Treatment of sensitized subjects for 7 days with oral sustained-release theophylline (6.5 mg/kg twice daily, producing mean serum concentrations of 18 µg/mL) causes significant protection against both the early and late asthmatic bronchoconstriction responses to inhaled TDI (70). In an interesting comparison, an inhaled corticosteroid (beclomethasone 1 mg twice daily for 7 days prior to TDI exposure) fails to suppress the immediate reaction while significantly inhibiting the late response (70). In spite of its protective effect against TDI-induced bronchoconstriction, theophylline does not prevent the induction of bronchial hyperresponsiveness to inhaled methacholine following TDI exposure—a finding reproduced in later studies with allergen (71,72)—while beclomethasone abolishes the increase in responsiveness. In a more recent study of allergen-induced bronchial hyperresponsiveness, however, the increase in methacholine reactivity 8 h after allergen inhalation was shown to be partially blocked by treatment with oral sustained-release theophylline (individually optimized to give mean serum theophylline concentrations of 13 μg/mL) (73). While it remains to be determined with certainty, therefore, whether theophylline has any effect on airway hyperresponsiveness, it is clear that any effect it may have is small. In asthmatic patients, airways responsiveness to inhaled histamine is reduced during a 3-week period of treatment with beclomethasone (800 μg/day), but no improvement is observed in patients receiving theophylline doses producing steady serum concentrations of 55–100 μM (10–20 μg/mL); when treatments are crossed over, patients receiving theophylline in place of the corticosteroid exhibit an increase in bronchial responsiveness, while those receiving beclomethasone in place of theophylline show a decrease (74).

In view of the ability of theophylline at serum concentrations below 10 μg/mL to protect against histamine- and exercise-induced bronchoconstriction (64,68), a study was undertaken of the effects of low doses of theophylline upon allergic asthmatic reactions. In this study, patients receiving oral sustained-release theophylline (200 mg twice daily) attained mean steady serum theophylline concentrations of 7.8 μg/mL and exhibited significant inhibition of late asthmatic reactions following inhalation of house dust mite extract (72). This observation demonstrates a protective effect against asthmatic reactions for a concentration at the lower end of the "therapeutic range" of bronchodilator serum concentrations. Analysis of the data for individual subjects in this study, however, revealed no statistically significant correlation between serum theophylline concentration and inhibition of late responses, so that more data must be collected to determine whether low doses of theophylline can consistently protect against allergic asthmatic reactions.

Thus, while theophylline's acute bronchodilator action may be fairly weak compared to that of β-adrenoceptor agonists, the drug does possess some potentially important bronchoprotective properties that are likely to be of therapeutic benefit in asthmatic patients. Theophylline's beneficial effects may be observable at lower serum concentrations than the target concentrations in clinical application of the drug. Since relatively low serum theophylline levels confer protection against exercise-induced asthmatic bronchoconstriction and the late asthmatic response to allergen, it will be interesting to see the effects of long-term treatment with low theophylline doses in clinical asthma. It is conceivable, however, that theophylline's protective effects ensue from a prolonged relaxant action on the airway smooth muscle. Recognizing this possibility, and notwithstanding the suggestion that they themselves may possess anti-inflammatory properties, the ability of long-acting β-adrenoceptor agonists such as salmeterol and formoterol to mimic the protective actions of theophylline must also be investigated thoroughly.

Actions on Pulmonary Vasculature

In addition to its actions on airway smooth muscle, theophylline also relaxes precontracted pulmonary artery smooth muscle in vitro at similar concentrations to those that inhibit PDE in tissue homogenates (58). 8-Phenyltheophylline does not relax pulmonary artery (58) while selective PDE3 and PDE5 inhibitors do (75), suggesting that the relaxation is mediated through PDE inhibition rather than adenosine antagonism.

Theophylline is less potent and less efficacious in relaxing pulmonary artery smooth muscle than bronchial smooth muscle in vitro. This difference may reflect differences in the nature of the musculature and also the fact that total PDE activity in pulmonary artery homogenates is approximately double that in bronchus (75).

As a pulmonary vasodilator, theophylline decreases mean pulmonary blood pressure in patients exhibiting pulmonary hypertension (76,77), and this property of theophylline has been proposed to contribute to its clinical effectiveness in the treatment of COPD (see Sec. IV.D).

Actions on Inflammatory Cells

Over the last 20 years, several studies have suggested that theophylline and other methylxanthines in use in clinical therapeutics might exert suppressive actions upon cells of the immune system that may contribute to the beneficial effects of these drugs. In the field of asthma research, many demonstrations have been made of suppression of asthmatic responses that cannot be accounted for fully by the drugs' bronchodilator actions and is assumed to represent an anti-inflammatory effect (78–80).

In the following sections, the pharmacology of alkylxanthine PDE inhibitors in cells of the immune system implicated in allergic airway inflammation and chronic airflow obstruction is described. Where appropriate, the relative contributions of adenosine receptor antagonism and PDE inhibition to these actions is discussed.

Lymphocytes

Immunoglobulin secretion from B lymphocytes in vitro can be reduced by high concentrations of theophylline and IBMX (81,82), and the secretion of

IgE from lymphocytes of patients with atopic dermatitis has specifically been demonstrated to be affected. The mechanism for these actions is unclear and, in fact, lower concentrations of theophylline—as well as other cyclic AMP–elevating agents—may enhance IgE production in mixed lymphocyte preparations, possibly through an inhibition of suppressor T-cell function (81,83).

Methylxanthines inhibit cell cycle progression and thereby proliferation of murine B cells induced by certain stimuli, including antigen, but they enhance progression in response to other stimuli (84,85). In T cells, whose function is clearly regulated by intracellular cyclic AMP (86,87), the situation is clearer. Antigen-induced proliferation of purified human peripheral blood lymphocytes is suppressed by pentoxifylline and proliferation of hamster lymph node cells has been shown to be inhibited by theophylline (88,89). These actions suggest the ability of methylxanthines to reduce proliferation of antigen-specific lymphocytes and thereby to retard the development of immune reactions. Proliferation of T lymphocytes from a number of species induced by anti-CD3 mitogenic plant lectins or phorbol esters can also be inhibited by theophylline (90–93), IBMX (94), and pentoxifylline (88,95–100). In contrast, theophylline and IBMX fail to inhibit interleukin-2 (IL-2)–induced proliferation of mouse thymocytes and cultured T cells, even though the proliferation of these cells in response to phorbol esters is profoundly suppressed by the drugs (90,94). The signaling pathways through which the different mitogens exert their action have not been fully elucidated, so the reason for the stimulus specificity of PDE inhibitors against T-cell proliferation remains unclear.

While many studies have utilized very high concentrations of methylxanthines, concentrations in the range of 50–500 μM (equivalent to 10–100 $\mu g/mL$) can be shown to inhibit colony formation of human peripheral blood mononuclear cells and of purified T cells (92,101). Furthermore, these actions appear to be largely or exclusively cyclic AMP–mediated and dependent upon PKA (97).

Theophylline inhibits phorbol ester–induced IL-2 release from mouse thymocytes and mitogen-induced IL-2 and tumor necrosis factor-β (TNF-β, lymphotoxin) release from human peripheral blood lymphocytes (90,92,102), while pentoxifylline has also been shown to suppress mitogen- or anti-CD3–induced release of TNF-α and interferon gamma (IFN-γ) but not of IFN-α or IL-1β (88,98,99,103). The release of TNF-α into the systemic circulation of mice in response to anti-CD3 in vivo is also reduced by pentoxifylline.

Concentrations of pentoxifylline that suppress T-cell TNF-α production in vitro are ineffective against spontaneous or induced IL-4 release; it was suggested that methylxanthine inhibition of cytokine elaboration is more marked in helper cells of the Th1 than the Th2 type (99), in keeping with the apparent preference of cyclic AMP for suppression of Th1 cell function (104). Th2 cells are regarded as being important in the pathophysiology of allergic diseases owing to their production of IL-4, which promotes IgE class switching (105); methylxanthines may, therefore, be less effective in allergy than in Th1 mediated reactions.

The adherence of T lymphocytes to endothelial and epithelial cells is an essential stage in their accumulation at sites of infection or inflammation. The phorbol ester–stimulated adherence of T cells to keratinocytes stimulated with IFN-γ or TNF-α is inhibited by pentoxifylline, which also suppresses TNF-α–induced expression of intercellular adhesion molecule 1 (ICAM-1) in human skin biopsies (106). It remains unclear whether pentoxifylline inhibits adhesion molecule expression on lymphocytes, endothelial cells, or both.

A reduction in the number of suppressor T cells in the circulation of asthmatic patients is observed and is reversed after a period of theophylline treatment (107) or provoked by withdrawal of theophylline from the patients' therapy (108), reflecting the ability of theophylline to enhance the suppression of autologous cell proliferation in mixed lymphocytes in vitro (109). Withdrawal of theophylline from asthmatic patients has also been shown to increase the numbers of T cells observed in bronchial biopsies in parallel with a decrease in T-cell numbers in the peripheral circulation, suggesting that theophylline may suppress a process of lymphocyte trafficking between the circulation and the airways (110). These effects were observed in patients whose mean serum theophylline concentrations prior to withdrawal were relatively low (5–10 μg/mL).

Neutrophils

Theophylline and IBMX exert actions on neutrophils that are broadly inhibitory. IBMX, for example, inhibits respiratory burst and lysosomal enzyme release by human neutrophils stimulated with the chemotactic tripeptide N-formylmethionyl-L-leucinyl-L-phenylalanine (fMLP), or the complement fragment C5a, although it is very poorly effective against phagocytosis-induced respiratory burst (111). At concentrations of theophylline within the therapeutic range of serum concentrations (20–100 μM), intracellular concentrations of cyclic AMP are elevated by 200% within 45 s of addition of the drug; this parallels an inhibition of reactive oxygen species generation (measured as lucigenin-enhanced chemiluminescence) and leukotriene B$_4$ (LTB$_4$) release induced by fMLP or calcium ionophores in the first 6 min following theophylline addition (112). Confirming the importance of cyclic AMP in these effects, the inhibition of the chemiluminescence response by isoprenaline, a β-adrenoceptor agonist, is enhanced by both theophylline and enprofylline (112,113). Theophylline antagonizes the inhibition of A23187-induced respiratory burst by adenosine while enprofylline causes a slight augmentation of adenosine's inhibitory action, presumably due to amplification by PDE inhibition of the cAMP elevation resulting from A_2-adenosine receptor activation (113). Another study showed fMLP-induced aggregation, superoxide anion (O_2^-) generation and degranulation to be inhibited only at higher concentrations of theophylline and IBMX (> 100 μM), while lower concentrations enhance the responses. The latter effect probably results from antagonism at adenosine A_2 receptors, since the enhancement is mimicked by adenosine deaminase or 8-phenyltheophylline (114) and is reversed by exogenous adenosine (115). These data are supported by the ability of enprofylline, in the concentration range 1–100 μM, to inhibit fMLP-induced O_2^- generation while theophylline, at the same concentrations, enhances the response. In the presence of adenosine deaminase, however, both drugs inhibit the response (116). Theophylline in the form of the water-soluble salt aminophylline (theophylline ethylenediamine) has also been demonstrated to cause a slight enhancement of fMLP-induced neutrophil chemotaxis and O_2^- generation at concentrations < 250 μM while inhibiting these functions at a millimolar concentration (117).

Inhibitory effects of theophylline on neutrophil function have also been observed *ex vivo* in cells obtained from the blood of human patients treated with theophylline. Chemotactic responsiveness of neutrophils (and monocytes) from chronically asthmatic children receiving regular oral theophylline is impaired compared to cells obtained from patients whose theophylline had been withdrawn 7 days prior to experimentation; the recovery of chemotactic responses after theophylline withdrawal was associated in this study with a mean 30% decrease in basal intracellular cyclic AMP levels (118). One week's treatment with oral theophylline, leading to a mean serum concentration of 9.4 μg/mL (approximately 50 μM), causes an increase in basal intracellular cAMP and enhances the ability of isoprenaline to stimulate cyclic AMP accumulation and to inhibit A23187-induced chemiluminescence (112). The correlation of cyclic AMP levels with suppression of neutrophil function remains unclear, however. Whilst IBMX enhances the inhibition of fMLP-induced neutrophil chemotaxis by isoprenaline, prostaglandin E_1 (PGE_1), or the adenylyl cyclase activator forskolin, the degree of elevation in intracellular cyclic AMP following these treatments does not correlate with the degree of functional inhibition. Furthermore, isoprenaline or PGE_1, in the presence of IBMX inhibits neutrophil chemotaxis in response to LTB_4, while forskolin, which causes a substantially greater elevation of cyclic AMP in the presence of IBMX, has no effect on this response (119). IBMX has also been demonstrated to cause a suppression of TNF-α receptor gene expression in neutrophil precursor cells that can be mimicked neither by forskolin nor by the stable cyclic AMP analogue $N^6,2'$-O-dibutyryladenosine $3':5'$-cyclic monophosphate (diBu-cAMP) (120).

Pentoxifylline inhibits fMLP-induced polymerization of globular actin to the filamentous F-actin form, although it does not affect the incorporation of actin into the neutrophil cytoskeleton (121,122), inhibits the formation of pseudopodia, and decreases the rigidity—and thereby the viscosity—of human neutrophils in vitro (123,124). These effects of pentoxifylline on microfilament assembly may underlie both the clinical effectiveness of the drug in reducing blood viscosity and its ability to inhibit the phagocytosis by neutrophils of latex or zymosan particles and bacteria (125,126). Concentrations of the drug that are effective against these cell functions increase intracellular cyclic AMP but also inhibit adenosine uptake, so that the increase in cyclic AMP cannot be said with certainty to result from PDE inhibition.

In vivo, pentoxifylline inhibits neutrophil-mediated lung, liver, and gastrointestinal injury associated with septicemia or ischemia/reperfusion in several species (127–132). It inhibits the increases in plasma levels of neutrophil elastase, lactoferrin, TNF-α, and I-L6 and, in bronchoalveolar lavage (BAL), levels of TNF-α and lysozyme occurring after intravenous bolus injection of *Escherichia coli* endotoxin in chimpanzees or aerosol administration of *Streptococcus pneumoniae* in rabbits, respectively (133,134), without having significant effects on neutrophil numbers in the general, hepatic, or gastric circulation or in the BAL (130,132–134). Surprisingly, proliferation of *S. pneumoniae* is reduced in the airways of pentoxifylline-treated rabbits despite the drug's lack of effect on neutrophil migration and its inhibition of some mechanisms thought to be involved in the cells' bactericidal action (134,135).

Eosinophils

As described above for neutrophils, theophylline and IBMX have been demonstrated to exert a range of actions on eosinophils both in vitro and in vivo. At millimolar concentrations, theophylline decreases the survival time of eosinophils cultured in the presence of IL-5 (136), apparently by inducing apoptosis (137). Such high concentrations, however, are unlikely to be achieved in vivo during theophylline therapy, so that the pharmacological significance of these observations is questionable. At concentrations at the upper end of the therapeutic serum concentration range, theophylline has been shown to inhibit partially the chemotaxis of eosinophils in response to a variety of stimuli in vitro (138), but within this concentration range theophylline enhances the generation of O_2^- in response to opsonized zymosan particles. The latter effect, like similar phenomena observed in neutrophils and platelets, is assumed to result from theophylline's antagonist action at A_2-adenosine receptors, since it can be mimicked by addition of adenosine deaminase or reversed by exogenous adenosine or A_2-receptor agonists (139). At 1 mM, theophylline exerts an inhibitory action on the zymosan-induced O_2^- generation. When oxygen radical generation is measured using luminol-enhanced chemiluminescence, the response induced by the anaphylotoxin C5a is inhibited concentration-dependently by theophylline with an IC_{50} of 525 μM (23); concentrations within the therapeutic range, therefore, cause somewhat less than 50% inhibition of this response. Similarly, inhibition of C5a-induced eosinophil degranulation, measured as the release of eosinophil-derived neurotoxin (EDN) or eosinophil cationic protein (ECP), reaches 50% only at concentrations above 300 μM (23). Leukotriene C_4 release induced by fMLP, however, is inhibited at lower concentrations of theophylline with an IC_{50} of only 50 μM, sixfold lower than the IC_{50} for PDE inhibition in the same study (140). In contrast to the cell responses listed above, antibody-dependent killing of schistosomula of the parasitic trematode helminth *Schistosoma mansoni* by human eosinophils is unaffected by theophylline at concentrations up to 550 μM (141).

IBMX exhibits a similar spectrum of actions to theophylline in vitro, inhibiting zymosan-stimulated oxygen radical generation in guinea pig peritoneal eosinophils (IC_{50} = 36 μM) (142) and fMLP-stimulated lucigenin-dependent chemiluminescence and C5a-induced degranulation in human peripheral blood eosinophils (IC_{50} = 16 μM and 50 μM, respectively) (23,29). Curiously, much higher concentrations of IBMX—almost identical to the necessary concentrations of theophylline— are required to suppress C5a-stimulated chemiluminescence (IC_{50} = 524 μM) (23).

Both theophylline and IBMX—as well as other cyclic AMP–elevating agents such as cholera toxin, β-adrenoceptor agonists, and prostaglandin E_2 (PGE_2)—inhibit degranulation of eosinophils stimulated with IgG or secretory IgA immunoglobulins (143). This suppressive effect is related to the magnitude of increases in intracellular cyclic AMP levels and the co-administration of IBMX with a β-agonist or PGE_2 leads to enhancement of both the rise in cyclic AMP and the inhibition of degranulation. Similarly, theophylline reduces the release of granulocyte-macrophase colony stimulating factor (GM-CSF) from eosinophils stimulated with IgA-coated sepharose beads (144).

In vivo, systemic administration of theophylline reduces the influx of eosinophils to inflammatory sites in the skin and lungs of experimental animals and humans. Substantial reduction in the accumulation of ^{111}In-labeled eosinophils in the skin of sensitized guinea pigs injected intradermally with zymosan-activated plasma (a source of C5a), PAF, or antigen is observed following treatment with theophylline (145). Eosinophil influx into the bronchoalveolar space of sensitized guinea pigs or rabbits following antigen inhalation is also reduced after theophylline pretreatment (146,147), although administration of theophylline up to 4 h after allergen inhalation does not prevent the late-phase eosinophil accumulation (148,149). Isbufylline also reduces eosinophil recruitment into the airways of sensitized guinea pigs following antigen inhalation (45). Six weeks' treatment with oral theophylline leads to decreased bronchial subepithelial eosinophil numbers observed following allergen inhalation in asthmatic humans (150); this effect occurs at serum theophylline concentrations below the normal therapeutic range (mean concentration = 6.6 μg/mL or 37 μM) and has been proposed to indicate a significant anti-inflammatory action of theophylline dissociated from the drug's bronchodilator action (79). It must be noted, however, that suppression by theophylline of airway eosinophil influx following antigen or PAF exposure in animals is associated with a reduction in neither acute bronchoconstriction nor bronchial hyperreactivity (146,147,151,152), although isbufylline has been shown to suppress PAF-induced bronchial responsiveness to intravenous histamine in guinea pigs (45).

Monocytes and Macrophages

Theophylline and IBMX have both been demonstrated to increase intracellular cyclic AMP concentrations in human peripheral blood monocytes (153,154) and alveolar macrophages (155,156), while IBMX also enhances isoprenaline-induced increases in macrophage cyclic AMP levels (155). Interestingly, the elevation of cyclic AMP by IBMX in alveolar macrophages in vitro is lower in cells obtained from asthmatic patients (156), suggesting that these cells may have a lower basal adenylyl cyclase activity or altered PDE enzymes.

Both the phagocytosis and the presentation of antigenic particles are inhibited by theophylline—which reduces the expression of the class II major histocompatibility complex (MHC) molecule HLA-DR, induced by bacterial lipopolysaccharide (LPS) in human monocytes (157)—and IBMX and pentoxifylline, which reduce the transcription of MHC II genes and expression of MHC II molecules in murine macrophages (100,158), whose phagocytic function is also inhibited by theophylline (159). The attachment of human monocytes to antibody-coated target cells is reduced by theophylline (160), and antibody-dependent cellular cytotoxicity (ADCC) of human monocytes is also reduced by theophylline and IBMX, although the magnitude of this inhibition does not correlate with the elevation in intracellular cyclic AMP, implying that theophylline may exert an additional action independent of PDE inhibition (160,161). The phagocytosis of protozoan parasites in vitro by mouse peritoneal macrophages is also inhibited by theophylline (162), while bacterial phagocytosis and intracellular killing *ex vivo* are reduced in alveolar macrophages obtained from human subjects treated with oral theophylline for 14 days (163).

The migration of monocytes to tissues, where they differentiate to macrophages, also appears to be under the influence of cyclic nucleotides and is inhibited by theophylline (164). This inhibition seems to represent interference with an early stage of cell activation as theophylline reduces chemoattractant-induced polarization of human monocytes and their chemotaxis in vitro (164). Guinea pig peritoneal macrophages exhibit a similar response, with the increased Ca^{2+} efflux and actin polymerization induced by fMLP being suppressed by theophylline (165). The effect of these drugs upon microfilaments appears to be to promote depolymerization of F-actin, since the level of monomeric actin in the cells increases while total actin content is unchanged (165). The expression of CD11b, the integrin α^M subunit, in response to LPS is reduced by theophylline in human monocytes (157), possibly interfering in the migration of monocytes to tissues. In vivo, the influx of macrophages to the airways of sensitized guinea pigs challenged by allergen aerosol is also inhibited by pretreatment of the animals with theophylline (166), although it is unclear whether this represents a direct effect on monocytes/macrophages or a diminished production of chemotactic factors at the site of challenge.

While theophylline and IBMX display a clear inhibition of the production of reactive oxygen species and arachidonic acid metabolites by human monocytes and alveolar macrophages in response to opsonized particles (167–171), theophylline has no effect upon granule enzyme release from either murine or human macrophages (170,172). The suppression of the human alveolar macrophage respiratory burst appears to be primarily if not exclusively mediated by PDE inhibition, since the inhibition of the cell function by theophylline is unaffected by addition of adenosine deaminase and is largely blocked by a selective inhibitor of PKA (171).

Cytokine production by monocytes and macrophages in response to bacterial LPS has been widely reported to be inhibited by methylxanthines. Release of TNF-α, as well as transcription of its gene, is suppressed by theophylline and IBMX in human and rat monocytes and in rat alveolar macrophages

(173,174), while pentoxifylline also reduces LPS-induced TNF-α production by cultured monocytes and decreases circulating TNF-α levels in humans during endotoxemia (175). IBMX has been reported to inhibit IL-1 release from human monocytes and a mouse peritoneal macrophage cell line (153,176), although other workers have found no effect of the drug on release of IL-1α or IL-1β from monocytes (173). In contrast, a small but significant stimulation of IL-6 production has been demonstrated in human monocytes treated with IBMX or pentoxifylline at concentrations that inhibit LPS-induced TNF-α production (103,173), a finding that concurs with reports that production of IL-6, which is induced by the adenylyl cyclase-activating receptor agonist, PGE$_1$, is increased by theophylline in a murine monocyte cell line (177).

That theophylline at concentrations as low as 10 μM should be effective in suppressing LPS-induced TNF-α production by human blood monocytes (174) is interesting, since this response is also inhibited potently by A$_2$-adenosine-receptor agonists (178). It appears likely, therefore, that endogenous adenosine does not play a major role in regulating the response and that theophylline exerts its actions through PDE inhibition.

Mast Cells and Basophils

In contrast to those from rodents, mucosal mast cells from primates appear to be sensitive to theophylline, which inhibits anti-IgE– or Con A–induced degranulation of mast cells from the intestinal mucosa of monkeys (179) and humans (180,181). That the suppressive actions of theophylline on mast-cell function are mediated by PDE inhibition is suggested by the elevation of intracellular cyclic AMP levels and the consequent activation of PKA evoked by concentrations of theophylline that inhibit anti-IgE– or 48/80-induced histamine release from rat peritoneal mast cells (182–184). Theophylline appears to exert an additional effect via adenosine receptor antagonism, since adenosine enhances histamine release in response to anti-IgE, and this enhancement is blocked by lower concentrations of theophylline than those which inhibit the anti-IgE response itself (55).

Most investigations of human mast-cell pharmacology have been undertaken using chopped skin or lung fragments. These preparations exhibit histamine release in response to anti-IgE, which is suppressed by theophylline and IBMX (180,185–188). In contrast to rodent "connective tissue" mast cells, the cells from human lung are poorly responsive to peptide secretagogues, while skin cells respond strongly to 48/80 and substance P (188,189). Human lung mast cells display heterogeneous density when isolated by centrifugation over Percoll density gradients, however, corresponding to varying granule histamine content, and the responsiveness of the cells to immunological stimuli and secretagogues varies among the subpopulations. Inhibition of anti-IgE–induced histamine release also varies among these separate populations, ranging from 30% inhibition by 300 µM IBMX to 60% (189).

Theophylline was demonstrated, more than 20 years ago, to elevate intracellular cyclic AMP levels and to suppress antigen-induced release of histamine and PAF from passively sensitized rabbit basophils (190), and similar effects have been observed in human cells in the intervening decades. Theophylline inhibits histamine release from human basophils stimulated by anti-IgE (187,188,191,192), allergen or complement factors (193,194), and substance P or 48/80 (187), while IBMX has also been observed to suppress histamine and LTC_4 release induced by anti-IgE or allergen (192,195,196). Both theophylline and enprofylline inhibit human basophil PDE activity and suppress immunologically evoked histamine release, with enprofylline exhibiting higher potency for both actions (197). The concentration dependence of intracellular cAMP elevation by IBMX or theophylline is very similar to that for inhibition of histamine release (192).

Basophils obtained from the peripheral blood of untreated asthmatic patients exhibit a spontaneous release of histamine in vitro that is higher than that observed with basophils from healthy or chronically medicated asthmatic subjects; this spontaneous degranulation is also inhibited by theophylline (198).

The eosinophil granule protein MBP, which is released into the extracellular medium at sites of eosinophilic inflammation, induces a Ca^{2+}- and calmodulin-dependent degranulation of human basophils that can be inhibited by theophylline (199). Similarly, histamine release from basophils stimulated with PAF is inhibited by IBMX (200). The ability of these drugs both to inhibit mediator release from inflammatory cells and to reduce their subsequent actions on other cells may be important in the study of the modulation of inflammatory conditions by PDE inhibitors. The influence of PDE inhibitors on cytokine secretion from mast cells has not been studied in detail, although IBMX has been demonstrated to enhance potently the release of IL-3 from anti-IgE-stimulated PB-3c murine mast cells, apparently by increasing the half-life of the cytokine's mRNA (201).

IV. Clinical Efficacy

Within the range of 5–20 µg/mL (28–110 µM), serum theophylline concentration exhibits a log-linear relationship to the drug's bronchodilator effect (Fig.

2). Reflecting this, the maintenance of serum theophylline concentrations at the upper end of this range has been demonstrated to produce maximal improvement in lung function in severe asthma (202). At lower serum levels, however, theophylline is effective against both exercise-induced bronchoconstriction and late asthmatic responses while causing little direct bronchodilation, as determined by improvement in baseline lung function (see Sec. III.B).

Theophylline may be administered enterally—by which route it is well absorbed—or parenterally (usually as intravenous aminophylline), and it is cleared by excretion in the urine or metabolism to monomethyl and dimethyl uric acids in the liver (202); these metabolites are very rapidly excreted, suggesting that they may be actively secreted by the renal tubules (202). The serum half-life of theophylline is approximately 8 h in adults and 3.6 h in children, but considerable variation is observed both between and within individuals. Changes in the rate of clearance of the drug frequently underlie the occurrence of toxicity (see Sec. V).

The capacity of theophylline to exert toxic effects at concentrations only slightly above the therapeutic range has led to great interest in the pharmacokinetics of the drug. The kinetics of theophylline clearance are generally linear, as a result of the balance between the diuretic action of high concentrations—leading to increased excretion of the unmetabolized drug— and the rapid excretion of the methyl uric acid metabolites, which account for a greater proportion of the excreted product at lower theophylline serum concentrations (202). Tolerance to the diuretic action of theophylline can occur after multiple doses, however, leading to a loss of first-order kinetics in clearance and an increase in the serum half-life. The development of sustained-release formulations of theophylline has allowed improved maintenance of serum concentrations with a single evening dose (or a one-third morning dose and a two-thirds evening dose), leading to serum concentrations that remain within the therapeutic range throughout the day and are at their highest during the early hours of the morning, when the risk of nocturnal attacks in severe asthma is greatest (12).

A range of N-7 substituted theophylline derivatives, including 7-(2,3-dihydroxypropyl) theophylline (also known as dyphylline, diprophylline, or glyphylline) and 7-(2-hydroxypropyl)theophylline (proxyphylline), have been developed and marketed for use in asthma therapy. These drugs, however, have the disadvantages of low bioavailability after oral dosing, rapid clearance, and low bronchodilator potency (16,202). Effects apart from bronchodilation are probably also reduced, since, in a study of exercise-induced bronchoconstriction, the addition of 300 mg each of proxyphylline and diprophylline to an intravenous dose of 200 mg theophylline caused a markedly smaller increase in protection against bronchoconstriction than was effected by elevating the theophylline dose by 150 mg (68).

Enprofylline is a more potent bronchodilator than theophylline but is very rapidly cleared, so that maintenance of adequate serum levels is more difficult. The potency of enprofylline is interesting, since it is more potent than theophylline in inhibiting PDE (197) but is a poor antagonist of most adenosine receptors (16,203), suggesting that the adenosine antagonistic capacity of xanthine derivatives does not, alone, account for their bronchodilator properties. It is also interesting to note that enprofylline exhibits similar effectiveness to theophylline in suppressing late asthmatic responses to allergen inhalation despite a fourfold lower steady-state serum concentration that results in a smaller inhibitory effect against the immediate bronchoconstrictor response to allergen (69).

Setting aside its demonstrated effectiveness against experimental asthmatic responses, theophylline has been used in the clinical treatment of asthma for several decades and remains the most widely prescribed antiasthma drug worldwide (14). Although theophylline has been relegated to a second- or third-line treatment in asthma therapy, often regarded as useful only when inhaled corticosteroids and inhaled β_2-adrenoceptor agonists fail to achieve therapeutic goals (204), the availability of sustained-release preparations and improved drug-monitoring techniques have allowed more reliable maintenance of serum theophylline concentrations, thereby permitting more precise control of drug actions and facilitating avoidance of toxic effects associated with excessive serum drug levels.

A. Acute Asthma

The bronchodilator action of theophylline underlies the use of intravenous aminophylline in the management of acute severe asthma, a condition in which it has been used effectively for over 50 years (14). Since theophylline, even by the intravenous route, is less effective than inhaled β_2-agonists in causing bronchodilation (205), this treatment is generally reserved for patients who fail to respond to β-agonists. Although coadministration of a β-agonist and theophylline can produce additive or even synergistic acute bronchodilation (202,206), no long-term benefit for symptom control has been demonstrated to result from administering intravenous aminophylline in conjunction with nebulized β-agonists to patients who respond to the latter drug alone (14,202). In fact, the addition of aminophylline to the treatment regimen can increase the incidence of side effects without producing any significant additional therapeutic benefit (207).

Patients undergoing acute asthma exacerbation who fail to exhibit satisfactory improvement in FEV_1 or PEFR after treatment with inhaled β-agonist may benefit from intravenous aminophylline. Rapid infusion of aminophylline can cause severe cardiac arrhythmias and, if the drug is to be used in acute asthma, it should be administered by slow infusion (recommended rate is 0.6 mg/kg lean body weight per hour) (205), with careful monitoring of serum concentrations.

B. Chronic Asthma

In the face of theophylline's weak acute bronchodilator action relative to β-agonists, the ability of the drug to prevent the symptoms of chronic asthma and to reduce the need for emergency medication appears to be more important from a clinical perspective (202). Therapeutic doses of theophylline that sustain a serum concentration above 10 μg/mL lead to an increased frequency of asymptomatic days and prolonged improvement of lung function in asthmatic patients (208) and reduce the need for short courses of daily corticosteroids (209).

In patients whose asthma is uncontrollable by bronchodilators alone and who, therefore, require chronic steroid therapy, the addition of theophylline to a treatment regimen including inhaled beclomethasone or alternate-day oral prednisolone leads to a reduction in the frequency of nocturnal symptoms, decreased use of inhaled β-agonists, and increased exercise tolerance (209), demonstrating that theophylline can exert therapeutic effects in addition to those conferred by regular corticosteroid use. Withdrawal of theophylline from a treatment regimen of oral and inhaled corticosteroids, inhaled β_2-agonists, inhaled anticholinergic drugs and cromoglycate and regular oral theophylline in a group of severe young asthmatics has been demonstrated to lead to a substantial deterioration in symptom control that cannot be rectified by increased steroid doses but responds to reintroduction of theophylline (210). Further studies of patients with severe chronic asthma have shown deterioration in lung function and symptom control in steroid-dependent asthmatics after theophylline withdrawal (14), and this deterioration appears to be accompanied by increased signs of airway inflammation. Theophylline appears, therefore, to have a role in the management of chronic asthma that is independent of its bronchodilator capacity. In particular, a set of severe asthmatics appears to benefit particularly from symptom control by theophylline that is not achievable with corticosteroids (210). The reason why some patients exhibit this requirement for theophylline remains unclear and requires further investigation (14). Since many bronchoprotective actions of theophylline are observed at serum concentrations below the bronchodilator range, it is feasible that theophylline at lower doses than those commonly prescribed may be of use in chronic asthma therapy, although research in this area is just beginning and a reevaluation of the role and appropriate dosages of theophylline must await the results of well-controlled studies.

C. Nocturnal Asthma

Patients with asthma exhibit circadian variations in airway tone and airway responsiveness such that, in more severe cases, the decreased caliber and increased responsiveness occurring during the night are manifested as nocturnal asthma attacks (211). Theophylline may be effective in the treatment of this condition, since administration of a sustained-release formulation of the drug at night controls nocturnal symptoms (212). Slow-release oral β_2-adrenoceptor agonists are less effective than theophylline against nocturnal asthma (213), but inhalation of the long-acting β_2-agonists salmeterol and formoterol improves lung function and decreases methacholine responsiveness over a 24-h period in asthmatic patients (214), while regular use of inhaled salmeterol attenuates the early morning decrease in PEFR in patients with nocturnal asthma symptoms (215). It remains unclear whether the actions of these drugs in nocturnal asthma reflect prolonged bronchodilation or a suppression of cyclical inflammatory processes in the airway wall (211).

D. COPD

Controversy has surrounded the use of theophylline in the treatment of diseases characterized by chronic obstruction of the airways. Theophylline has a number of demonstrable actions that may be of clinical benefit in chronic airway obstruction and that should be considered in decisions on individual treatment programs; the lack of short-term bronchodilation does not necessarily indicate that no benefit can be gained by the patient from regular long-term use of the drug. The effects of withdrawal of theophylline from COPD patients receiving optimized bronchodilator therapy suggest that theophylline is important in the control of symptoms in a substantial proportion of patients and that individual responses need to be assessed in order to determine the patients' requirement for theophylline treatment (216,217).

Although bronchodilation may often be unobservable after theophylline administration in patients with COPD (202), a bronchodilating effect of theophylline can be associated with prolonged therapy in patients with chronic, stable COPD (218). Additive bronchodilation can be achieved by combining theophylline and β_2-adrenoceptor agonists, although it is difficult to draw firm conclusions from these studies, which employed suboptimal doses of β-agonists (218–220).

The predominant complaint of COPD patients is dyspnea accompanied by reduced exercise tolerance (221); this symptom has also been shown to be controlled by theophylline in some studies (see Ref. 222). Improvement in dyspnea ratings can be observed in the absence of significant measurable bronchodilation, although the ability to demonstrate effectiveness of theophylline in relieving dyspnea depends to some extent upon the sensitivity of the dyspnea index used for assessment (216–219,221). Studying changes in symptom score (indicating cough, sputum production, and dyspnea) and transition dyspnea index in COPD patients upon theophylline withdrawal or continuance reveals significant worsening of dyspnea in a majority of patients after withdrawal of long-term theophylline treatment (217). An accompanying decrease in exercise tolerance, measured by the 6-min walking test, is observable after theophylline withdrawal (217), while exercise tolerance has also been shown to be increased by the introduction of theophylline to the treatment schedule of COPD patients (223,224). The increased respiratory muscle performance that may underlie improved exercise tolerance in patients treated with theophylline (see below) (218,225) appears to be associated with a reduction in trapped gas volume (224); the reduction in hyperinflation and increased muscle performance might account, at least in part, for the improvement in lung function conferred by theophylline (218).

Theophylline has a well-characterized ability to increase diaphragmatic contractility; this is more pronounced in fatigued (hypoxic) diaphragm than under normal conditions (218). This action leads to pronounced increases in maximal transdiaphragmatic or pleural pressure and in ventilatory endurance in COPD patients with marked hypoxia/hypercapnia (225,226), while increases are insignificant in patients with mild hypoxia (227,228). Hypoventilation in some COPD patients, which is thought to result from depressed central nervous system respiratory drive, may also be overcome by theophylline (229), although the importance of this mechanism is not fully understood.

As stated above (Sec. III.B), theophylline decreases pulmonary arterial pressure and pulmonary vascular resistance as a result of pulmonary vasodilation and partly because of the drug's positive inotropic action. Hypoxia in severe COPD is associated with reflex pulmonary vasoconstriction and increased pulmonary arterial resistance; these symptoms have been shown to be diminished by oral (sustained-release) or intravenous theophylline in COPD patients without cor pulmonale, who display increased cardiac output, oxygen consumption, and oxygen saturation (230). Patients with cor pulmonale, a pos-

sible complication of COPD, appear to receive much less hemodynamic benefit from theophylline. While improvements in pulmonary hemodynamics may
account for some of the improvements in dyspnea and exercise tolerance, this
remains to be confirmed; the lack of hemodynamic improvement in patients
exhibiting cor pulmonale does not necessarily imply that no improvement in
lung function or relief of dyspnea can be achieved with theophylline treatment.

V. Systemic Effects

Concerns over the side effects of theophylline have been voiced widely, and
theophylline, as well as other methylxanthines, does indeed have numerous
extrapulmonary actions that complicate the use of such drugs in the treatment
of obstructive lung disease (16,231). After enteral administration, methylxanthines are absorbed rapidly and distributed throughout all body compartments
(16), where their nonselective PDE inhibitory action, along with other actions
such as adenosine-receptor antagonism, leads to a broad range of effects. In
addition to theophylline's side effects at serum concentration within the therapeutic range, several toxic effects of the drug are exhibited at serum concentrations above this range.

     Acute toxicity is rare and is almost always associated with very high
serum concentrations of theophylline (>40 µg/mL) (232), well above the
range of effective bronchodilator concentrations ($5-20$ µg/mL) (231). Within
the therapeutic concentration range, an average of 56% of theophylline is
bound to plasma proteins; at higher concentrations, the protein binding is satu-
rated, resulting in disproportionate increases in free drug concentrations and
increased risk of toxicity (16). Chronic overdosing is a more common cause
of adverse effects, although severe toxicity is infrequent and the mortality rate
is higher in acute overdosing (232). The severity of toxicity in acute overdosing correlates closely with serum concentration, and most deaths in these cases
occur while serum levels are still very high (>100 µg/mL); the correlation
of toxicity with serum levels is less clear in chronic overmedication (232).

     Theophylline toxicity can result from a variety of causes, including pa-
tient or practitioner error (232), impaired drug metabolism resulting from infection or liver disease (which also reduces theophylline binding to plasma
proteins) (16), and heart failure or drug interactions (231), which may reduce
the clearance of theophylline (16,202,232,233). It is particularly important
to note that theophylline exhibits interactions with erythromycin and certain
histamine H_2 antagonists: use of both of these drugs may be indicated in
asthma and chronic obstructive pulmonary disease, where upper respiratory
tract infection is common and corticosteroid use is often associated with gas-

tric ulceration. The most common manifestations of theophylline toxicity are cardiovascular and gastrointestinal reactions, although a small number of cases may exhibit central nervous system effects, which are more often associated with chronic than acute overdosing. Electrolyte imbalances are observed frequently in acute overdose but are less common in cases of chronic overdose.

A. Cardiovascular Effects

The most common cardiovascular effects of theophylline are sinus tachycardia and runs of premature ventricular beats. Arrhythmias have also been noted less frequently, although acute toxicity resulting from rapid intravenous administration of the soluble theophylline salt aminophylline (theophylline ethylenediamine) has resulted in sudden death due to cardiac arrhythmias (16). Therapeutic serum concentrations of theophylline rarely induce tachycardia or ectopic beats, even in patients with chronic ventricular arrhythmia (202). The combination of a small net increase in force of contraction with a decreased preload resulting from vasodilation leads to a modest increase in the cardiac output of patients treated with intravenous aminophylline (234).

The adverse effects of high concentrations of theophylline on cardiac rhythm appear to result directly from its PDE-inhibitory action. Since cyclic AMP itself has demonstrable arrhythmogenic properties, resulting from increased cytosolic calcium concentrations in the cardiac muscle (235), the reduced survival observed in groups of patients treated for congestive heart failure with the selective PDE3 inhibitor milrinone may be due to the increased incidence of cyclic AMP–dependent arrhythmias, particularly fast atrial fibrillation (236–238). In view of this phenomenon, it would appear that PDE inhibitors acting upon cardiac cyclic AMP–hydrolyzing enzymes must inevitably induce tachycardia as a side effect (235), and it is interesting to note that derivatives of theophylline containing a large alkyl substituent at the N-3 position (such as enprofylline) exhibit both increased bronchodilator potency and increased risk of tachycardia (17). However, since adenosine has a negative chronotropic action, the adenosine antagonistic action of theophylline may contribute to the effects of theophylline on heart rate (239).

B. Gastrointestinal Effects

Nausea and emesis are frequent side effects in the early stages of theophylline treatment; gastric discomfort and diarrhea may also occur. These effects are poorly correlated with serum theophylline concentration and often diminish during long-term therapy (202). Gastrointestinal effects occur most frequently in patients receiving high theophylline dosages for severe asthma but can also be associated with relatively low doses in chronic treatment. In animal studies, the emetic side effects of xanthine bronchodilators correlate closely with the drugs' potency as PDE inhibitors but only weakly with their adenosine antagonistic activity (240), suggesting that this adverse effect is also an inherent feature of PDE inhibitory drugs. Since nausea and vomiting are recognized side effects of selective inhibitors of PDE4 (241), inhibition of this isoenzyme in particular may mediate the emetic actions of methylxanthines.

Theophylline and caffeine stimulate gastric secretion (acid and pepsin) and may induce discomfort or (rarely) gastric bleeding. Relaxation of the lower esophageal sphincter may also occur, and the two conditions together can favor gastroesophageal reflux (17). The stimulation of gastric secretion is likely to be mediated by adenosine antagonism, since this action is not exhibited by enprofylline, while relaxation of the sphincter is a property shared by theophylline and enprofylline and probably results from PDE inhibition.

C. Central Nervous System Effects

Theophylline and caffeine stimulate the central nervous system (CNS) at relatively low concentrations in vivo, since the drugs are concentrated in the cerebrospinal fluid (239). Actions of methylxanthines in the CNS include a beneficial increase in ventilatory drive and a general increase in alertness and lessening of fatigue, but they also account for the risk of tremor and seizures during theophylline therapy.

In addition to headache and dizziness, CNS stimulation leading to tension, anxiety, restlessness, and dysphoria is induced by ingestion of high doses of caffeine or theophylline (16). Seizures can occur in patients with no previous indication of neurological disorder when high serum concentrations of theophylline (usually >50 μg/mL) are reached (232,242). This severe and life-threatening toxic effect has been observed in the absence of minor adverse effects and can only be predicted by measurement of serum theophylline levels (202). Theophylline-induced seizures are occasionally resistant to treatment with conventional anticonvulsants (16), and the mechanism through which the seizures occur remains unclear, although the ability of theophylline to cause significant reductions in cerebral blood flow and oxygenation may be important (243). The induction of seizures is proposed to be mediated by adenosine receptor antagonism, but a recent report has shown no beneficial effects of adenosine A_1-receptor agonists against convulsions induced by toxic concentrations of theophylline in mice (244). Other CNS actions of theophylline, such as the reversal of benzodiazepine sedation, also appear to be mediated by adenosine antagonism (239).

D. Electrolyte Effects

Theophylline has long been recognized as a diuretic, this action resulting at least in part from increased renal blood flow and glomerular filtration rate. However, theophylline also exerts direct actions on the renal tubules, leading to increased Na^+ and Cl^- excretion without any significant change in urinary H^+ concentration (245), apparently through inhibition of solute resorption (246). In vivo, theophylline treatment can cause electrolyte disturbances, with hypokalemia being a particular problem (247). Hypokalemia is exhibited in most cases of acute theophylline toxicity (248) and is probably due to a direct effect on the renal tubules. Severe hypokalemia is less common in chronic theophylline overdosing, although increased risk of electrolyte disturbances—including hypokalemia, hyponatremia, and hypophosphatemia—has been demonstrated for a therapeutic range of serum theophylline concentrations from 5.5–110 μM (approximately 1–20 μg/mL) after oral theophylline dosing (249). Intravenous theophylline administration in patients suffering from recurrent asthmatic attacks leads to increased excretion of magnesium, calcium, and sodium and depresses serum potassium concentrations (250). These side effects may be mediated by PDE inhibition, since the selective PDE4 inhibitor rolipram also induces acute reductions in plasma osmolality and sodium concentration, although levels return to normal within 1 week of regular rolipram use (251). While enprofylline is commonly reported to lack theophylline's diuretic action (17), diminished adenosine antagonism may not abolish the electrolyte disturbances caused by PDE-inhibiting methylxanthines, although further research is required in this area.

VI. Summary

Theophylline has long been regarded as a weak bronchodilator and its value in the therapy of asthma has been debated since the introduction of highly effective bronchodilators such as $β_2$-adrenoceptor agonists. It remains apparent, however, that many asthmatic patients benefit from theophylline treatment despite receiving maximally effective doses of β-agonists. A large body of evidence has accumulated for an anti-inflammatory action of theophylline and related alkylxanthine PDE inhibitors, from both in vitro experiments with inflammatory cells and in vivo experiments in models of allergic and autoimmune diseases. The observation that theophylline withdrawal has deleterious effects in steroid-dependent asthmatic patients suggests that theophylline plays a role in disease control, while the demonstration of inflammatory changes in the airways of asthmatic patients after theophylline withdrawal shows this to be an anti-inflammatory role. The degree of significance of theophylline's anti-inflammatory actions remains a subject for discussion, although recent clinical trials in which the ability of theophylline to complement the actions of corticosteroids in asthma has been addressed may provide additional support to theophylline's unique anti-inflammatory role (see Chap. 5).

In COPD, theophylline appears to exert beneficial effects in all areas of disease pathology, although its effects are of varying magnitude and difficult to quantify. However, while novel therapeutic agents for the treatment of this common and debilitating condition are developed, the bronchodilation and relief of dyspnea obtained with theophylline treatment in some patients will remain important. As the pathology of COPD becomes better understood, therapy based on theophylline in combination with other drugs such as corticosteroids should be fully optimized (see Chap. 6).

References

1. Salter H. On some points in the treatment and clinical history of asthma. Edinb Med J 1859; 4:1109–1115.
2. Kossel A. Über das Theophyllin, einen neuen Bestandteil des Thees. Z Physiol Chemie 1889; 13;298–308.
3. Fischer E, Ach L. Neue Synthese der Harnsäure und ihrer Methylderivate. Berichte Deutsch Chem Gesellschaft 1985; 28:2473–2480.
4. Hirsch S. Klinischer und experimenteller Beitrag zur krampflösenden Wirkung der Purinderivate. Klin Wochenschr 1922; 1:615–618.
5. Minkowski O. Ueber Theocin (Theophyllin) als Diureticum. Ther Gegenwart 1902; 43:490–493.
6. Guggenheimer H. Euphyllin intravenös als Herzmittel. Ther Halbmonatshefte 1921; 35:566–572.
7. Hermann G, Aynesworth MB, Martin J. Successful treatment of persistent extreme dyspnea "status asthmaticus": use of theophylline ethylene diamine (aminophylline, USP) intravenously. J Lab Clin Med 1937; 23:135–148.
8. Hendeles L, Amarshi N, Weinberger M. A clinical and pharmacokinetic basis for the selection and use of slow release theophylline products. Clin Pharmacokinet 1984; 9:95–135.
9. Götz J, Sauter R, Steinijans VW, Jonkman JHG. Steady-state pharmacokinetics of a once-daily theophylline formulation (Euphylong) when given twice daily. Int J Clin Pharmacol Ther Toxicol 1994; 32:168–173.
10. David-Wang AS, Scarth B, Freeman D, Chapman KR. A rapid monoclonal

antibody blood theophylline assay: lack of cross-reactivity with enprofylline. Ther Drug Monit 1994; 16:323–326.

11. Steinijans VW, Schulz H-U, Beier W, Radtke HW. Once daily theophylline: multiple-dose comparison of an encapsulated micro-osmotic system (Euphylong) with a tablet (Uniphyllin). Int J Clin Pharmacol Ther Toxicol 1986; 24:438–447.

12. Steinijans VW, Trautmann H, Johnson E, Beier W. Theophylline steady-state pharmacokinetics: recent concepts and their application in chronotherapy of reactive airway diseases. Chronobiol Int 1987; 4:331–347.

13. Barnes PJ. New drugs for asthma. Eur Respir J 1992; 5:1126–1136.

14. Barnes PJ, Pauwels R. Theophylline in the management of asthma: time for reappraisal? Eur Respir J 1994; 7:579–591.

15. Persson CGA, Karlsson J-A. In vitro responses to bronchodilator drugs. In: Jenne JW, Murphy S, eds. Drug Therapy for Asthma: Research and Clinical Practice (Lung Biology in Health and Disease, Vol. 31). New York: Marcel Dekker, 1987:129–176.

16. Rall TW. Drugs used in the treatment of asthma: the methylxanthines, cromolyn sodium, and other agents. In: Gilman AG, Rall TW, Nies AS, Taylor P, eds. Goodman and Gilman's The Pharmacological Basis of Therapeutics. New York: Pergamon, 1990:618–637.

17. Persson CGA. Development of safer xanthine drugs for treatment of obstructive airways disease. J Allergy Clin Immunol 1986; 78:817–824.

18. Erhardt PW. Second-generation phosphodiesterase inhibitors: structure-activity relationships and receptor models. In: Beavo J, Houslay MD, eds. Cyclic Nucleotide Phosphodiesterases: Structure, Regulation and Drug Action. Chichester: Wiley, 1990:317–332.

19. Cortijo J, Bou J, Beleta J, Cardelus I, Llenas J, Morcillo E, Gristwood RW. Investigation into the role of phosphodiesterase IV in bronchorelaxation, including studies with human bronchus. Br J Pharmacol 1993; 108:562–568.

20. Rabe KF, Tenor H, Dent G, Schudt C, Liebig S, Magnussen H. Phosphodiesterase isoenzymes modulating inherent tone in human airways: identification and characterization. Am J Physiol 1993; 264:L458–L464.

21. Dent G, Rabe KF. Effects of theophylline and non-selective xanthine derivatives on PDE isoenzymes and cellular function. In: Schudt C, Dent G, Rabe KF, eds. Phosphodiesterase Inhibitors. London: Academic Press, 1996: 41–64.

22. Schudt C, Winder S, Müller B, Ukena D. Zardaverine as a selective inhibitor of phosphodiesterase isozymes. Biochem Pharmacol 1991; 42:153–162.

23. Hatzelmann A, Tenor H, Schudt C. Differential effects of non-selective and selective phosphodiesterase inhibitors on human eosinophil functions. Br J Pharmacol 1995; 114:821–831.

24. Beavo JA. Multiple isozymes of cyclic nucleotide phosphodiesterase. Adv Second Messenger Phosphoprotein Res 1988; 22:1–38.

25. Schudt C, Winder S, Eltze M, Kilian U, Beume R. Zardaverine: a cyclic AMP specific PDE III/IV inhibitor. Agents Actions 1991; 34(suppl):379–402.

26. Ukena D, Schudt C, Sybrecht GW. Adenosine receptor-blocking xanthines as inhibitors of phosphodiesterase isozymes. Biochem Pharmacol 1993;45:847–851.

27. Shahid M, Van Amsterdam RGM, de Boer J, ten Berge RE, Nicholson CD, Zaagsma J. The presence of five cyclic nucleotide phosphodiesterase isoenzymes activities in bovine tracheal smooth muscle and the functional effects of selective inhibitors. Br J Pharmacol 1991; 104:471–477.

28. Galvan M, Schudt C. Actions of the phosphodiesterase inhibitor zardaverine on guinea-pig ventricular muscle. Naunyn Schmiedebergs Arch Pharmacol 1990; 342:221–227.

29. Bray KM, Mueller T. Inhibition of phosphodiesterase type IV attenuates the oxidative burst in human isolated eosinophils. Br J Pharmacol 1994; 113:88P.

30. Schudt C, Winder S, Forderkunz S, Hatzelmann A, Ullrich V. Influence of selective phosphodiesterase inhibitors on human neutrophil functions and levels of cAMP and Ca. Naunyn Schmiedebergs Arch Pharmacol 1991; 344: 682–690.

31. Nicholson CD, Challiss RAJ, Shahid M. Differential modulation of tissue function and therapeutic potential of selective inhibitors of cyclic nucleotide phosphodiesterase isoenzymes. Trends Pharmacol Sci 1991; 12:19–27.

32. Buckle DR, Arch JRS, Connolly BJ, Fenwick AE, Foster KA, Murray KJ, Readshaw SA, Smallridge M, Smith DG. Inhibition of cyclic nucleotide phosphodiesterase by derivatives of 1,3-bis(cyclopropylmethyl)xanthine. J Med Chem 1994; 37:476–485.

33. Palfreyman MN. Phosphodiesterase type IV inhibitors as antiinflammatory agents. Drugs Fut 1995; 20:793–804.

34. Dent G, Giembycz MA. Interaction of PDE4 inhibitors with enzymes and cell functions. In: Schudt C, Dent G, Rabe KF, eds. Phosphodiesterase Inhibitors. London: Academic Press, 1996: 111–126.

35. Bowman WC, Rand MJ. Textbook of Pharmacology. Oxford: Blackwell, 1980.

36. Persson CGA. Overview of effects of theophylline. J Allergy Clin Immunol 1986; 78:780–787.

37. Torphy TJ. β-Adrenoceptors, cAMP and airway smooth muscle relaxation: challenges to the dogma. Trends Pharmacol Sci 1994; 15:370–374.

38. Butcher RW, Sutherland EW. Adenosine-3′,5′-phosphate in biological materials: I. Purification and properties of cyclic 3′,5′-nucleotide phosphodiesterase and use of this enzyme to characterize adenosine 3′,5′-phosphate in human urine. J Biol Chem 1962; 237:1244–1250.

39. Loughney K, Ferguson K. Identification and quantification of PDE isoenzymes and subtypes by molecular biological methods. In: Schudt C, Dent G, Rabe KF, eds. Phosphodiesterase Inhibitors. London: Academic Press, 1996:1–19.

40. Soderling SH, Bayuga SJ, Beavo JA. Cloning and characterization of a cAMP-

specific cyclic nucleotide phosphodiesterase. Proc Natl Acad Sci USA 1998; 95:8991–8996.

41. Giembycz MA, Raeburn D. Current concepts on mechanisms of force generation and maintenance in airways smooth muscle. Pulm Pharmacol 1992; 5:279–297.

42. Diamond J. Role of cyclic GMP in airway smooth muscle relaxation. Agents Actions 1993; 43(suppl):13–26.

43. Edwards G, Weston AH. Potassium channel openers and vascular smooth muscle relaxation. Pharmacol Ther 1990; 48:237–258.

44. Manzini S, Meini S, Giachetti A, Beani L, Borea PA, Antonelli T, Ballati L, Bacciarelli C. Pharmacodynamic profile of isbufylline, a new antibronchospastic xanthine devoid of central excitatory actions. Arzneimittelforschung 1990; 40:1205–1213.

45. Manzini S, Perretti F, Abelli L, Evangelista S, Seeds EA, Page CP. Isbufylline, a new xanthine derivative, inhibits airway responsiveness and airway inflammation in guinea pigs. Eur J Pharmacol 1993; 249:251–257.

46. Magnussen H, Jörres R, Hartmann V. Bronchodilator effect of theophylline preparations and aerosol fenoterol in stable asthma. Chest 1986; 90:722–725.

47. Schultze-Werninghaus G, Debelic M. Asthma: Grundlagen-Diagnostik-Therapie. Berlin: Springer-Verlag, 1988.

48. Sakai R, Konno K, Yamamoto Y, Sanai F, Takagi K, Hasegawa T, Iwasaki N, Kakiuchi M, Kato H, Miyamoto K. Effects of alkyl substitutions of xanthine skeleton on bronchodilation. J Med Chem 1992; 35:4039–4044.

49. Dent G, Rabe KF. Adenosine. In: Leff AR, ed. Pulmonary and Critical Care Pharmacology and Therapeutics. New York: McGraw-Hill, 1996:173–180.

50. Cushley MJ, Tattersfield AE, Holgate ST. Inhaled adenosine and guanosine on airway resistance in normal and asthmatic subjects. Br J Clin Pharmacol 1983; 15:161–165.

51. Björck T, Gustafsson LE, Dahlén S-E. Isolated bronchi from asthmatics are hyperresponsive to adenosine, which apparently acts indirectly by liberation of leukotrienes and histamine. Am Rev Respir Dis 1992; 145:1087–1091.

52. Joad JP, Kott KS. Effect of adenosine receptor ligands on cAMP content in human airways and peripheral lung. Am J Respir Cell Mol Biol 1993; 9:134–140.

53. Fredholm BB, Abbracchio MP, Burnstock G, Daly JW, Harden TK, Jacobson KA, Leff P, Williams M. Nomenclature and classification of purinoceptors. Pharmacol Rev 1994; 46:143–156.

54. Linden J. Cloned adenosine A_3 receptors: pharmacological properties, species differences and receptor functions. Trends Pharmacol Sci 1994; 15:298–306.

55. Sydbom A, Fredholm BB. On the mechanism by which theophylline inhibits histamine release from rat mast cells. Acta Physiol Scand 1982; 114:243–251.

56. Cushley MJ, Tattersfield AE, Holgate ST. Adenosine-induced bronchoconstric-

tion in asthma: antagonism by inhaled theophylline. Am Rev Respir Dis 1984; 129:380–384.

57. Mann JS, Holgate ST. Specific antagonism of adenosine-induced bronchoconstriction in asthma by oral theophylline. Br J Clin Pharmacol 1985; 19:685–692.

58. Rabe KF, Magnussen H, Dent G. Theophylline and selective PDE inhibitors as bronchodilators and smooth muscle relaxants. Eur Respir J 1995; 8:637–642.

59. Mitenko PA, Ogilvie RI. Rational intravenous doses of theophylline. N Engl J Med 1973; 289:600–603.

60. Rabe KF, Dent G. Theophylline. In: Barnes PJ, Grunstein MM, Leff AR, Woolcock AJ, eds. Asthma. Philadelphia: Lippincott-Raven, 1997:1535–1554.

61. Qian Y, Naline E, Karlsson J-A, Raeburn D, Advenier C. Effects of rolipram and siguazodan on the human isolated bronchus and their interaction with isoprenaline and sodium nitroprusside. Br J Pharmacol 1993; 109:774–778.

62. Torphy TJ, Undem BJ, Cieslinski LB, Luttmann MA, Reeves ML, Hay DWP. Identification, characterization and functional role of phosphodiesterase isozymes in human airway smooth muscle. J Pharmacol Exp Ther 1993; 265: 1213–1223.

63. Finney MJB, Karlsson J-A, Persson CGA. Effects of bronchoconstriction and bronchodilation on a novel human small airway preparation. Br J Pharmacol 1985; 85:29–36.

64. Magnussen H, Reuss G, Jörres R. Theophylline has a dose-related effect on the airway response to inhaled histamine and methacholine in asthmatics. Am Rev Respir Dis 1987; 136:1163–1167.

65. McWilliams BC, Menendez R, Kelly WH, Howick J. Effects of theophylline on inhaled methacholine and histamine in asthmatic children. Am Rev Respir Dis 1984; 130:193–197.

66. Cartier A, Lemire I, L'Archeveque J, Ghezzo H, Martin RR, Malo J-L. Theophylline partially inhibits bronchoconstriction caused by inhaled histamine in subjects with asthma. J Allergy Clin Immunol 1986; 77:570–575.

67. Pollock J, Kiechel F, Cooper D, Weinberger M. Relationship of serum theophylline concentration to inhibition of exercise-induced bronchospasm and comparison with cromolyn. Pediatrics 1977; 60:840–846.

68. Magnussen H, Reuss G, Jörres R. Methylxanthines inhibit exercise-induced bronchoconstriction at low serum theophylline concentration and in a dose-dependent fashion. J Allergy Clin Immunol 1988; 81:531–537.

69. Pauwels R, van Renterghem D, van der Straeten M, Johannesson N, Persson CGA. The effect of theophylline and enprofylline on allergen-induced bronchoconstriction. J Allergy Clin Immunol 1985; 76:583–590.

70. Mapp C, Boschetto P, Dal Vecchio L, et al. Protective effect of antiasthma drugs on late asthmatic reactions and increased airway responsiveness induced by toluene diisocyanate in sensitized subjects. Am Rev Respir Dis 1987; 136: 1403–1407.

71. Cockcroft DW, Murdock KY, Gore BP, O'Byrne PM, Manning P. Theophyl-

line does not inhibit allergen-induced increase in airway responsiveness to methacholine. J Allergy Clin Immunol 1989; 83:913–920.

72. Ward AJM, McKenniff M, Evans JM, Page CP, Costello JF. Theophylline—an immunomodulatory role in asthma? Am Rev Respir Dis 1993; 147:518–523.

73. Crescioli S, Spinnazzi A, Plebani M, Pozzani M, Mapp CE, Boschetto P, Fabri LM. Theophylline inhibits early and late asthmatic reactions induced by allergens in asthmatic subjects. Ann Allergy 1991; 66:245–251.

74. Dutoit JI, Salome CM, Woolcock AJ. Inhaled corticosteroids reduce the severity of bronchial hyperresponsiveness in asthma but oral theophylline does not. Am Rev Respir Dis 1987; 136:1174–1178.

75. Rabe KF, Tenor H, Dent G, Schudt C, Nakashima M, Magnussen H. Identification of PDE isozymes in human pulmonary artery and the effect of selective PDE inhibitors. Am J Physiol 1994; 266:L536–L543.

76. Harris MN, Daborn AK, O'Dwyer JP. Milrinone and the pulmonary vascular system. Eur J Anaesthesiol 1992; 5(suppl):27–30.

77. Grützmacher J, Schicht R, Schlaeger R, Sill V. Plasma level-dependent hemodynamic effects of theophylline in patients with chronic obstructive lung disease and pulmonary hypertension. Semin Respir Med 1985; 7:171–174.

78. Persson CGA, Erjefält I, Gustafsson B. Xanthines—symptomatic or prophylactic in asthma? Agents Actions 1988; 23(suppl):137–155.

79. Banner KH, Page CP. Theophylline and selective phosphodiesterase inhibitors as anti-inflammatory drugs in the treatment of bronchial asthma. Eur Respir J 1995; 8:996–1000.

80. Banner KH, Page CP. Immunomodulatory actions of xanthines and isoenzyme selective phosphodiesterase inhibitors. Monaldi Arch Chest Dis 1995; 50:286–292.

81. Strannegard O, Strannegard IL. Effect of cyclic AMP-elevating agents on human spontaneous IgE synthesis in vitro. Int Arch Allergy Appl Immunol 1984; 74:9–14.

82. Shearer WT, Patke CL, Gilliam EB, Rosenblatt HM, Barron KS, Orson FM. Modulation of a human lymphoblastoid B cell line by cyclic AMP: Ig secretion and phosphatidylcholine metabolism. J Immunol 1988; 141:1678–1686.

83. Shah TP, Lichtenstein LM, Undem B, MacDonald SM. Effects of cyclic-AMP on human IgE synthesis in vitro. J Allergy Clin Immunol 1991; 89:173.

84. Cohen DP, Rothstein TL. Adenosine 3',5'-cyclic monophosphate modulates the mitogenic responses of murine B lymphocytes. Cell Immunol 1989; 121:113–124.

85. Muthusamy N, Baluyut AR, Subbarao B. Differential regulation of surface Ig- and Lyb2-mediated B cell activation by cyclic AMP: I. Evidence for alternative regulation of signaling through two different receptors linked to phosphatidylinositol hydrolysis in murine B cells. J Immunol 1991; 147:2483–2492.

86. Mary D, Aussel C, Ferrua B, Fehlmann M. Regulation of interleukin 2 synthesis by cAMP in human T cells. J Immunol 1987; 139:1179–1184.

87. Giembycz MA, Corrigan CJ, Seybold J, Newton R, Barnes PJ. Identification
     of cyclic AMP phosphodiesterases 3, 4 and 7 in human CD4$^+$ and CD8$^+$ T-
     lymphocytes: role in regulating proliferation and the biosynthesis of interleu-
     kin-2. Br J Pharmacol 1996; 118:1945–1958.

88. Tilg H, Eibl B, Pichl M, Gachter A, Herold M, Brankova J, Huber C, Nieder-
     wieser D. Immune response modulation by pentoxifylline in vitro. Transplanta-
     tion 1993; 56:196–201.

89. Hart DA. Lithium potentiates antigen-dependent stimulation of lymphocytes
     only under suboptimal conditions. Int J Immunopharmacol 1988; 10:153–
     160.

90. Novogrodsky A, Patya M, Rubin AL, Stenzel KH. Agents that increase cellular
     cAMP inhibit production of interleukin-2, but not its activity. Biochem Biophys
     Res Commun 1983; 114:93–98.

91. Crosti F, Secchi A, Ferrero E, Falqui L, Inverardi L, Pontiroli AE, Ciboddo GF,
     Pavoni D, Protti P, Rugarli C. Impairment of lymphocyte-suppressive system
     in recent-onset insulin-dependent diabetes mellitus: correlation with metabolic
     control. Diabetes 1986; 35:1053–1057.

92. Scordamaglia A, Ciprandi G, Ruffoni S, Caria M, Paolieri F, Venuti D, Can-
     onica GW. Theophylline and the immune response: in vitro and in vivo effects.
     Clin Immunol Immunopathol 1988; 48:238–246.

93. Kotecki M, Pawlak AL, Wiktorowicz KE. The inhibitory effect of theophylline
     on cell cycle kinetics of human lymphocytes in vitro. Arch Immunol Ther Exp
     (Warsaw) 1989; 37:725–733.

94. Goto Y, Takeshita T, Sugamura K. Adenosine 3′,5′-cyclic monophosphate
     (cAMP) inhibits phorbol ester-induced growth of an IL-2-dependent T cell line.
     FEBS Lett 1988; 239:165–168.

95. Bessler H, Gilgal R, Zahavi I, Djaldetti M. Effect of pentoxifylline on E-rosette
     formation and on the mitogenic response of human mononuclear cells. Biomed
     Pharmacother 1987; 41:439–441.

96. Rao KM, Currie MS, McCachren SS, Cohen HJ. Pentoxifylline and other
     methyl xanthines inhibit interleukin-2 receptor expression in human lympho-
     cytes. Cell Immunol 1991; 135:314–325.

97. Rosenthal LA, Taub DD, Moors MA, Blank KJ. Methylxanthine-induced inhi-
     bition of the antigen- and superantigen-specific activation of T and B lympho-
     cytes. Immunopharmacology 1992; 24:203–217.

98. Singer JW, Bianco JA, Takahashi G, Simrell C, Petersen J, Andrews DF III.
     Effect of methylxanthine derivatives on T cell activation. Bone Marrow Trans-
     plant 1992; 10:19–25.

99. Rott O, Cash E, Fleischer B. Phosphodiesterase inhibitor pentoxyfylline, a se-
     lective suppressor of T-helper type 1- but not type 2-associated lymphokine
     production, prevents induction of experimental autoimmune encephalomyelitis
     in Lewis rats. Eur J Immunol 1993; 23:1745–1751.

100. Hecht M, Muller M, Lohmann-Matthes ML, Emmendörffer A. In vitro and in

vivo effects of pentoxifylline on macrophages and lymphocytes derived from autoimmune MRL-lpr/lpr mice. J Leukoc Biol 1995; 57:242–249.

101. Ghio R, Scordamaglia A, D'Elia P, et al. Inhibition of the colony-forming capacity of human T-lymphocytes exerted by theophylline. Int J Immunopharmacol 1988; 10:299–302.

102. Prieur AM, Granger GA. The effect of agents which modulate levels of the cyclic nucleotides on human lymphotoxin secretion and activity in vitro. Transplanation 1975; 20:331–337.

103. Schandené L, Vandenbussche P, Crusiaux A, Alegre ML, Abromowicz D, Dupont E, Content J, Goldman M. Differential effects of pentoxifylline on the production of tumour necrosis factor-alpha (TNF-α) and interleukin-6 (IL-6) by monocytes and T cells. Immunology 1992; 76:30–34.

104. Novak TJ, Rothenberg EV. Cyclic AMP inhibits induction of interleukin 2 but not of interleukin 4 in T cells. Proc Natl Acad Sci USA 1990; 87:9353–9357.

105. Anderson GP, Coyle AJ. T_H2 and ''T_H2-like'' cells in allergy and asthma: pharmacological perspectives. Trends Pharmacol Sci 1994; 15:324–332.

106. Bruynzeel I, van der Raaij LM, Stoof TJ, Willemze R. Pentoxifylline inhibits T-cell adherence to keratinocytes. J Invest Dermatol 1995; 104:1004–1007.

107. Shohat B, Volovitz B, Varsano I. Induction of suppressor T cells in asthmatic children by theophylline treatment. Clin Allergy 1983; 13:487–493.

108. Fink G, Mittelman M, Shohat B, Spitzer SA. Theophylline-induced alterations in cellular immunity in asthmatic patients. Clin Allergy 1987; 17:313–316.

109. Zocchi MR, Pardi R, Gromo G, et al. Theophylline induced nonspecific suppressor activity in human peripheral blood lymphocytes. J Immunopharmacol 1985; 7:217–234.

110. Kidney JC, Dominguez M, Taylor PM, Rose M, Chung KF, Barnes PJ. Immunomodulation by theophylline in asthma: demonstration by withdrawal of therapy. Am J Respir Crit Care Med 1995; 151:1907–1914.

111. Wright CD, Kuipers PJ, Kobylarz-Singer D, Devall LJ, Klinkefus BA, Weishaar RE. Differential inhibition of human neutrophil functions: role of cyclic AMP–specific, cyclic GMP–insensitive phosphodiesterase. Biochem Pharmacol 1990; 40:699–707.

112. Nielson CP, Crowley JJ, Morgan ME, Vestal RE. Polymorphonuclear leukocyte inhibition by therapeutic concentrations of theophylline is mediated by cyclic-3′,5′-adenosine monophosphate. Am Rev Respir Dis 1988; 137:25–30.

113. Nielson CP, Crowley JJ, Cusack BJ, Vestal RE. Therapeutic concentrations of theophylline and enprofylline potentiate catecholamine effects and inhibit leukocyte activation. J Allergy Clin Immunol 1986; 78:660–667.

114. Dianzani C, Brunelleschi S, Viano I, Fantozzi R. Adenosine modulation of primed human neutrophils. Eur J Pharmacol 1994; 263:223–226.

115. Schmeichel CJ, Thomas LL. Methylxanthine bronchodilators potentiate multiple human neutrophil functions. J Immunol 1987; 138:1896–1903.

116. Kaneko M, Suzuki K, Furui H, Takagi K, Satake T. Comparison of theophylline

and enprofylline effects on human neutrophil superoxide production. Clin Exp Pharmacol Physiol 1990; 17:849–859.

117. Llewellyn-Jones CG, Stockley RA. The effects of β_2-agonists and methylxanthines on neutrophil function in vitro. Eur Respir J 1994; 7:1460–1466.

118. Condino-Neto A, Vilela MM, Cambiucci EC, et al. Theophylline therapy inhibits neutrophil and mononuclear cell chemotaxis from chronic asthmatic children. Br J Clin Pharmacol 1991; 32:557–561.

119. Harvath L, Robbins JD, Russell AA, Seamon KB. cAMP and human neutrophil chemotaxis: elevation of cAMP differentially affects chemotactic responsiveness. J Immunol 1991; 146:224–232.

120. Lindvall L, Lantz M, Gullberg U, Olsson I. Modulation of the constitutive gene expression of the 55 kD tumor necrosis factor receptor in hematopoietic cells. Biochem Biophys Res Commun 1990; 172:557–563.

121. Rao KM, Crawford J, Currie MS, Cohen HJ. Actin depolymerization and inhibition of capping induced by pentoxifylline in human lymphocytes and neutrophils. J Cell Physiol 1988; 137:577–582.

122. Freyburger G, Belloc F, Boisseau MR. Pentoxifylline inhibits actin polymerization in human neutrophils after stimulation by chemoattractant factor. Agents Actions 1990; 31:72–78.

123. Armstrong M Jr, Needham D, Hatchell DL, Nunn RS. Effect of pentoxifylline on the flow of polymorphonuclear leukocytes through a model capillary. Angiology 1990; 41:253–262.

124. Wong PM, Schmid-Schonbein GW. Attenuation of spontaneous pseudopod formation in human neutrophils by pentoxifylline. Cell Biophys 1991; 18:203–215.

125. Bessler H, Gilgal R, Djaldetti M, Zahavi I. Effect of pentoxifylline on the phagocytic activity, cAMP levels, and superoxide anion production by monocytes and polymorphonuclear cells. J Leukoc Biol 1986; 40:747–754.

126. Hand WL, Butera ML, King-Thompson NL, Hand DL. Pentoxifylline modulation of plasma membrane functions in human polymorphonuclear leukocytes. Infect Immun 1989; 57:3520–3526.

127. Welsh CH, Lien D, Worthen GS, Weil JV. Pentoxifylline decreases endotoxin-induced pulmonary neutrophil sequestration and extravascular protein accumulation in the dog. Am Rev Respir Dis 1988; 138:1106–1114.

128. Lilly CM, Sandhu JS, Ishizaka A, Harada H, Yonemaru M, Larrick JW, Shi TX, O'Hanley PT, Raffin TA. Pentoxifylline prevents tumor necrosis factor–induced lung injury. Am Rev Respir Dis 1989; 139:1361–1368.

129. Hoffmann H, Hatherill JR, Crowley J, Harada H, Yonemaru M, Zheng H, Ishizaka A, Raffin TA. Early post-treatment with pentoxifylline or dibutyryl cAMP attenuates *Escherichia coli*-induced acute lung injury in guinea pigs. Am Rev Respir Dis 1991; 143:289–293.

130. Hewett JA, Jean PA, Kunkel SL, Roth RA. Relationship between tumor necrosis factor-alpha and neutrophils in endotoxin-induced liver injury. Am J Physiol 1993; 265:G1011–G1015.

131. Reignier J, Mazmanian M, Detruit H, Chapelier A, Weiss M, Libert JM, Herve P. Reduction of ischemia-reperfusion injury by pentoxifylline in the isolated rat lung. Paris-Sud University Lung Transplantation Group. Am J Respir Crit Care Med 1994; 150:342–347.

132. Santucci L, Fiorucci S, Giansanti M, Brunori PM, Di Matteo FM, Morelli A. Pentoxifylline prevents indomethacin induced acute gastric mucosal damage in rats: role of tumour necrosis factor alpha. Gut 1994; 35:909–915.

133. van Leenen D, van der Poll T, Levi M, ten Cate H, van Deventer SJ, Hack CE, Aarden LA, ten Cate JW. Pentoxifylline attenuates neutrophil activation in experimental endotoxemia in chimpanzees. J Immunol 1993; 151:2318–2325.

134. Mah MP, Aeberhard EE, Gilliam MB, Sherman MP. Effects of pentoxifylline on in vivo leukocyte function and clearance of group B streptococci from preterm rabbit lungs. Crit Care Med 1993; 21:712–720.

135. Andres DW, Kutkoski GJ, Quinlan WM, Doyle NA, Doerschuk CM. Effect of pentoxifylline on changes in neutrophil sequestration and emigration in the lungs. Am J Physiol 1995; 268:L27–L32.

136. Hossain M, Okubo Y, Sekiguchi M. Effects of various drugs (staurosporine, herbimycin A, ketotifen, theophylline, FK506 and cyclosporin A) on eosinophil viability. Arerugi 1994; 43:711–717.

137. Ohta K, Sawamoto S, Nakajima M, et al. The prolonged survival of human eosinophils with interleukin-5 and its inhibition by theophylline via apoptosis. Clin Exp Allergy 1996; 26(suppl 2):10–15.

138. Numao T, Fukuda T, Akutsu I, Makino S. Effects of anti-asthmatic drugs on human eosinophil chemotaxis. Nippon Kyobu Shikkan Gakkai Zasshi 1991; 29:65–71.

139. Yukawa T, Kroegel C, Chanez P, et al. Effect of theophylline and adenosine on eosinophil function. Am Rev Respir Dis 1989; 140:327–333.

140. Tenor H, Shute JK, Church MK, Hatzelmann A, Schudt C. Inhibition of human peripheral blood eosinophil LTC4 production by PDE inhibitors. Eur Respir J 1995; 8:9s.

141. Thorne KJI, Richardson BA, Butterworth AE, Hay I, Higenbottam TW. Effect of drugs used in the treatment of asthma on the production of eosinophil-activating factor by monocytes. Int Arch Allergy Appl Immunol 1988; 85:257–259.

142. Dent G, Giembycz MA, Rabe KF, Barnes PJ. Inhibition of eosinophil cyclic nucleotide PDE activity and opsonised zymosan-stimulated respiratory burst by "type IV"-selective PDE inhibitors. Br J Pharmacol 1991; 103:1339–1346.

143. Kita H, Abu-Ghazaleh RI, Gleich GJ, Abraham RT. Regulation of Ig-induced eosinophil degranulation by adenosine 3′,5′-cyclic monophosphate. J Immunol 1991; 146:2712–2718.

144. Shute JK, Lindley I, Peichl P, Holgate ST, Church MK, Djukanović R. Mucosal IgA is an important moderator of eosinophil responses to tissue-derived chemoattractants. Int Arch Allergy Immunol 1995; 107:340–341.

145. Teixeira MM, Rossi AG, Williams TJ, Hellewell PG. Effects of phosphodiester-

ase isoenzyme inhibitors on cutaneous inflammation in the guinea-pig. Br J Pharmacol 1994; 112:332–340.

146. Sanjar S, Aoki S, Kristersson A, Smith D, Morley J. Antigen challenge induces pulmonary airway eosinophil accumulation and airway hyperreactivity in sensitized guinea-pigs: the effect of anti-asthma drugs. Br J Pharmacol 1990; 99: 679–686.

147. Gozzard N, Herd CM, Page CP. Effect of theophylline on antigen-induced airway responses in the neonatally immunised rabbit. Br J Pharmacol 1995; 115: 155P.

148. Tarayre JP, Aliaga M, Barbara M, Malfetes N, Vieu S, Tisne-Versailles J. Theophylline reduces pulmonary eosinophilia after various types of active anaphylactic shock in guinea-pigs. J Pharm Pharmacol 1991; 43:877–879.

149. Chand N, Harrison JE, Rooney SM, et al. Allergic bronchial eosinophilia: a therapeutic approach for the selection of potential bronchial anti-inflammatory drugs. Allergy 1993; 48:624–626.

150. Sullivan P, Bekir S, Jaffar Z, Page C, Jeffery P, Costello J. Anti-inflammatory effects of low-dose oral theophylline in atopic asthma. Lancet 1994; 343:1006–1008.

151. Sanjar S, Aoki S, Boubekeur K, et al. Inhibition of PAF-induced eosinophil accumulation in pulmonary airways of guinea pigs by anti-asthma drugs. Jpn J Pharmacol 1989; 51:167–172.

152. Sanjar S, Aoki S, Boubekeur K, et al. Eosinophil accumulation in pulmonary airways of guinea-pigs induced by exposure to an aerosol of platelet-activating factor: effect of anti-asthma drugs. Br J Pharmacol 1990; 99:267–272.

153. Kassis S, Lee JC, Hanna N. Effects of prostaglandins and cAMP levels on monocyte IL-1 production. Agents Actions 1989; 27:274–276.

154. Nokta MA, Pollard RB. Human immunodeficiency virus replication: modulation by cellular levels of cAMP. AIDS Res Hum Retroviruses 1992; 8:1255–1261.

155. Hjemdahl P, Larsson K, Johansson M-C, Zetterlund A, Eklund A. β-Adrenoceptors in human alveolar macrophages isolated by elutriation. Br J Clin Pharmacol 1990; 30:673–682.

156. Bachelet M, Vincent D, Havet N, et al. Reduced responsiveness of adenylate cyclase in alveolar macrophages from patients with asthma. J Allergy Clin Immunol 1991; 88:322–328.

157. McLeish KR, Wellhausen SR, Dean WL. Biochemical basis of HLA-DR and CR3 modulation on human peripheral blood monocytes by lipopolysaccharide. Cell Immunol 1987; 108:242–248.

158. Figueiredo F, Uhing RJ, Okonogi K, et al. Activation of the cAMP cascade inhibits an early event involved in murine macrophage Ia expression. J Biol Chem 1990; 265:12317–12323.

159. Hisadome M, Terasawa M, Goto K, Kawazoe Y, Okumoto T. Stimulation of phagocytic activity of leukocytes and macrophages by traxanox sodium in mice and rats. Jpn J Pharmacol 1989; 49:275–284.

160. Herlin T, Kragballe K. Divergent effects of methylxanthines and adenylate cyclase agonists on monocyte cytotoxicity and cyclic AMP levels. Eur J Clin Invest 1982; 12:293–299.

161. Herlin T, Kragballe K. Facilitation of cAMP increments during ADCC mediated by monocytes pretreated with cAMP-elevating agents. Int Arch Allergy Appl Immunol 1983; 72:1–5.

162. Wirth JJ, Kierszenbaum F. Inhibitory action of elevated levels of adenosine-3':5' cyclic monophosphate on phagocytosis: effects on macrophage-*Trypanosoma cruzi* interaction. J Immunol 1982; 129:2759–2762.

163. O'Neill SJ, Sitar DS, Klass DJ, Taraska VA, Kepron W, Mitenko PA. The pulmonary disposition of theophylline and its influence on human alveolar macrophage bactericidal function. Am Rev Respir Dis 1986; 134:1225–1228.

164. Stephens CG, Snyderman R. Cyclic nucleotides regulate the morphologic alterations required for chemotaxis in monocytes. J Immunol 1982; 128:1192–1197.

165. Hamachi T, Hirata M, Koga T. Effect of cAMP-elevating drugs on Ca^{2+} efflux and actin polymerization in peritoneal macrophages stimulated with *N*-formyl chemotactic peptide. Biochim Biophys Acta 1984; 804:230–236.

166. Santing RE, Olymulder CG, Van der Molen K, Meurs H, Zaagsma J. Phosphodiesterase inhibitors reduce bronchial hyperreactivity and airway inflammation in unrestrained guinea pigs. Eur J Pharmacol 1995; 275:75–82.

167. Godfrey RW, Manzi RM, Gennaro DE, Hoffstein ST. Phospholipid and arachidonic acid metabolism in zymosan-stimulated human monocytes: modulation by cAMP. J Cell Physiol 1987; 131:384–392.

168. Wiik P. Vasoactive intestinal peptide inhibits the respiratory burst in human monocytes by a cyclic AMP-mediated mechanism. Regul Pept 1989; 25:187–197.

169. Calhoun WJ, Stevens CA, Lambert SB. Modulation of superoxide production of alveolar macrophages and peripheral blood mononuclear cells by β-agonists and theophylline. J Lab Clin Med 1991; 117:514–522.

170. Baker AJ, Fuller RW. Effect of cyclic adenosine monophosphate, 5'-(N-ethylcarboxamido)-adenosine and methylxanthines on the release of thromboxane and lysosomal enzymes from human alveolar macrophages and peripheral blood monocytes in vitro. Eur J Pharmacol 1992; 211:157–161.

171. Dent G, Giembycz MA, Rabe KF, Wolf B, Barnes PJ, Magnussen H. Theophylline suppresses human alveolar macrophage respiratory burst through phosphodiesterase inhibition. Am J Respir Cell Mol Biol 1994; 10:565–572.

172. Ackerman NR, Beebe JR. Effects of pharmacologic agents on release of lysosomal enzymes from alveolar mononuclear cells. J Pharmacol Exp Ther 1975; 193:603–613.

173. Bailly S, Ferrua B, Fay M, Gougerot-Pocidalo MA. Differential regulation of IL 6, IL 1 A, IL 1 beta and TNF alpha production in LPS-stimulated human monocytes: role of cyclic AMP. Cytokine 1990; 2:205–210.

174. Spatafora M, Chiappara G, Merendino AM, D'Amico D, Bellia V, Bonsignore

G. Theophylline suppresses the release of tumour necrosis factor-α by blood monocytes and alveolar macrophages. Eur Respir J 1994; 7:223–228.

175. Zabel P, Schade FU, Schlaak M. Inhibition of endogenous TNF formation by pentoxifylline. Immunobiology 1993; 187:447–463.

176. Brandwein SR. Regulation of interleukin 1 production by mouse peritoneal macrophages: effects of arachidonic acid metabolites, cyclic nucleotides, and interferons. J Biol Chem 1986; 261:8624–8632.

177. Dendorfer U, Oettgen P, Libermann TA. Multiple regulatory elements in the interleukin-6 gene mediate induction by prostaglandins, cyclic AMP, and lipopolysaccharide. Mol Cell Biol 1994; 14:4443–4454.

178. Prabhakar U, Brooks DP, Lipshlitz D, Esser KM. Inhibition of LPS-induced TNFα production in human monocytes by adenosine (A_2) receptor selective agonists. Int J Immunopharmacol 1995; 17:221–224.

179. Barrett KE, Metcalfe DD. The histologic and functional characterization of enzymatically dispersed intestinal mast cells of nonhuman primates: effects of secretagogues and anti-allergic drugs on histamine secretion. J Immunol 1985; 135:2020–2026.

180. Fox CC, Wolf EJ, Kagey-Sobotka A, Lichtenstein LM. Comparison of human lung and intestinal mast cells. J Allergy Clin Immunol 1988; 81:89–94.

181. Liu WL, Boulos PB, Lau HY, Pearce FL. Mast cells from human gastric mucosa: a comparative study with lung and colonic mast cells. Agents Actions 1991; 33:13–15.

182. Sullivan TJ, Parker KL, Eisen SA, Parker CW. Modulation of cyclic AMP in purified rat mast cells: II. Studies on the relationship between intracellular cyclic AMP concentrations and histamine release. J Immunol 1975; 114:1480–1485.

183. Holgate ST, Winslow CM, Lewis RA, Austen KF. Effects of prostaglandin D_2 and theophylline on rat serosal mast cells: discordance between increased cellular levels of cyclic AMP and activation of cyclic AMP-dependent protein kinase. J Immunol 1981; 127:1530–1533.

184. Ishizaka T, Hirata F, Sterk AR, Ishizaka K, Axelrod JA. Bridging of IgE receptors activates phospholipid methylation and adenylate cyclase in mast cell plasma membranes. Proc Natl Acad Sci USA 1981; 78:6812–6816.

185. Peters SP, Schulman ES, Schleimer RP, MacGlashan DW Jr, Newball HH, Lichtenstein LM. Dispersed human lung mast cells: pharmacologic aspects and comparison with human lung tissue fragments. Am Rev Respir Dis 1982; 126:1034–1039.

186. Peachell PT, MacGlashan DW Jr, Lichtenstein LM, Schleimer RP. Regulation of human basophil and lung mast cell function by cyclic adenosine monophosphate. J Immunol 1988; 140:571–579.

187. Louis RE, Radermecker MF. Substance P-induced histamine release from human basophils, skin and lung fragments: effect of nedocromil sodium and theophylline. Int Arch Allergy Appl Immunol 1990; 92:329–333.

188. Louis R, Bury T, Corhay JL, Radermecker M. LY 186655, a phosphodiesterase

inhibitor, inhibits histamine release from human basophils, lung and skin fragments. Int J Immunopharmacol 1992; 14:191–194.

189. Schulman ES, Post TJ, Vigderman RJ. Density heterogeneity of human lung mast cells. J Allergy Clin Immunol 1988; 82:78–86.

190. Bussolino F, Benveniste J. Pharmacological modulation of platelet-activating factor (PAF) release from rabbit leucocytes: I. Role of cAMP. Immunology 1980; 40:367–376.

191. Spirer Z, Zakuth V, Diamant S, Stabinsky Y, Fridkin M. Studies on the activity of phorbol myristate acetate on the human polymorphonuclear leukocytes. Experientia 1979; 35:830–831.

192. Peachell PT, Undem BJ, Schleimer RP, et al. Preliminary identification and role of phosphodiesterase isozymes in human basophils. J Immunol 1992; 148: 2503–2510.

193. Grant JA, Dupree E, Goldman AS, Schultz DR, Jackson AL. Complement-mediated release of histamine from human leukocytes. J Immunol 1975; 114: 1101–1106.

194. Grant JA, Settle L, Whorton EB, Dupree E. Complement-mediated release of histamine from human basophils: II. Biochemical characterization of the reaction. J Immunol 1976; 117:450–456.

195. Marone G, Kagey-Sobotka A, Lichtenstein LM. IgE-mediated histamine release from human basophils: differences between antigen and anti-IgE-induced secretion. Int Arch Allergy Appl Immunol 1981; 65:339–348.

196. Warner JA, MacGlashan DW, Peters SP, Kagey-Sobotka A, Lichtenstein LM. The pharmacologic modulation of mediator release from human basophils. J Allergy Clin Immunol 1988; 82:432–438.

197. Toll JBC, Andersson RGG. Effects of enprofylline and theophylline on purified human basophils. Allergy 1984; 39:515–520.

198. Akagi K, Kohi F, Trivedi R, Townley RG. Pharmacologic modulation of spontaneous histamine release. Ann Allergy 1989; 63:39–46.

199. Thomas LL, Zheutlin LM, Gleich GJ. Pharmacological control of human basophil histamine release stimulated by eosinophil granule major basic protein. Immunology 1989; 66:611–615.

200. Columbo M, Horowitz EM, McKenzie-White J, Kagey-Sobotka A, Lichtenstein LM. Pharmacologic control of histamine release from human basophils induced by platelet-activating factor. Int Arch Allergy Immunol 1993; 102: 383–390.

201. Hahn S, Moroni C. Modulation of cytokine expression in PB-3c mastocytes by IBMX and PMA. Lymphokine Cytokine Res 1994; 13:247–252.

202. Hendeles L, Weinberger M. Theophylline: a "state of the art" review. Pharmacotherapy 1983; 3:2–44.

203. Torphy TJ, Undem BJ. Phosphodiesterase inhibitors: new opportunities for the treatment of asthma. Thorax 1991; 46:512–523.

204. Project IA. International consensus report on diagnosis and management of asthma. Eur Respir J 1992; 5:601–641.

205. National Heart, Lung, and Blood Institute National Asthma Education Program Expert Panel: guidelines for the diagnosis and management of asthma. J Allergy Clin Immunol 1991; 88:425–534.

206. Jenne JW. Physiology and pharmacology of the xanthines. In: Jenne JW, Murphy S, eds. Drug Therapy for Asthma: Research and Clinical Practice (Lung Biology in Health and Disease, vol. 31). New York: Marcel Dekker, 1987: 297–334.

207. Siegel D, Sheppard D, Gelb A, Weinberg PF. Aminophylline increases the toxicity but not the efficacy of an inhaled β-adrenergic agonist in the treatment of acute exacerbations of asthma. Am Rev Respir Dis 1985; 132:283–286.

208. Hambleton G, Weinberger M, Taylor J, et al. Comparison of cromoglycate (cromolyn) and theophylline in controlling symptoms of chronic asthma: a collaborative study. Lancet 1977; 1:381–385.

209. Nassif EG, Weinberger M, Thompson R, Huntley W. The value of maintenance theophylline in steroid-dependent asthma. N Engl J Med 1981; 304:71–75.

210. Brenner M, Berkowitz R, Marshall N, Strunk RC. Need for theophylline in severe steroid requiring asthmatics. Clin Allergy 1988; 18:143–150.

211. Busse WW. Pathogenesis and pathophysiology of nocturnal asthma. Am J Med 1988; 85(suppl 1B):24–29.

212. Barnes PJ, Greening AP, Neville L, Timmers J, Poole GW. Single dose slow-release aminophylline at night prevents nocturnal asthma. Lancet 1982; 1:299–301.

213. Heins M, Kurtin L, Oellerich M, Maes R, Sybrecht GW. Nocturnal asthma: slow-release terbutaline versus slow-release theophylline therapy. Eur Respir J 1988; 1:306–310.

214. Rabe KF, Jörres R, Nowak D, Behr N, Magnussen H. Comparison of the effects of salmeterol and formoterol on airway tone and responsiveness over 24 hours in bronchial asthma. Am Rev Respir Dis 1993; 147:1436–1441.

215. Fitzpatrick MF, Mackay T, Driver H, Douglas NJ. Salmeterol in nocturnal asthma: a double-blind, placebo-controlled trial of a long acting inhaled β_2-agonist. BMJ 1990; 301:1365–1368.

216. Mahler DA, Matthay RA, Snyder PE, Wells CK, Loke J. Sustained-release theophylline reduces dyspnea in nonreversible obstructive airway disease. Am Rev Respir Dis 1985; 131:22–25.

217. Kirsten DK, Wegner RE, Jörres RA, Magnussen H. Effects of theophylline withdrawal in severe chronic obstructive pulmonary disease. Chest 1993; 104: 1101–1107.

218. Vaz Fragoso CA, Miller MA. Review of the clinical efficacy of theophylline in the treatment of chronic obstructive pulmonary disease. Am Rev Respir Dis 1993; 147:S40–S47.

219. Dullinger D, Kronenberg R, Niewoehner DE. Efficacy of inhaled metaproterenol and orally administered theophylline in patients with chronic airflow obstruction. Chest 1986; 89:171–173.

220. Thomas P, Pugsley JA, Stewart JH. Theophylline and salbutamol improve pul-

monary function in patients with irreversible chronic obstructive pulmonary disease. Chest 1992; 101:160–165.

221. Wegner RE, Jörres RA, Kirsten DK, Magnussen H. Factor analysis of exercise capacity, dyspnoea ratings and lung function in patients with severe COPD. Eur Respir J 1994; 7:725–729.

222. Rabe KF, Dent G, Magnussen H. Theophylline in the treatment of bronchial asthma and chronic obstructive pulmonary disease. In: Leff AR, ed. Pulmonary and Critical Care Pharmacology and Therapeutics. New York: McGraw-Hill, 1996:525–534.

223. Guyatt GH, Townsend M, Pugsley SO, et al. Bronchodilators in chronic airflow limitation. Am Rev Respir Dis 1987; 135:1069–1074.

224. Chrystyn H, Mulley BA, Peake MD. Dose response relation to oral theophylline in severe chronic obstructive airways disease. BMJ 1988; 297:1506–1510.

225. Murciano D, Auclair M-H, Pariente R, Aubier M. A randomized, controlled trial of theophylline in patients with severe chronic obstructive pulmonary disease. N Engl J Med 1989; 320:1521–1525.

226. Murciano D, Aubier M, Lecocguic Y, Pariente R. Effects of theophylline on diaphragmatic strength in patients with chronic obstructive pulmonary disease. N Engl J Med 1984; 311:349–353.

227. Foxworth JW, Reisz GR, Knudson SM, Cuddy PG, Pyszcznski DR, Emory CE. Theophylline and diaphragmatic contractility. Am Rev Respir Dis 1988; 138:1532–1534.

228. Kongragunta VR, Druz WS, Sharp JT. Dyspnea and diaphragmatic fatigue in patients with chronic obstructive pulmonary disease. Am Rev Respir Dis 1988; 137:662–667.

229. Aubier M, Murciano D, Fournier M, Milic-Emili J, Pariente R, Derenne JP. Central respiratory drive in acute respiratory failure of patients with chronic obstructive pulmonary disease. Am Rev Respir Dis 1980; 122:191–199.

230. Parker JO, Ashekian PB, Di Giorgi S, West RO. Hemodynamic effects of aminophylline in chronic obstructive pulmonary disease. Circulation 1967; 35: 365–372.

231. Milgrom H, Bender B. Current issues in the use of theophylline. Am Rev Respir Dis 1993; 147:S33–S39.

232. Sessler CN. Theophylline toxicity: clinical features of 116 consecutive cases. Am J Med 1990; 88:567–576.

233. Greenberger PA, Cranberg JA, Ganz MA, Hubler GL. A prospective evaluation of elevated serum theophylline concentrations to determine if high concentrations are predictable. Am J Med 1991; 91:67–73.

234. Ogilvie RI, Fernandez PG, Winsberg F. Cardiovascular response to increasing theophylline concentrations. Eur J Clin Pharmacol 1977; 12:409–414.

235. Lubbe WF, Podzuweit T, Opie LH. Potential arrhythmogenic role of cyclic adenosine monophosphate (AMP) and cytosolic calcium overload: implications for prophylactic effects of beta blockers in myocardial infarction and pro-

arrhythmic effects of phosphodiesterase inhibitors. J Am Coll Cardiol 1992; 19:1622–1633.

236. Cruickshank JM. Phosphodiesterase III inhibitors: long-term risks and short-term benefits. Cardiovasc Drugs Ther 1993; 7:655–660.

237. Feneck RO. Intravenous milrinone following cardiac surgery: I. Effects of bolus infusion followed by variable dose maintenance infusion: the European Milrinone Multicentre Trial Group. J Cardiothorac Vasc Anesth 1992; 6:554–562.

238. Varriale P, Ramaprasad S. Aminophylline induced atrial fibrillation. Pacing Clin Electrophysiol 1993; 16:1953–1955.

239. Sullivan P, Page CP, Costello JF. Xanthines. In: Page CP, Metzger WJ, eds. Drugs and the Lung. New York: Raven Press, 1994:69–99.

240. Howell RE, Muehsam WT, Kinnier WJ. Mechanism for the emetic side effect of xanthine bronchodilators. Life Sci 1990; 46:563–568.

241. Lowe JA III, Cheng JB. The PDE IV family of calcium-independent phosphodiesterase enzymes. Drugs Fut 1992; 17:799–807.

242. Zwillich CW, Sutton FD, Neff TA, Cohn WM, Matthay RA, Weinberger MM. Theophylline-induced seizures in adults: correlation with serum concentrations. Ann Intern Med 1975; 82:784–787.

243. Nishimura M, Yoshioka A, Yamamoto M, Akiyama Y, Miyamoto K, Kawakami Y. Effect of theophylline on brain tissue oxygenation during normoxia and hypoxia in humans. J Appl Physiol 1993; 74:2724–2728.

244. Hornfeldt CS, Larson AA. Adenosine receptors are not involved in theophylline-induced seizures. J Toxicol Clin Toxicol 1994; 32:257–265.

245. Weiner IM. Diuretics and other agents employed in the mobilization of edema fluid. In: Gilman AG, Rall TW, Nies AS, Taylor P, eds. Goodman & Gilman's The Pharmacological Basis of Therapeutics. New York: Pergamon, 1990:713–731.

246. Brater DC, Kaojaren S, Chennavasin P. Pharmacodynamics of the diuretic effects of aminophylline and acetazolamide alone and combined with furosemide in normal subjects. J Pharmacol Exp Ther 1983; 227:92–97.

247. Sigurd B, Olesen KH. Comparative natriuretic and diuretic efficacy of theophylline ethylenediamine and of bendroflumethiazide during long-term treatment with the potent diuretic bumetanide: permutation trial tests in patients with congestive heart failure. Acta Med Scand 1978; 203:113–119.

248. Shannon M. Hypokalemia, hyperglycemia and plasma catecholamine activity after severe theophylline intoxication. J Toxicol Clin Toxicol 1994; 32:41–47.

249. Flack JM, Ryder KW, Strickland D, Whang R. Metabolic correlates of theophylline therapy: a concentration-related phenomenon. Ann Pharmacother 1994; 28:175–179.

250. Knutsen R, Bohmer T, Falch J. Intravenous theophylline-induced excretion of calcium, magnesium and sodium in patients with recurrent asthmatic attacks. Scand J Clin Lab Invest 1994; 54:119–125.

251. Sturgess I, Searle GF. The acute toxic effect of the phosphodiesterase inhibitor rolipram on plasma osmolality. Br J Clin Pharmacol 1990; 29:369–370.

4

Leukotriene Modifiers

MICHAEL E. WECHSLER and JEFFREY M. DRAZEN

Brigham and Women's Hospital
Harvard Medical School
Boston, Massachusetts

I. Introduction

In recent years, several medications that selectively inhibit the formation or action of leukotrienes have been introduced as new therapy in asthma. Known as leukotriene modifiers, these medications include both 5-lipoxygenase inhibitors such as zileuton as well as leukotriene receptor antagonists such as pranlukast, zafirlukast, and montelukast. All of these medications have been found to play an important role in mediating the airway inflammation and bronchoconstriction in patients with asthma. This chapter addresses the history, pharmacology, clinical efficacy, and safety of these important, novel therapeutic agents for asthma.

II. Historical Perspective

Purified in the late 1970s, leukotrienes were so named because they were initially isolated from leukocytes and because their carbon backbone contained

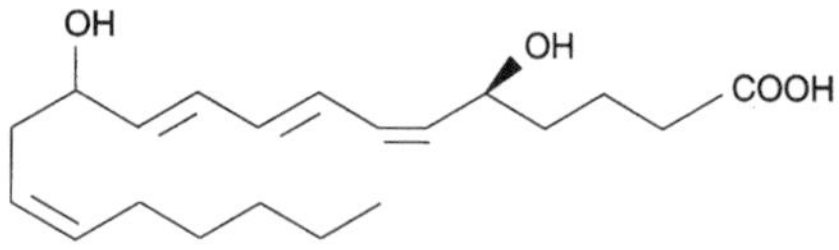

Leukotriene B_4

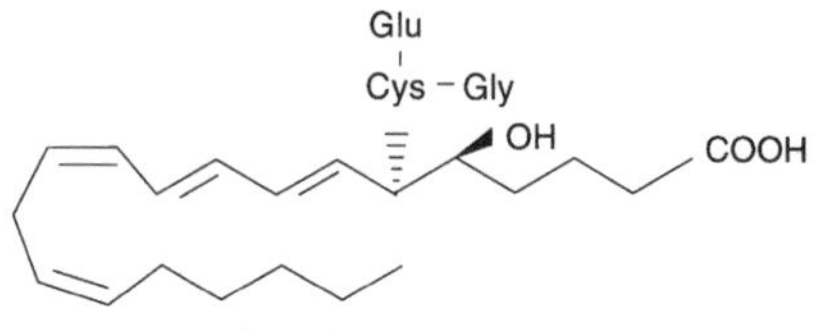

Leukotriene C_4

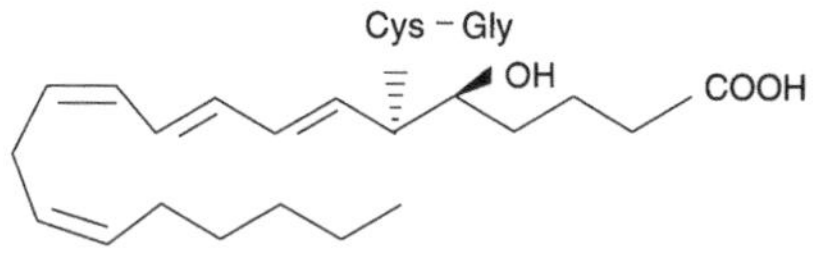

Leukotriene D_4

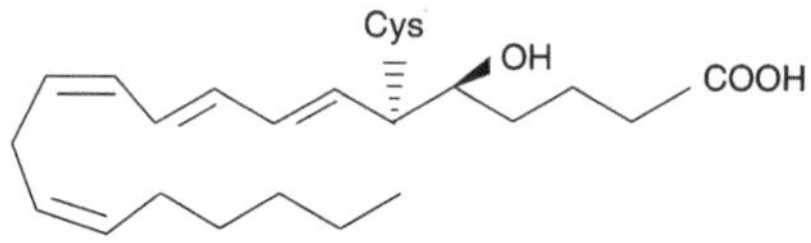

Leukotriene E_4

Figure 1 Structure of leukotrienes B_4, C_4, D_4, and E_4. Leukotrienes C_4, D_4, and E_4 all have cysteine residues and are potent mediators that induce smooth muscle contraction, airway edema, mucus secretion, and eosinophil recruitment into the airway. Leukotriene B_4 does not have a cysteine residue but is a potent chemotactic factor for neutrophils and eosinophils.

three double bonds in series, constituting a triene. However, several decades before they were chemically defined, these molecules were recognized as distinct biological entities. A role in asthma pathogenesis was first implicated after Feldberg and Kellaway noted in 1938 that cobra venom caused a slow-onset, sustained contraction of smooth muscle in guinea pig lung perfusate (1). Such substances became known as the slow-reacting substances of anaphylaxis (SRS-A) 2 years later, when Kellaway and Trethewie revealed that the time course of this contraction was distinct from that caused by histamine (2). A role in asthma was further suggested in the 1960s, when it was found that SRS-A was released from lung fragments of a subject with asthma exposed to allergen (3), and in the following decade, when Drazen and Austen demonstrated the effect on pulmonary mechanics after the intravenous administration of SRS-A to guinea pigs (4). By 1980, SRS-A was finally chemically characterized as three specific cysteinyl leukotriene products of the 5-lipoxygenase (5-LO) pathway, whose chemical structures were elucidated as 5(S)-hydroxy-6(R)-glutathionyl-7,9-*trans*-11,14-*cis*-eicosatetraenoic acid and its cysteinyl-glycyl and cysteinyl congeners (leukotriene C_4, D_4 and E_4, respectively) (5) (Fig. 1). Since its structure was elucidated, researchers have further demonstrated its potency in smooth muscle constriction in both human and animal models, in vitro and in vivo and have also shown that 5-LO products may stimulate smooth muscle proliferation (6–8) and eosinophil recruitment and activation; they may also cause tissue edema (9–12). Potentially invoked as the causative agents in a host of inflammatory conditions such as inflammatory bowel disease, psoriasis, rheumatoid arthritis, and glomerulonephritis (13), the attributes of leukotrienes are particularly implicated in the airway inflammatory pathway of asthma. In the 1990s, several medications directed at the 5-LO pathway have been developed to treat asthma; currently, one 5-LO inhibitor and three distinct cysteinyl leukotriene receptor antagonists are available throughout the world and marketed as treatment for asthma.

III. Pharmacological Mechanisms

A. Leukotriene Biosynthetic Pathways

Leukotrienes are fatty acids derived from arachidonic acid, the ubiquitous 20-carbon fatty acid membrane constituent. They are members of a larger group of biomolecules known as eicosanoids, which encompasses 5-LO products such as the leukotrienes; cyclooxygenase products such as prostaglandins, thromboxanes, and prostacyclin; products of 12- or 15-LO (the lipoxins); and 5- and 15-LO (14,15). The synthesis of leukotrienes is initiated following trauma, infection, and inflammation. The initial step in this pathway is a receptor-mediated influx of calcium ions that cause translocation to the cell membrane of cytosolic phospholipase A2, a phospholipase enzyme, which selectively cleaves arachidonic acid from perinuclear cell membranes. Arachidonic acid is converted sequentially to 5-hydroperoxyeicosatetraenoic acid (5-

HPETE) and then to leukotriene A_4 (5,6-oxido-7,9-*trans* 11,14-*cis*-eicosate-traenoic acid, or LTA_4) by a catalytic complex consisting of 5-LO and the 5-LO activating protein (FLAP) in the presence of increased calcium levels. FLAP is a hydrophobic membrane protein that binds arachidonic acid and is critical to leukotriene synthesis (16). LTA_4 is unstable and may be transformed through the action of the bifunctional enzyme LTA_4 epoxide hydrolase in poly-morphonuclear leukocytes into leukotriene B_4 (LTB_4), which is involved in eosinophil and neutrophil chemotaxis. Alternatively, in the presence of leuko-triene C_4 (LTC_4) synthase, glutathione is adducted to the C6 position of LTA_4 in eosinophils, mast cells, and alveolar macrophages to yield the molecule known as LTC_4. Once exported from the cytosol to the extracellular microen-vironment, the glutamic acid moiety of LTC_4 is cleaved by γ-glutamyltrans-peptidase to form the active entity leukotriene D_4 (LTD_4). Cleavage of the glycine moiety from LTD_4 by a variety of dipeptidases results in the formation of leukotriene E_4 (LTE_4). LTC_4, LTD_4, and LTE_4 are all known as the cysteinyl leukotrienes, as each one contains a cysteine. Together, these three molecules make up the biological mixture formerly known as SRS-A. While each of these cysteinyl leukotrienes have similar biological effects, LTE_4 is the least potent.

   All of these reactions take place in mast cells, eosinophils, and alveolar macrophages (17,18–20), all of which have been implicated as critical effector cells in the pathobiology of asthma. Airway epithelial cells (21,22) and pulmo-nary vascular endothelial cells (23) may also produce leukotrienes via transcel-lular metabolism (24,25). A variety of physical, chemical, and immunological stimuli have been shown to activate these cells so that they can produce leuko-trienes. These stimuli include the activation of mast-cell antigen-specific IgE bound to F_c receptors (26,27), hyperventilation of cold, dry air (28), aspirin ingestion by aspirin-intolerant individuals (29–31), hypoxia (32), hyperoxia (33), and exposure to platelet activating factor (34). Macrophages and mono-cytes can release both LTB_4 and LTD_4 after being exposed to nonimmunologi-cal stimuli (such as the calcium ionophore A23187) or to immunological stim-uli such as the interaction with various immunoglobulins (35–37). Eosinophils and mast cells secrete primarily LTC_4, whereas neutrophils primarily release LTB_4 (38).

B. LT Degradation

The cysteinyl leukotrienes are rapidly catabolized in the extracellular space and the liver to inactive products through three major mechanisms: the forma-tion of the *N*-acetyl derivative of LTE_4, the interaction of the leukotriene and hypochlorous acid to form the respective leukotriene sulfoxide and LTB_4, and the ω-oxidation and β-elimination with progressive shortening of the ω-portion of the molecule. Each of these conversions is associated with a loss of bioactivity (39–41). As for LTB_4, it is degraded by multiple pathways, including cytochrome P-450 (CYP4F4 and CYP4F5) and 12-hydroxyeicosanoid dehydrogenase (42), in multiple tissues primarily by ω-oxidation and β-elimination, resulting in hydroxylation, carboxylation, and the progressive shortening of the ω-portion of the molecule, all of which result in a loss of bioactivity in some but not all assay systems (44–48).

C. Leukotriene Receptors

Leukotrienes exert their biological activities by binding to specific receptors that have been characterized functionally through comparisons of the activity of various agonists and antagonists. LTB_4 binds to the B leukotriene receptor (BLT), a seven-membrane-spanning G protein–coupled receptor whose structure has been elucidated by molecular cloning. It is a 60-kDa cell-surface protein that predominantly transduces chemotaxis and cellular activation (49–52). It is found in two states, high affinity and low affinity, and is found predominantly on leukocytes. While LTB_4 is the preferred ligand for this receptor, other agents, such as 20-OH-LTB_4 and 12 R-HETE, can transduce signals via this receptor, albeit with less potency (53–58).

The cysteinyl leukotrienes bind to two distinct receptors that have been identified pharmacologically as $CysLT_1$ and $CysLT_2$, but only the former has been cloned (43). Previously known as the LTD_4 receptor LTR_D, $CysLT_1$ is a G-protein-coupled seven-transmembrane-spanning receptor found in airway smooth muscle. Stimulation of this receptor occurs by phosphoinositide-stimulated signal transduction and leads to smooth muscle constriction (59–62). LTD_4 is the preferred ligand, but LTC_4 and LTE_4 also bind to this receptor, albeit with less biopotency (63–66). The *CysLT₂* receptor was previously known as the LTC_4 receptor, or LTR_c. Stimulation of this pulmonary vascular smooth muscle receptor results in smooth muscle constriction and chemotaxis.

IV. Biological Effects of Leukotrienes

A. LTB_4

LTB_4 secretion by myeloid cells and binding to its receptor leads to a host of cellular and molecular responses that contribute to mediation of the inflammatory response. Most notably, LTB_4 is probably the most potent neutrophil chemotactic agent produced by the arachidonic acid cascade. Its chemokinetic effects are substantially stronger than those of other lipoxygenase by-products such as 5-, 12-, and 15-hydroxyeicosatetraenoic acid or 5-, 12-, and 15-hydro-peroxyeicosatetraenoic acid (67). Intratracheal instillation of LTB_4 induces selective recruitment of functionally active neutrophils into BAL fluid in humans, and subcutaneous injection of LTB_4 into humans causes neutrophils to accumulate rapidly in the affected tissue (68,69). LTB_4 may also play a pivotal role in the induction of neutrophil-endothelial cell adherence: the topical application of LTB_4 to the vascular network within the hamster cheek pouch results in immediate and reversible adherence of neutrophils to venular endothelial cells. LTB_4 also plays a role in induction of neutrophil degranulation and lysosomal enzyme release: at nanomolar concentrations, LTB_4 releases substantial quantities of glucoronidase and lysozyme from neutrophils, although less effectively than the chemotactic fragment of the complement component C5 (70,71). LTB_4 also is important in immune modulation: it stimulates myelopoiesis by human bone marrow cells; it augments IL-6 production in human monocytes by increasing IL-6 gene transcription and messenger RNA stabilization; it may modulate the production of other cytokines by stimulating gene transcription of the proto-oncognes *c-jun* and *c-fos* in mononuclear cells (57); and it may exert a proliferative effect on T lymphocytes through the stimulation of IL-2 secretion (72). Finally, it can replace IL-2 in the induction of interferon gamma (INF-γ) by T cells (73).

B. Cysteinyl Leukotrienes

The biological activity of the cysteinyl leukotrienes differs from that of LTB_4. While their roles in the inflammatory process also include increasing vasopermeability, enhancing mucus secretion, and acting as immunomodulatory agents, LTC_4, LTD_4, and LTE_4 are best known for their capacity to induce airway, gastrointestinal, and mesangial smooth muscle contraction, akin to the initially described activity of the SRS-A (74). The cysteinyl leukotrienes produce vigorous prolonged contraction and bronchoconstriction in both human and animal tissues. In vitro studies have involved both animal and human bronchial specimens, and in vivo studies have demonstrated potent and sustained bronchoconstriction approximately 1000 times that of histamine or prostaglandin $F_{2\alpha}$ following inhalation of leukotrienes (75,76). In addition to their role in smooth muscle contraction, the cysteinyl leukotrienes play an important role in the modulation of vascular permeability and vasoconstriction; they are felt to drive the permeability of the venular endothelium so as to allow proinflammatory cells to migrate to the site of inflammation, with concomitant leakage of plasma components into extravascular tissue and the development of edema. This has been demonstrated in vivo when the application of cysteinyl leukotrienes to the buccal mucosa of hamsters resulted in submucosal edema (77) and when subcutaneous application in humans resulted in dermal edema with a wheal-and-flare reaction within 2 min of injection (68). In terms of vasoconstriction, it appears that the smooth muscle constrictive effect of cysteinyl leukotrienes extends to vascular smooth muscle. LTC_4 and LTD_4 induce local vasoconstriction in several different animal models (77,78) and human models (68,69), but they may also exert profound systemic circulatory effects: infusion of LTC_4 or LTD_4 into the systemic circulation of rats produced coronary and renal vasoconstriction (79,80).

Other functions of the cysteinyl leukotrienes include enhancement of mucus secretion in airways (they are potent mucus secretagogues in human tracheal explants and in animal tracheas in vivo) and modulation of several components of the immune system. For example, LTC_4 and LTD_4 stimulate the expansion of myeloid colonies treated with colony-stimulating factor (81) are involved in glomerular epithelial cell and fibroblast proliferation, enhance IL-1 production by human monocytes and can induce INF-γ secretion by T lymphocytes (82–84). The cysteinyl leukotrienes have also been found to be potent and specific chemoattractants for human eosinophils both in vitro (85) and in vivo: inhaled LTD_4 has been shown to increase the number of eosinophils in induced sputum specimens from asthmatics and inhaled LTE_4 has been shown to markedly increase numbers of eosinophils in biopsy specimens from the airways of asthmatics (11). This property is one of the links between leukotrienes and the eosinophilia that accompanies asthma.

V. Role of Leukotrienes in Asthma

As asthma is a disease that is clinically characterized by many effects reminiscent of those of the leukotrienes—namely bronchoconstriction, hyperresponsiveness, increased microvascular permeability with tissue edema, hypersecretion of mucus, and recruitment of eosinophils—these substances have been strongly implicated as mediators of the airway obstruction of asthma. This relationship has been hypothesized since the original description of the slow-reacting substances of anaphylaxis, which were found to be generated during antigenic challenge of sensitized lung. Further evidence of this relationship has since been provided through numerous studies that analyzed the effects of administration of leukotrienes in both asthmatics and controls as well as through the measurement of leukotrienes in biological fluids in patients with asthma.

Early in vitro studies comparing the contractility of surgically removed lung tissue following administration of various bronchoconstrictor agents demonstrated that LTC_4 and LTD_4 were at least 1000 times more potent in terms of contractility than histamine and 10 times more potent than LTE_4 (63,64,86,87). Subsequent in vivo studies involved administration of leukotrienes to human subjects. In normal individuals, inhaled LTC_4 and LTD_4 resulted in airways obstruction as manifested by decreased specific airway conductance (S_{Gaw}) and decreased flow rates (88). Leukotrienes C_4 and D_4 were approximately 1000 times as potent as histamine in causing such bronchoconstriction and had a longer duration of action; they were 10 times as potent as LTE_4, but LTE_4's duration of action was longer. However, while bronchoconstriction from LTD_4 and LTE_4 was noted within 4 to 6 min of administration, LTC_4 took 10 min to take effect, suggesting that it is first metabolized to LTD_4 to take effect (89). No significant difference was noted in bronchi of different sizes, suggesting that both small and large airways respond to leukotriene-induced bronchoconstriction. After these effects were characterized in normal subjects, Bisgaard et al. demonstrated that asthmatic subjects were 100 to 1000 times more responsive to LTD_4 than controls (90). They were also found to have increased airway hyperresponsiveness to both inhaled LTC_4 and LTD_4 and responded at lower doses of inhaled leukotrienes compared with equivalent doses of histamine or methacholine. Subsequent studies demonstrated that prior inhalation of leukotrienes caused an increase in airway responsiveness to both histamine and methacholine that lasted as long as 1 week.

A. Leukotrienes in Body Fluids

Much of our understanding of the role of leukotrienes in asthma comes from measurement of leukotrienes from various body fluids. Despite their rapid metabolism and degradation, leukotrienes have been identified in plasma, nasal and BAL fluids, and urine. LTC_4 and LTD_4 have been found in increased levels in the plasma and BAL fluids of patients with stable asthma as compared with controls (91,92), and Lam et al. identified LTC_4 and LTB_4 in the sputum of patients with asthma but not in that of patients with other lung diseases (93). Following endobronchial allergen challenge of asthmatic subjects, BAL LTC_4 levels are increased, as are urine LTE_4 levels (92,94,95). Urine LTE_4 levels are also increased among many (but not all) patients having spontaneous asthma attacks (96) as well as those subjects with nocturnal asthma (97), exercise-induced asthma, and asthma induced by aspirin administration (98,99). At baseline, urinary LTE_4 levels are approximately sixfold higher in aspirin-sensitive asthmatics than in aspirin-tolerant asthmatics; this population also has increased levels of LTC_4 in nasal lavage and demonstrates a fourfold increase in urinary LTE_4 at 6 h after aspirin challenge; similar findings are not seen in aspirin-tolerant asthmatics (36,100).

VI. Leukotriene Modifiers and Asthma

The strongest evidence for the role of leukotrienes as mediators of airway obstruction in asthma comes from studies with pharmacological agents that interfere with the synthesis or action of 5-LO products. A number of agents with the capacity to interrupt the 5-LO pathway have been developed and are now available in many countries around the world as novel treatments for

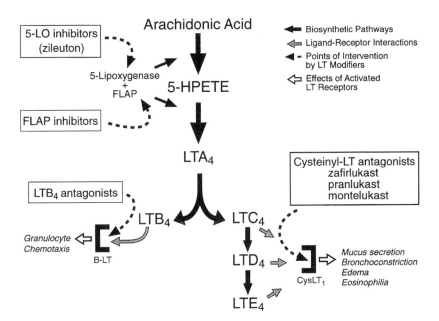

Figure 2 Leukotriene biosynthesis, their effects, and points of therapeutic interruption. Leukotrienes are synthesized from arachidonic acid via the action of 5-lipoxygenase (5-LO) and 5-lipoxygenase activating protein (FLAP) and play important roles in mediating airway inflammation. Leukotriene modifiers include 5-LO inhibitors, FLAP inhibitors, cysteinyl leukotriene antagonists, and LTB_4 antagonists. (From Ref. 172.)

asthma. These agents belong to one of three general classes: (1) agents that inhibit the interaction of arachidonic acid and the FLAP (BAY x 1005, MK-886); (2) agents that inhibit catalysis by 5-LO itself (zileuton, ABT-761); and (3) agents that prevent the action of cysteinyl leukotrienes at their receptor (montelukast, zafirlukast, and pranlukast) (Fig. 2). Collectively, these medications are referred to as leukotriene modifiers. These agents have been studied in three distinct types of asthma: laboratory-induced asthma, asthmatic bronchoconstriction, and chronic persistent asthma.

VII. Leukotriene Modifiers in Laboratory-Induced Asthma

Laboratory-induced asthma includes asthma that is induced by LTD_4 inhalation, cold-air challenge, exercise challenge, aspirin challenge, or antigen challenge. In each of these, leukotriene modifiers have reduced the bronchoconstriction associated with the trigger.

A. Inhaled LTD_4 Challenge

Several leukotriene receptor antagonists have been shown to effectively inhibit the bronchoconstrictive response to inhaled LTD_4 in both asthmatic and normal subjects. Zafirlukast caused a 90- to 100-fold shift in the provocative concentration of LTD_4 required to produce a 20% reduction in FEV_1 (101) and had significant antagonism maintained for 24 h. It did so in a dose-related fashion, as would be expected with a competitive antagonist. MK-571 shifted the curve 30- to 40-fold, (102) and 200 mg of MK-076 completely inhibited the LTD_4 challenge in all six mild asthmatics participating in that trial (103). Similarly, pranlukast almost completely blocked the LTD_4 induced obstruction in normal volunteers (104). These studies all demonstrate that cysteinyl leukotriene receptor antagonists specifically oppose the inflammatory effects of inhaled leukotriene D_4.

B. Exercise and Cold-Air Challenge

Asthma and bronchoconstriction may be provoked by exercise or a cold-air stimulus in certain predisposed individuals; over 70% of asthmatics develop exercise-induced bronchospasm (105). Bronchoconstriction in these patients in mediated through the release of bronchoconstrictor substances from inflammatory cells in the airway wall and, as evidenced by numerous studies with leukotriene modifiers that were able to inhibit exercise and cold-induced asthma, leukotrienes seem to play a particularly important role in modulating airway bronchospasm in these patients. The receptor antagonists zafirlukast and MK-571, given orally or by inhalation, were effective in inhibiting the maximal bronchoconstrictor response after exercise by 50–70% and completely inhibited any bronchoconstrictor response in 30–50% of asthmatics studied (106,107). When zafirlukast was given 30 min before cycle ergometry in patients with exercise-induced airway obstruction, the maximal percentage fall in FEV_1 was 14.5% after medication compared with 30.2% with placebo. The median time to recovery was 20 min, versus 60 min with placebo (106,107). When the long-lasting potent receptor antagonist cinalukast was administered, more than 80% of asthmatic patients had reduced bronchoconstriction that lasted for more than 8 h (108). Similarly, patients with exercise-induced asthma treated with zileuton demonstrated a maximum decrease of 15.6% in FEV_1, compared with 28% in the placebo group (109). It is also important to note that when subjects with exercise-induced asthma use inhaled β-agonists as a regular preventative therapy for this form of bronchospasm, there is a loss of bronchoprotective effect with time (110). However, it has recently been shown that the bronchoprotective effects of cinalukast and montelukast are maintained over many weeks of treatment (108,111). In the most recent trial, which involved 110 patients with documented 20% reduction in FEV_1 in response to exercise, montelukast treatment offered significantly greater protection against exercise-induced bronchoconstriction than placebo and resulted in a quicker return to baseline. Tolerance and rebound worsening were not seen (112).

In terms of cold-air challenge, which is thought to induce bronchospasm by a mechanism similar to exercise, Israel and coworkers effectively demonstrated that zileuton attenuated the bronchoconstrictor response to cold air (113). Other agents, including the FLAP inhibitor BAY x 1005 and the cysteinyl leukotriene receptor antagonist zafirlukast, have been shown to similarly attenuate cold-induced bronchospasm (114,115). Fischer et al. demonstrated that regular treatment with zileuton for 13 weeks improved airway responsiveness to cold air for as long as 10 days after completion of treatment (116), much longer than the expected duration of zileuton's pharmacological action, suggesting that inhibition of leukotriene generation can improve airway hyperresponsiveness. As it appears that leukotriene modifiers are effective in both exercise- and cold-induced asthma, one proposed mechanism suggests that the cooling and drying of the airways provoked by these challenges results in the generation of leukotrienes, which, in turn, results in bronchoconstriction. However, the heterogenic response to leukotriene modifiers among some subjects subject to cold air but not others and the fact that urinary leukotrienes are elevated in some subjects but not others during exercise (117–119) suggest that cold- and exercise-induced bronchospasm may not necessarily be primarily leukotriene-mediated in all subjects with this form of airway narrowing.

C. Aspirin-Induced Asthma

Leukotrienes appear to play an important role in aspirin-induced asthma, which affects 5–8% of asthmatics and may cause profound, life-threatening bronchospasm (120) as well as naso-ocular and gastrointestinal symptoms. These subjects often have elevated urinary leukotriene excretion at baseline and increased levels following aspirin challenge. When they are exposed to aerosols of lysine aspirin, aspirin-sensitive individuals only develop bronchospasm. When the cysteinyl leukotriene receptor antagonist pobilukast edamine was used for pretreatment, many patients tolerated all doses of lysine aspirin that had previously caused a bronchospastic reaction, and urinary leukotriene levels were not altered (121). Similarly, when zileuton and aspirin were given, not only bronchospasm but also nasal, gastrointestinal, and dermal symptoms were ablated and urinary LTE_4 levels were reduced by 68% (30). Further evidence pointing to a causal relationship between the cysteinyl leukotrienes and aspirin-sensitive asthma comes from Dahlen et al., who demonstrated that administration of the $CysLT_1$ receptor antagonist MK-679 to subjects with aspirin-sensitive asthma resulted in improved lung function even in the absence of aspirin provocation, and the magnitude of FEV_1 improvement increased with decreasing urinary LTE_4 levels (31). Based on these studies, it appears that the bronchospasm associated with aspirin-related asthma is leukotriene-mediated and that leukotriene modifiers are the treatment of choice for these patients.

D. Allergen-Induced Asthma

Inhalation of environmental allergens may provoke both an early (15–120 min) and a late (3–24 h) asthmatic response with bronchoconstriction and airway hyperresponsiveness. The role of leukotrienes in allergen-induced asthma has been partly elucidated by studying these patients in the laboratory and exposing them to aerosols containing the agent to which they are allergic. Urinary leukotrienes have been found to be elevated during the early asthmatic response, and the magnitude of the elevation correlates with the magnitude of the early response. While each leukotriene receptor antagonist studied has inhibited the early phase of antigen-induced bronchoconstriction by as much as 58–84%, more potent LTD_4 receptor antagonists also inhibit the late-phase antigen response (122–125). Some studies with 5-LO inhibitors and FLAP inhibitors have had mixed results, however; in one trial, zileuton's effect on the early-phase response was insignificant and there was no effect on the late phase. Similarly, in a study in which a selective antagonist of LTB_4, which has no effects on the $CysLT_1$ receptor, was given to patients before allergen challenge, the cellular infiltrate associated with the early asthmatic response was diminished, but there was no effect on the physiological response (126). While these studies suggest that there is at least a partial role of leukotrienes in modulating the asthmatic allergic response (particularly the early response), none of the agents studied to date has resulted in a total prevention of the bronchoconstrictor response (particularly the late response) elicited by antigen stimulation. Other mediators are clearly involved, however, as a recent study demonstrated that patients with allergen-induced bronchospasm who were treated with both an antihistamine (loratidine) and a leukotriene receptor antagonist (zafirlukast) demonstrated enhanced inhibition of early- and late-phase effects compared with that observed with zafirlukast alone (127).

VIII. Leukotriene Modifiers in Asthmatic Bronchoconstriction and Hyperresponsiveness

The spontaneous reversible bronchoconstriction that may develop in mild-to-moderate asthmatics who withhold bronchodilator therapy has been another focus of studies involving leukotriene modifiers. To assess the role of leukotrienes in the spontaneous airway narrowing of asthma, several leukotriene modifiers have been administered to patients with varying degrees of asthma, and spirometry has been performed. Gaddy et al. have shown that intravenously administered MK-571 resulted in acute bronchodilatation that was additive to the effect of salbutamol in patients with mild to moderate asthma (128). A similar study involved giving the LTD_4 receptor antagonist ICI204219 to subjects with moderately severe asthma: FEV_1 improved by 5–10% within 1–3 h of administration. While inhalation of a β-agonist increased the FEV_1 by 20–30%, the effects of the β-agonist were also additive to that of the LTD_4 receptor antagonist, suggesting that distinct contractile mechanisms are involved in each response (129). Similar sustained improvements in FEV_1 occurred with other leukotriene receptor antagonists, such as zafirlukast (130), and also with the 5-LO inhibitor zileuton (131). Because similar studies of nonasthmatic subjects have shown no reversal of airway tone, the reversal of asthmatic bronchoconstriction by leukotriene modifiers suggests that a significant component of asthmatic bronchoconstriction and basal airway tone is mediated by the effect of leukotrienes at their receptors and also by ongoing leukotriene synthesis by 5-LO.

Of note, these drugs also have a significant effect on bronchial hyperresponsiveness. In one study, pranlukast was given orally for 1 week to patients with stable asthma. It produced a small but significant reduction in bronchial hyperresponsiveness to methacholine (132). In another study, pranlukast given twice daily was associated with improvement in clinical symptoms as well as improved histamine reactivity by bronchial challenge at 12 and 24 weeks posttreatment. This suggests that cysteinyl leukotrienes are involved in hyperresponsiveness in chronic asthma as well as asthma induced after allergen challenge.

IX. Leukotriene Modifiers in Chronic Persistent Asthma

There is now a substantial body of literature addressing the efficacy of leukotriene modifiers in patients with chronic persistent asthma. There have been various studies of patients whose asthma was characterized by average FEV_1 values of 60–80% of predicted, moderate daytime or nocturnal symptoms, and the use of inhaled medium-acting β-agonists as their only asthma medication other than study drug; these have demonstrated that when such patients were treated with each of the approved leukotriene modifiers (pranlukast, zafirlukast, montelukast, and zileuton), their asthma improved, such that there was an improvement in airway obstruction, a decreased need for rescue treatment with β-agonists, relief of asthma symptoms, and a decreased frequency of asthma exacerbations requiring systemic corticosteroid therapy (101,111,131, 133–138).

A. Short-Term Studies (1–2 Months)

In short-term studies of 4–6 weeks duration, patients with moderate asthma (mean FEV_1 of 65% predicted) treated only with β-agonists were given placebo in a single-blind manner for a run-in period that lasted from 7–14 days, followed by an active treatment period of 4–6 weeks (followed in some cases by a withdrawal period). In most of the trials, during the first month of treatment, the FEV_1 improved significantly by 10–15%, and the degree of improvement was statistically significant with active agent when compared with placebo. This was associated with a decrease in asthma symptoms, a decrease in nighttime awakenings, improvement in morning and evening peak flow rates, and a decrease β-agonist use. In the trials with zileuton (131) and zafirlukast (101), patients receiving higher doses of either drug had significantly greater increases in FEV$_1$ than did patients receiving placebo, and those patients receiving lower doses had increases of intermediate magnitude (101,131,133, 139).

B. Long-Term Studies (3–6 Months)

Long-term studies with each of the leukotriene modifiers have demonstrated similar findings. For instance, when 401 patients were randomized in a double-blind fashion to 3 months of therapy with placebo or with one of two doses of zileuton, there was a significant increase in FEV$_1$ with zileuton compared with placebo (16% with zileuton 600 mg four times a day vs. 8% with placebo), a significant decrease in asthma symptoms, a decrease in β-agonist use, and a significantly lower percentage of patients who required treatment with corticosteroids (6 vs. 16%). Furthermore, 6 months of treatment with zileuton reduced peripheral eosinophil counts by more than 20% (Fig. 3) (136). Al-

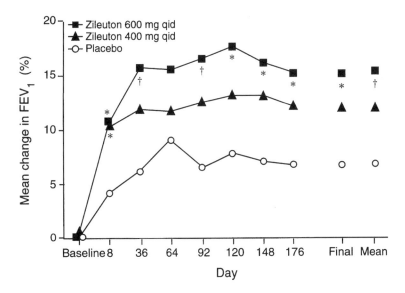

Figure 3 Comparison of chronic trough effects of zileuton 600 mg and 400 mg four times daily with those of placebo four times daily. *$p \leq 0.05$; †$p \leq 0.01$. (From Ref. 136.)

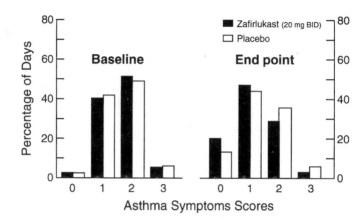

Figure 4 Distribution of daytime asthma symptom scores reported at baseline and at endpoint for patients in the zafirlukast twice-daily and placebo groups. Asthma symptom rating scale: 0 = no symptoms, 1 = mild symptoms that did not interfere with activities, 2 = moderate symptoms that interfered with some activities, and 3= severe symptoms that interfered with many activities. (From Ref. 142.)

though most of the improvement in airway function occurs within 2–4 weeks after the initiation of drug therapy, the improvement in FEV_1 was maintained over the course of the trial, extending previous findings that patients do not become tolerant of the effects of 5-LO inhibition or blockade.

The effect on FEV_1 also appears to be greater in patients with more severe airway obstruction: zafirlukast improved FEV_1 by only 40 mL in patients whose baseline FEV_1 was more than 80% predicted, compared with an increase of 800 mL in those whose FEV_1 was less than 45% predicted (101). Among patients using inhaled corticosteroids, pranlukast allowed a 50% reduction in the dose of inhaled corticosteroid compared to placebo without loss of asthma control (140). Other benefits of these agents were reported by Suissa et al. (141), who demonstrated in a prospective manner that zafirlukast use was associated with fewer days lost from school or work, fewer unscheduled medical care episodes, and fewer days with asthma symptoms (142) (Fig. 4).

Treatment once daily with montelukast appears to confer the same benefit as treatment on a more frequent basis with other agents (Fig. 5) (111). Furthermore, among these agents, only montelukast has been studied in children between the ages of 6 and 12. In this group, administration of a 5-mg chewable montelukast tablet at bedtime was associated with an improvement

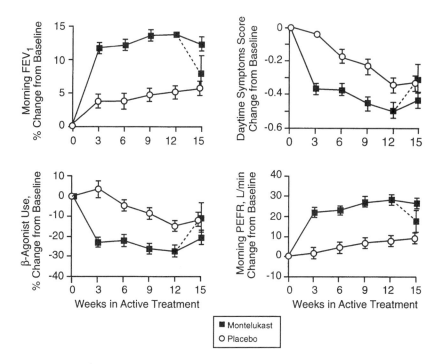

Figure 5 The effect of montelukast and placebo on FEV_1, daytime symptom score, β-agonist use, and morning peak flow during a 12-week active treatment period and a 3-week placebo washout period. Montelukast, compared with placebo, caused significant improvement in all endpoints. (From Ref. 111.)

in lung function and asthma symptoms in those with moderate persistent asthma, many of whom were also receiving inhaled steroids as antiasthma treatment (143,144).

C. FLAP Inhibitors and Asthma

While no 5-LO activating protein (FLAP) inhibitors are currently approved for use with patients, these drugs have been evaluated in clinical studies. For instance, MK-0591 was given to patients with moderately severe asthma who required treatment with inhaled corticosteroids, and those who received 125 mg of the drug twice daily had a significantly greater rise in mean FEV_1 and peak flow rates than those receiving placebo and also had fewer asthma symptoms and no adverse events (145). Similarly, when BAYx1005 was given to 67 patients with moderate chronic asthma receiving corticosteroids, there were small but significant increases in FEV_1 after 4 weeks of treatment (146). These are promising drugs that may contribute significantly to asthma therapy in the future.

D. Efficacy of Leukotriene Modifiers Compared with Other Asthma Medications

While leukotriene modifiers have been demonstrated to decrease doses and need for corticosteroids, there have been limited published reports to date comparing the efficacy of leukotriene modifiers directly with that of corticosteroids. While these studies suggest that inhaled corticosteroids show greater improvement in FEV_1 and peak flow compared with leukotriene modifiers, no significant difference in exacerbation rates over a 3-month period was demonstrated (147,148). Furthermore, compliance studies with oral versus inhaled asthma medications suggest that oral medications such as the leukotriene modifiers may lead to greater long-term compliance compared with that of inhaled corticosteroids (149). In terms of other asthma therapy, when zileuton was compared with twice-daily theophylline in a 3-month trial, the two drugs resulted in similar increases in FEV_1, but treatment with theophylline resulted in somewhat greater symptomatic relief in the first 2 months of the trial (150). A double-blind study comparing the long-acting β-agonist salmeterol with zafirlukast over 4 weeks in 301 patients with persistent asthma (mean $FEV_1 = 66\%$) revealed that salmeterol was more effective than zafirlukast in improving pulmonary function and symptom control, although exacerbation rates and adverse event profiles were similar between the two drugs (151). When zafirlukast and cromolyn were compared with each other and with placebo, both medications were found to be superior to placebo but comparable to each other in terms of symptom scores and β-agonist usage (152,153). As there have been only a few limited studies comparing leukotriene modifiers with other asthma medications, the relative importance of each drug in asthma therapy remains unclear and further studies are warranted.

E. Leukotriene Modifiers and COPD

Leukotriene modifier agents have been studied only in patients with asthma, yet many physicians have prescribed leukotriene-modifying medications to patients with chronic obstructive pulmonary disease. While there might be some theoretical and anecdotal basis for their use in some patients with an inflammatory component of COPD, particularly chronic bronchitis, there have been no clinical trials to date documenting its efficacy or safety in this population and no drugs involved in the 5-LO pathway are currently approved for this use.

X. Systemic Effects of Leukotriene Modifiers

In the clinical trials leading to the approval of zileuton, zafirlukast, montelukast, and pranlukast, the drugs were very well tolerated and had side-effect profiles similar to those of placebo. The most common side effects included headache, dyspepsia, nausea, diarrhea, nonspecific pain and myalgia (154). As the number of patients taking these medications has increased, several reports of systemic adverse effects have been reported with these medications (see Table 1).

A. Liver Function Abnormalities

Long-term safety studies of zileuton have revealed that approximately 5% of patients receiving the drug had clinically significant increases in transaminases within the first few months of therapy, while 2% of patients in the usual-care group had an increase. These effects reversed with drug withdrawal, but it is generally felt that patients receiving the drug require monitoring of liver function tests at the onset of treatment and periodically thereafter. This complication does not occur with zafirlukast when given at the recommended dose of 20 mg twice daily, but it does occur at an appreciable frequency when higher doses are given. There has been no report of elevated liver function tests with montelukast therapy (155).

B. Eosinophilic Vasculitis and the Churg-Strauss Syndrome

Within 6 months after the release of zafirlukast, eight patients who received the drug for moderate to severe asthma developed eosinophilia, pulmonary infiltrates, cardiomyopathy, and other signs of vasculitis, which are characteristic of the Churg-Strauss syndrome (156). All of the patients had discontinued high-dose corticosteroid use within 3 months of presentation, and all devel-

Table 1 Drug Interactions with Leukotrienes

Generic/Trade Name	Dose	Lab Tests Needed	Drug Interaction
Zileuton/Zyflo	600 qid	Liver function tests	Warfarin, theophylline
Zafirlukast/Accolate	20 bid		Warfarin, theophylline
Montelukast/Singulair	10 qd		Phenobarbital, erythromycin

oped the syndrome within 4 months of zafirlukast initiation; the syndrome dramatically improved in each patient upon reinitiation of corticosteroid therapy. Since that report, multiple similar cases have been reported to Zeneca and to federal drug regulatory agencies (157–159) with regard to zafirlukast, and there have now been several case reports in association with montelukast (160–162). Many potential mechanisms for the association between zafirlukast and montelukast and the Churg-Strauss syndrome have been postulated, including increased syndrome reporting due to bias, potential for allergic drug reaction, and leukotriene imbalance resulting from leukotriene receptor blockade (156,163). However, careful analysis of all reported cases suggests that the Churg-Strauss syndrome developed only in those patients taking zafirlukast or montelukast who had an underlying eosinophilic disorder that was being masked by corticosteroid treatment and unmasked by leukotriene receptor antagonist–mediated steroid withdrawal, similar to the "forme fruste" of the Churg-Strauss syndrome (164). While recent studies suggest that previous reports underestimated the incidence of Churg-Strauss syndrome in the asthma population compared with that of the general population (64.4 vs. 1.8 cases per million patient years) (165); as the incidence of this syndrome with the leukotriene modifiers is also about 60 cases per million patient years, it appears that neither drug is directly causative of this rare syndrome. There has, however, been one report of drug-induced lupus with zafilukast (166). Of note, while there have been only a few reports to the United States Food and Drug Administration of cases of Churg-Strauss syndrome in association with zileuton use, the distribution of this drug is much less than that of the two cysteinyl leukotriene receptor antagonists (167).

In the 3 years since pranlukast was introduced in Japan, there has been at least one case report of the Churg-Strauss syndrome in association with pranlukast use (168). Although it is generally felt to be safe, with minimal reports of adverse effects or laboratory abnormalities, there has been one published case report of a patient who developed acute tubulointerstitial nephritis that subsequently resolved while taking the drug during a clinical trial (169).

C. Interactions with Other Medications

Each of the leukotriene modifiers has been administered with other therapies routinely used in the prophylaxis and treatment of asthma, with no apparent increase in adverse reactions. However, it is important to be wary of possible interactions with these medications and to understand how they may affect levels of other drugs. For instance, coadministration of either zileuton or zafirlukast with warfarin results in increased half-life of this anticoagulant and leads to increase prothrombin time. In these patients, prothrombin time should be followed closely and anticoagulant levels adjusted appropriately. As montelukast has been shown to have no clinically significant interaction with warfarin, montelukast may be a better asthma treatment option for those patients who require anticoagulant therapy (170). No formal drug interactions have been reported with zafirlukast or with zileuton and other drugs metabolized by the cytochrome P-450 system (phenytoin, carbamazepine, calcium channel blockers, and cyclosporine); however, careful monitoring of patients taking these drugs simultaneously is recommended. While zafirlukast does not affect the pharmacokinetics of azithromycin nor clarithromycin (171), it is important to note that zafirlukast levels are reduced when zafirlukast is taken in conjunction with theophylline and erythromycin, hence close monitoring of asthma symptoms during coadministration with these agents is appropriate. Treatment with zileuton results in an increase in theophylline levels, hence it is important to monitor patients taking this combination of drugs closely and to follow each patient clinically and with theophylline levels. Similar drug interactions with montelukast have not been reported except with phenobarbital, which reduces montelukast levels. No dosage adjustment is recommended, however (154).

XI. Conclusions and Future Directions

Leukotriene modifiers represent the newest class of asthma pharmacotherapy and have emerged as safe, potent medications that are effective in controlling the bronchoconstriction and inflammation of asthma. Both cysteinyl leukotriene receptor antagonists and 5-lipoxygenase inhibitors are particularly effective in treating patients with exercise and aspirin-induced asthma and may be useful in controlling the early and late allergic response. In terms of chronic, stable asthma, these medications have clearly demonstrated a bronchodilatory effect that is additive to yet distinct from that caused by β-adrenergic agonists. They improve lung function, result in fewer asthma symptoms particularly at night, decrease the frequency of asthma exacerbations, and yield excellent compliance due to their oral bioavailability. These drugs are useful as corticosteroid-sparing agents and represent an alternative to inhaled steroids for mild patients who are using β-agonists as their primary asthma treatment. Despite their capacity for superb asthma control, the role of these drugs with respect to current asthma guidelines needs to be clarified and their role as an alternative to corticosteroids needs to be investigated formally before they can be considered first-line therapy in appropriate patients.

Future directions of therapy with leukotriene modifiers will include the search for new medications that target specific areas of the 5-LO cascade and may involve the use of PLA_2 inhibitors, novel FLAP inhibitors, LTB_4 receptor antagonists, and other cysteinyl leukotriene receptor antagonists. Trials with these agents in patients with COPD are currently lacking; although widely used in these patients, no data exist with regard to their safety and efficacy. As we learn more about leukotrienes and their functions through further investigation, we will undoubtedly uncover much about the pathobiology of asthma and other inflammatory conditions.

References

1. Feldberg W, Kellaway CH. Liberation of histamine and formation of lysocithin-like substances by cobra venom. J Physiol 1938; 94:187–191.
2. Kellaway CH, Trethewie ER. The liberation of a slow-reacting smooth muscle stimulating substance in anaphylaxis. Q J Exp Physiol 1940; 30:121–145.
3. Brocklehurst WE. The release of histamine and the formation of a slow-reacting substance (SRS-A) during anaphylactic shock. J Physiol (Lond) 1960; 151: 416–435.
4. Drazen JM, Austen KF. Effects of intravenous administration of slow-reacting substance of anaphylaxis, histamine, bradykinin, and prostaglandin F_2alpha on pulmonary mechanics in the guinea pig. J Clin Invest 1974; 53:1679–1685.
5. Samuelsson B, Dahlen SE, Lindgren JA, Rouzer CA, Serhan CN. Leukotrienes and lipoxins: structures, biosynthesis, and biological effects. Science 1987; 237: 1171–1176.
6. Pasquale D, Chikkappa G. Lipoxygenase products regulate proliferation of granulocyte-macrophage progenitors. Exp Hematol 1993; 21:1361–1365.
7. Porreca E, Difebbo C, Disciullo A, Angelucci D, Nasuti M, Vitullo P, Reale M, Conti P, Cuccurullo F, Poggi A. Cysteinyl leukotriene D_4 induced vascular smooth muscle cell proliferation: a possible role in myointimal hyperplasia. Thromb Haemost 1996; 76:99–104.
8. Cohen P, Noveral JP, Bhala A, Nunn SE, Herrick DJ, Grunstein MM. Leukotriene D_4 facilitates airway smooth muscle cell proliferation via modulation of the IGF axis. Am J Physiol 1995; 13:L151–L157.
9. Hui KP, Lotvall J, Chung KF, Barnes PJ. Attenuation of inhaled allergen-induced airway microvascular leakage and airflow obstruction in guinea pigs by a 5-lipoxygenase inhibitor (A-63162). Am Rev Respir Dis 1991; 143:1015–1019.
10. Wasserman MA, Welton AF, Renzetti LM. Synergism exhibited by LTD_4 and PAF receptor antagonists in decreasing antigen-induced airway microvascular leakage. Prostaglandins Rel Comp 1995; 23:273.

11. Laitinen LA, Laitinen A, Haahtela T, Vilkka V, Spur BW, Lee TH. Leukotriene-E(4) and granulocytic infiltration into asthmatic airways. Lancet 1993; 341:989–990.

12. Munoz NM, Leff AR. Blockade of eosinophil migration by 5-lipoxygenase and cyclooxygenase inhibition in explanted guinea pig trachealis. Am J Physiol 1995; 12:L446–L454.

13. Lewis RA, Austen KF, Soberman RJ. Leukotrienes and other products of the 5-lipoxygenase pathway: biochemistry and relation to pathobiology in human diseases. N Eng J Med 1990; 323:645–655.

14. Samuelsson B. Leukotrienes: mediators of immediate hypersensitivity reactions and inflammation. Science 1983; 220:568–575.

15. Samuelsson B, Dahlen SE, Lindgren JA, Rouzer CA, Serhan CN. Leukotrienes and lipoxins: structures, biosynthesis, and biological effects. Science 1987; 237: 1171–1176.

16. Woods JW, Evans JF, Ethier D, Scott S, Vickers PJ, Hearn L, Heibein JA, Charleson S, Singer II. 5-Lipoxygenase and 5-lipoxygenase activating protein are localized in the nuclear envelope of activated human leukocytes. J Exp Med 1993; 178:1935–1946.

17. Schleimer RP, MacGlashan DW Jr, Peters SP, Pinckard RN, Adkinson NF Jr, Lichtenstein LM. Characterization of inflammatory mediator release from purified human lung mast cells. Am Rev Respir Dis 1986; 133:614–617.

18. Weller PF, Lee CW, Foster DW, Corey EJ, Austen KF, Lewis RA. Generation and metabolism of 5-lipoxygenase pathway leukotrienes by human eosinophils: predominant production of leukotriene C4. Proc Natl Acad Sci USA 1983; 80: 7626–7630.

19. Rankin JA, Hitchcock M, Merrill W, Bach MK, Brashler JR, Askenase PW. IgE-dependent release of leukotriene C4 from alveolar macrophages. Nature 1982; 297:329–331.

20. Schonfeld W, Schluter B, Hilger R, Konig W. Leukotriene generation and metabolism in isolated human lung macrophages. Immunology 1988; 65:529–536.

21. Holtzman MJ. Arachidonic acid metabolism in airway epithelial cells. Annu Rev Physiol 1992; 54:303–329.

22. Eling TE, Danilowicz RM, Henke DC, Sivarajah K, Yankaskas JR, Boucher RC. Arachidonic acid metabolism by canine tracheal epithelial cells: product formation and relationship to chloride secretion. J Biol Chem 1986; 261: 12841–12849.

23. Feinmark SJ, Cannon PJ. Endothelial cell leukotriene C4 synthesis results from intercellular transfer of leukotriene A4 synthesized by polymorphonuclear leukocytes. J Biol Chem 1986; 261:16466–16472.

24. Jackson RM, Chandler DB, Fulmer JD. Production of arachidonic acid metabolites by endothelial cells in hyperoxia. J Appl Physiol 1986; 61:584–591.

25. Piper PJ, Galton SA. Generation of leukotriene B4 and leukotriene E4 from porcine pulmonary artery. Prostaglandins 1984; 28:905–914.

26. Bjorck T, Dahlen SE. Evidence indicating that leukotrienes C4, D4 and E4 are major mediators of contraction induced by anti-IgE in human bronchi. Agents Actions 1989; 26:87–89.

27. Orning L, Hammarstrom S. Inhibition of leukotriene C and leukotriene D biosynthesis. J Biol Chem 1980; 255:8023–8026.

28. Togias AG, Naclerio RM, Peters SP, Nimmagadda I, Proud D, Kagey-Sobotka A, Adkinson NF Jr, Norman PS, Lichtenstein LM. Local generation of sulfidopeptide leukotrienes upon nasal provocation with cold, dry air. Am Rev Respir Dis 1986; 133:1133–1137.

29. Knapp HR, Sladek K, Fitzgerald GA. Increased excretion of leukotriene-E4 during aspirin-induced asthma. J Lab Clin Med 1992; 119:48–51.

30. Israel E, Fischer AR, Rosenberg MA, Lilly CM, Callery JC, Shapiro J, Cohn J, Rubin R, Drazen JM. The pivotal role of 5-lipoxygenase products in the reaction of aspirin-sensitive asthmatics to aspirin. Am Rev Respir Dis 1993; 148:1447–1451.

31. Dahlen B, Margolskee DJ, Zetterstrom O, Dahlen SE. Effect of the leukotriene receptor antagonist MK-0679 on baseline pulmonary function in aspirin sensitive asthmatic subjects. Thorax 1993; 48:1205–1210.

32. Morganroth ML, Stenmark KR, Zirrolli JA, Mauldin R, Mathias M, Reeves JT, Murphy RC, Voelkel NF. Leukotriene C4 production during hypoxic pulmonary vasoconstriction in isolated rat lungs. Prostaglandins 1984; 28:867–875.

33. Taniguchi H, Taki F, Takagi K, Satake T, Sugiyama S, Ozawa T. The role of leukotriene B4 in the genesis of oxygen toxicity in the lung. Am Rev Respir Dis 1986; 133:805–808.

34. Taylor IK, Ward PS, Taylor GW, Dollery CT, Fuller RW. Inhaled PAF stimulates leukotriene and thromboxane-A2 production in humans. J Appl Physiol 1991; 71:1396–1402.

35. Goldyne ME, Burrish GF, Poubelle PE, Borgeat P. Arachidonic acid metabolism among human mononuclear leukocytes: lipoxygenase-related pathways. J Biol Chem 1984; 259:8815–8819.

36. Ferreri NR, Howland WC, Stevenson DD, Spiegelberg HL. Release of leukotrienes, prostaglandins, and histamine into nasal secretions of aspirin-sensitive asthmatics during reaction to aspirin. Am Rev Respir Dis 1988; 137:847–854.

37. Williams JD, Czop JK, Austen KF. Release of leukotrienes by human monocytes on stimulation of their phagocytic receptor for particulate activators. J Immunol 1984; 136:4188–4193.

38. Henderson WR, Kleber FX. Leukotriene production and inactivation by normal, chronic granulomatous disease and myeloperoxidase-deficient neutrophils. J Biol Chem 1983; 258:13522–13527.

39. Denzlinger C, Guhlmann A, Scheuber PH, Wilker D, Hammer DK, Keppler D. Metabolism and analysis of cysteinyl leukotrienes in the monkey. J Biol Chem 1986; 261:15601–15606.

40. Lee CW, Lewis RA, Tauber AI, Mehrotra M, Corey EJ, Austen KF. The mye-loperoxidase-dependent metabolism of leukotrienes C4, D4, and E4 to 6-trans-leukotriene B4 diastereoisomers and the subclass-specific S-diastereoisomeric sulfoxides. J Biol Chem 1983; 258:15004–15010.

41. Stene DO, Murphy RC. Metabolism of leukotriene E4 in isolated rat hepato-cytes: identification of beta-oxidation products of sulfidopeptide leukotrienes. J Biol Chem 1988; 263:2773–2778.

42. Kawashima H, Kusunose E, Thompson CM, Strobel HW. Protein expression, characterization, and regulation of CYP4F4 and CYP4F5 cloned from rat brain. Arch Biochem Biophys 1997; 347:148–154.

43. Lynch KR, O'Neil GP, Liu Q, Im DS, Sawyer N, Melters KM, Coulombe N, Abramovitz M, Figueroa DJ, Zeng Z, Connolly BM, Bal C, Austin CP, Cha-teauneuf A, Stocco R, Greig GM, Kargman S, Hooks SB, Hosfield E, Williams Jr DL, Ford-Hutchinson AW, Caskey CT, Evans JF. Characterization of the human CysLT₁ receptor. Nature 1999; 399:789–793.

44. Coleman RA, Eglen RM, Jones RL, Narumiya S, Shimizu T, Smith WL, Dahlen SE, Drazen JM, Gardiner PJ, Jackson WT, Jones TR, Krell RD, Nicosia S. Prostanoid and leukotriene receptors: a progress report from the IUPHAR work-ing parties on classification and nomenclature. Prostaglandins Rel Comp 1995; 23:285.

45. Yokomizo T, Izumi T, Chang K, Takuwa Y, Shimizu T. A G-protein-coupled receptor for leukotriene B₄ that mediates chemotaxis. Nature 1997; 387:620–624.

46. Piper PJ. Pharmacology of leukotrienes. Br Med Bull 1983; 39:255–259.

47. Serhan CN, Haeggstrom JZ, Leslie CC. Lipid mediator networks in cell signal-ing: update and impact of cytokines. FASEB J 1996; 10:1147–1158.

48. Lewis RA, Austen KF, Drazen JM, Clark DA, Marfat A, Corey EJ. Slow re-acting substances of anaphylaxis: identification of leukotrienes C-1 and D from human and rat sources. Proc Natl Acad Sci USA 1980; 77:3710–3714.

49. Goldman DW, Gifford LA, Young RN, Marotti T, Cheung MK, Goetzl EJ. Affinity labeling of the membrane protein-binding component of human poly-morphonuclear leukocyte receptors for leukotriene B4. J Immunol 1991; 146: 2671–2677.

50. Slipetz DM, Scoggan KA, Nicholson DW, Metters KM. Photoaffinity labelling and radiation inactivation of the leukotriene B4 receptor in human myeloid cells. Eur J Pharmacol 1993; 244:161–173.

51. Ford-Hutchinson AW. Leukotriene B4 in inflammation. Crit Rev Immunol 1990; 10:1–12.

52. Rola-Pleszczynski M, Thivierge M, Gagnon N, Lacasse C, Stankova J. Differ-ential regulation of cytokine and cytokine receptor genes by PAF, LTB4 and PGE2. J Lipid Med 1993; 6:175–181.

53. Miki I, Watanabe T, Nakamura M, Seyama Y, Ui M, Sato F, Shimizu T. Solubi-lization and characterization of leukotriene B4 receptor–GTP binding protein

complex from porcine spleen. Biochem Biophys Res Commun 1990; 166:342–348.

54. Kriesle RA, Parker CW, Griffin GL, Senior RM, Stenson WF. Studies of leukotriene B4-specific binding and function in rat polymorphonuclear leukocytes: absence of a chemotactic response. J Immunol 1985; 134:3356–3363.

55. O'Flaherty J, Kosfeld S, Nishihira J. Binding and metabolism of leukotriene B4 by neutrophils and their subcellular organelles. J Cell Physiol 1986; 126:359–370.

56. Dahinden CA, Clancy RM, Hugli TE. Stereospecificity of leukotriene B4 and structure-function relationships for chemotaxis of human neutrophils. J Immunol 1984; 133:1477–1482.

57. Britton J. Airway hyperresponsiveness and the clinical diagnosis of asthma—histamine or history. J Allergy Clin Immunol 1992; 89:19–22.

58. Evans JF, Leblanc Y, Fitzsimmons BJ, Charleson S, Nathaniel D, Leveille C. Activation of leukocyte movement and displacement of [3H] leukotriene B4 from leukocyte membrane preparations by (12R)- and (12S)-hydroxyeicosatetraenoic acid. Biochim Biophys Acta 1987; 917:406–410.

59. Mong S, Wu HL, Miller J, Hall RF, Gleason JG, Crooke ST. SKF 104353, a high affinity antagonist for human and guinea pig lung leukotriene D4 receptor, blocked phosphatidylinositol metabolism and thromboxane synthesis induced by leukotriene D4. Mol Pharmacol 1987; 32:223–229.

60. Mong S, Hoffman K, Wu HL, Crooke ST. Leukotriene-induced hydrolysis of inositol lipids in guinea pig lung: mechanism of signal transduction for leukotriene-D4 receptors. Mol Pharmacol 1987; 31:35–41.

61. Crooke ST, Mattern M, Sarau HM, Winkler JD, Balcarek J, Wong A, Bennett CF. The signal transduction system of the leukotriene D4 receptor. Trend Pharmacol Sci 1989; 10:103–107.

62. Crooke ST, Sarau H, Saussy D, Winkler J, Foley J. Signal transduction processes for the LTD4 receptor. Adv Prost Thromb Leukot Res 1990; 20:127–137.

63. Buckner CK, Krell RD, Laravuso RB, Coursin DB, Bernstein PR, Will JA. Pharmacological evidence that human intralobar airways do not contain different receptors that mediate contractions to leukotriene C4 and leukotriene D4. J Pharmacol Exp Ther 1986; 237:558–562.

64. Jones TR, Davis C, Daniel EE. Pharmacological study of the contractile activity of leukotriene C4 and D4 on isolated human airway smooth muscle. Can J Physiol Pharmacol 1982; 60:638–643.

65. Davis C, Kannan MS, Jones TR, Daniel EE. Control of human airway smooth muscle: in vitro studies. J Appl Physiol 1982; 53:1080–1087.

66. Muccitelli RM, Tucker SS, Hay DW, Torphy TJ, Wasserman MA. Is the guinea pig trachea a good in vitro model of human large and central airways? Comparison on leukotriene-, methacholine-, histamine- and antigen-induced contractions. J Pharmacol Exp Ther 1987; 243:467–473.

67. Palmer RM, Stepney RJ, Higgs GA, Eakins KE. Chemokinetic activities of arachidonic and lipoxygenase products on leukocytes of different species. Prostaglandins 1980; 20:411–418.

68. Soter NA, Lewis RA, Corey EJ, Austen KF. Local effects of synthetic leukotrienes (LTC4, LTD4, LTE4 and LTB4) in human skin. J Invest Dermatol 1983; 80:119.

69. Camp RD, Coutts AA, Greaves MW, Kay AB, Walport MJ. Responses of human skin to intradermal injection of leukotriene C4, D4, and B4. Br J Pharmacol 1983; 80:497–502.

70. Bass DA, Thomas MJ, Goetzl EJ, DeChatelet LR, Mccall CE. Lipoxygenase-derived products of arachidonic acid mediate stimulation of hexose reuptake in human polymorphonuclear leukocytes. Biochem Biophys Res Commun 1981; 100:1–7.

71. Sha'afi RI, Naccache PH, Molski TF, Borgeat P, Goetzl EJ. Cellular regulatory role of leukotriene B4: its effects on cation homeostasis in rabbit neutrophils. J Cell Physiol 1981; 108:401–408.

72. Jackson WT, Boyd RJ, Froelich LL, Mallett BE, Gapinski DM. Specific inhibition of leukotriene-B(4)-induced neutrophil activation by LY223982. J Pharmacol Exp Ther 1992; 263:1009–1014.

73. Silbaugh SA, Stengel PW, Cockerham SL, Roman CR, Saussy DLJ, Spaethe SM, Goodson T Jr, Herron DK, Fleisch JH. Pulmonary actions of LY255283, a leukotriene B4 receptor antagonist. Eur J Pharmacol 1992; 223:57–64.

74. Labaudiniere R, Dereu N, Cavy F, Guillet MC, Marquis O, Terlain B. Omega-[(4,6-diphenyl-2-pyridyl)oxy]alkanoic acid derivatives: a new family of potent and orally active LTB4 antagonists. J Med Chem 1992; 35:4315–4324.

75. Wetmore LA, Gerard NP, Herron DK, Bollinger NG, Baker SR, Feldman HA, Drazen JM. Leukotriene receptor on U-937 cells: discriminatory responses to leukotrienes C4 and D4. Am J Physiol 1991; 261:L164–L171.

76. Mong S, Wu HL, Scott MO, Lewis MA, Clark MA, Weichman BM, Kinzig CM, Gleason JG, Crooke ST. Molecular heterogeneity of leukotriene receptors: correlation of smooth muscle contraction and radioligand binding in guinea-pig lung. J Pharmacol Exp Ther 1985; 234:316–325.

77. Dahlen SE, Bjork J, Hedqvist P, Arfors KE, Hammarstrom S, Lindgren JA, Samuelsson B. Leukotrienes promote plasma leakage and and leukocyte adhesion in postcapillary venules: in vivo effects with relevance to the acute inflammatory response. Proc Natl Acad Sci USA 1981; 78:3887–3891.

78. Huang FC, Chan WK, Warus JD, Morrissette MM, Moriarty KJ, Chang MN, Travis JJ, Mitchell LS, Nuss GW, Sutherland CA. 4-[2-[Methyl(2-phenethyl)amino]-2-oxoethyl]-8-(phenylmethoxy)-2-naphthalenecarboxylic acid: a high affinity, competitive, orally active leukotriene B4 receptor antagonist. J Med Chem 1992; 35:4253–4255.

79. Michelassi F, Landa L, Hill RD, Lowenstein E, Watkins WD, Petkau AJ, Zapol

WM. Leukotriene D4: a potent coronary artery vasoconstrictor associated with impaired ventricular contraction. Science 1982; 217:841–843.

80. Badr KF, Baylis C, Pfeffer JM, Pfeffer MA, Soberman RJ, Lewis RA, Austen KF, Corey EJ, Brenner BM. Renal and systemic hemodynamic responses to intravenous infusion of leukotriene C4 in the rat. Circ Res 1984; 54:492–499.

81. Miller AM, Weiner RS, Ziboh VA. Evidence for the role of leukotriene C4 and D4 as essential intermediates in CSF-stimulated human myeloid colony formation. Exp Hematol 1986; 14:760–765.

82. Baud L, Sraer J, Perez J, Nivez MP, Ardaillou R. Leukotriene C4 binds to human glomerular epithelial cells and promotes their proliferation in vitro. J Clin Invest 1985; 76:374–377.

83. Baud L, Perez J, Denis M, Ardaillou R. Modulation of fibroblast proliferation by sufidopeptide leukotrienes:effect of indomethacin. J Immunol 1999; 138: 1190–1195.

84. Johnson HM, Russell JK, Torres BA. Second mesenger role of arachidonic acid and it metabolites in interferon-gamma production. J Immunol 1986; 137: 3053–3056.

85. Spada CS, Nieves AL, Krauss AH, Woodward DF. Comparison of leukotriene B4 and D4 effects on human eosinophil and neutrophil motility in vitro. J Leukoc Biol 1994; 55:183–191.

86. Dahlen SE, Hedqvist P, Hammarstrom S, Samuelsson B. Leukotrienes are potent constrictors of human bronchi. Nature 1980; 288:484–486.

87. Hanna CJ, Bach MK, Pare PD, Schellenberg RR. Slow-reacting substances (leukotrienes) contract human airway and pulmonary vascular smooth muscle in vitro. Nature 1981; 290:343–344.

88. Drazen JM. Inhalation challenge with sulfidopeptide leukotrienes in human subjects. Chest 1986; 89:414–419.

89. Barnes NC, Piper PJ, Costello JF. Comparative effects of inhaled leukotriene C4, leukotriene D4, and histamine in normal human subjects. Thorax 1984; 39: 500–504.

90. Bisgaard H, Groth S, Madsen F. Bronchial hyperreactivity to leucotriene D4 and histamine in exogenous asthma. BMJ 1985; 290:1468–1471.

91. Okubo T, Takahashi H, Sumitomo M, Shindoh K, Suzuki S. Plasma levels of leukotrienes C4 and D4 during wheezing attack in asthmatic patients. Int Arch Allergy Appl Immunol 1987; 84:149–155.

92. Wenzel SE, Larsen GL, Johnston K, Voelkel NF, Westcott JY. Elevated levels of leukotriene C4 in bronchoalveolar lavage fluid from atopic asthmatics after endobronchial allergen challenge. Am Rev Respir Dis 1990; 142:112–119.

93. Lam S, Chan H, LeRiche JC, Chan-Yeung M, Salari H. Release of leukotrienes in patients with bronchial asthma. J Allergy Clin Immunol 1988; 81:711–717.

94. Wenzel SE, Trudeau JB, Kaminsky DA, Cohn J, Martin RJ, Westcott JY. Effect of 5-lipoxygenase inhibition on bronchoconstriction and airway inflammation in nocturnal asthma. Am J Respir Crit Care Med 1995; 152:897–905.

95. Sladek K, Dworski R, Fitzgerald GA, Buitkus KL, Block FJ, Marney SR, Jr., Sheller JR. Allergen-stimulated release of thromboxane A2 and leukotriene E4 in humans. Effect of indomethacin. Am Rev Respir Dis 1990; 141:1441–1445.

96. Drazen JM, Obrien J, Sparrow D, Weiss ST, Martins MA, Israel E, Fanta CH. Recovery of leukotriene-E4 from the urine of patients with airway obstruction. Am Rev Respir Dis 1992; 146:104–108.

97. Bellia V, Bonanno A, Cibella F, Cuttitta G, Mirabella A, Profita M, Vignola AM, Bonsignore G. Urinary leukotriene E_4 in the assessment of nocturnal asthma. J Allerg Clin Immunol 1996; 97:735–741.

98. Kumlin M, Dahlen B, Bjorck T, Zetterstrom O, Granstrom E, Dahlen SE. Urinary excretion of leukotriene-E4 and 11-dehydro-thromboxane-B2 in response to bronchial provocations with allergen, aspirin, leukotriene-D4, and histamine in asthmatics. Am Rev Respir Dis 1992; 146:96–103.

99. Sladek K, Szczeklik A. Leukotriene overproduction and mast cell activation during aspirin provoked bronchoconstriction in aspirin-induced asthma (abstr). Am Rev Respir Dis 1992; 145:A17.

100. Christie PE, Tagari P, Fordhutchinson AW, Charlesson S, Chee P, Arm JP, Lee TH. Urinary leukotriene-E4 concentrations increase after aspirin challenge in aspirin-sensitive asthmatic subjects. Am Rev Respir Dis 1991; 143:1025–1029.

101. Spector SL, Smith LJ, Glass M, Birmingham BK, Bronsky EA, Dunn KD, Fish JE, Grossman J, Howland W, Minkwitz MC, Larsen JS, Nathan RA, Rennard SI, Schulman ES, Segal A, Seltzer LM. Effects of 6 weeks of therapy with oral doses of ICI 204, 219, a leukotriene D_4 receptor antagonist, in subjects with bronchial asthma. Am J Respir Crit Care Med 1994; 150:618–623.

102. Spector SL. Leukotriene inhibitors and antagonists in asthma. Ann Allergy Asthma Immunol 1995; 75:463–473.

103. Botto A, Delepeleire I, Rochette F, Reiss TF, Zhang J, Kundu S, Decramer M. MK-0476 causes prolonged potent LTD4 receptor antagonism in the airways of asthmatics (abstr). Am J Respir Crit Care Med 1994; 149:A465.

104. Nakagawa T, Mizushima Y, Ishii A, Nambu F, Mutoishi M, Yui Y, Shida T, Miyamoto T. Effect of a leukotriene antagonist on experimental and clinical bronchial asthma. Adv Prost Thromb Leukot Res 1990; 21:465–468.

105. Anderson SD. Exercise-induced asthma: the state of the art. Am Rev Respir Dis 1985; 87S:191–195.

106. Manning PJ, Watson RM, Margolskee DJ, Williams VC, Schwartz JI, O'Byrne PM. Inhibition of exercise-induced bronchoconstriction by MK-571, a potent leukotriene D4-receptor antagonist. N Engl J Med 1990; 323:1736–1739.

107. Makker HK, Lau LC, Thomson HW, Binks SM, Holgate ST. The protective effect of inhaled leukotriene-D_4 receptor antagonist ICI-204,219 against exercise-induced asthma. Am Rev Respir Dis 1993; 147:1413–1418.

108. Adelroth E, Inman MD, Summers E, Pace D, Modi M, Obyrne PM. Prolonged

protection against exercise-induced bronchoconstriction by the leukotriene D_4-receptor antagonist cinalukast. J Allergy Clin Immunol 1997; 99:210–215.

109. Meltzer SS, Rechsteiner EA, Johns MA, Cohn J, Bleecker ER. Inhibition of exercise-induced asthma by zileuton, a 5-lipoxygenase inhibition (abstr). Am J Respir Crit Care Med 1994; 149:A215.

110. Inman MD, O'Byrne PM. The effect of regular inhaled albuterol on exercise-induced bronchoconstriction. Am J Respir Crit Care Med 1996; 153:65–69.

111. Reiss TF, Chervinsky P, Dockhorn RJ, Shingo S, Seidenberg B, Edwards TB. Montelukast, a once-daily leukotriene receptor antagonist in the treatment of chronic asthma. Arch Intern Med 1998; 158:1213–1220.

112. Leff JA, Busse WW, Pearlman D, Bronsky EA, Kemp J, Hendeles L, Dockhorn R, Kundu S, Zhang J, Seidenberg B, Reiss TF. Montelukast, a leukotriene receptor antagonist, for the treatment of mild asthma and exercise-induced bronchoconstriction. N Engl J Med 1998; 339:147–152.

113. Israel E, Dermarkarian R, Rosenberg M, Sperling R, Taylor G, Rubin P, Drazen JM. The effects of a 5-lipoxygenase inhibitor on asthma induced by cold, dry air. N Engl J Med 1990; 323:1740–1744.

114. Fischer AR. Chronic inhibition of 5-lipoxygenase decreases airway reactivity to cold, dry air independent of the acute inhibition of 5-lipoxygenase (abstr). Am J Respir Crit Care Med 1994; 149:A1056.

115. Christie PE, Smith CM, Lee TH. The potent and selective sulfidopeptide leukotriene antagonist, SK&F 104353, inhibits aspirin-induced asthma. Am Rev Respir Dis 1991; 144:957–958.

116. Fischer AR, Mcfadden CA, Frantz R, Awni WM, Cohn J, Drazen JM, Israel E. Effect of chronic 5-lipoxygenase inhibition on airway hyperresponsiveness in asthmatic subjects. Am J Respir Crit Care Med 1995; 152:1203–1207.

117. Kikawa Y, Miyanomae T, Inoue Y, Saito M, Nakai A, Shigematsu Y, Hosoi S, Sudo M. Urinary leukotriene E4 after exercise challenge in children with asthma. J Allergy Clin Immunol 1992; 89:1111–1119.

118. Reiss TF, Hill JB, Harman E, Zhang J, Tanaka WK, Bronsky E, Guerreiro D, Hendeles L. Increased urinary excretion of LTE4 after exercise and attenuation of exercise-induced bronchospasm by montelukast, a cysteinyl leukotriene receptor antagonist (abstr). Thorax 1997; 52:1030–1035.

119. Taylor IK, Wellings R, Taylor GW, Fuller RW. Urinary leukotriene-E4 excretion in exercise-induced asthma. J Appl Physiol 1992; 73:743–748.

120. Stevenson DD, Hankammer MA, Mathison DA, Christiansen SC, Simon RA. Aspirin desensitization treatment of aspirin-sensitive patients with rhinosinusitis-asthma: long-term outcomes. J Allergy Clin Immunol 1996; 98:751–758.

121. Christie L, Lee TH. The effects of SKF104353 on aspirin induced asthma. Am Rev Respir Dis 1991; 144:957–958.

122. Fuller RW, Black PN, Dollery CT. Effect of the oral leukotriene D4 antagonist LY171883 on inhaled and intradermal challenge with antigen and leukotriene D4 in atopic subjects. J Allergy Clin Immunol 1989; 83:939–944.

123. Rasmussen JB, Margolskee DJ, Eriksson LO, Williams VC, Andersson KE. Leukotriene (LT) D4 is involved in antigen-induced asthma: a study with the LTD4 receptor antagonist, MK-571. Ann NY Acad Sci 1991; 629:436–436.

124. Taylor IK, O'Shaughnessy KM, Fuller RW, Dollery CT. Effect of cysteinyl-leukotriene receptor antagonist ICI 204.219 on allergen-induced bronchoconstriction and airway hyperreactivity in atopic subjects. Lancet 1991; 337:690–694.

125. Dahlen SE, Dahlen B, Eliasson E, Johansson H, Bjorck T, Kumlin M, Boo K, Whitney J, Binks S, King B. Inhibition of allergic bronchoconstriction in asthmatics by the leukotriene-antagonist ICI-204,219. Adv Prost Thromb Leukot Res 1991; 21A:461–464.

126. Evans DJ, Barnes PJ, Spaethe SM, Vanalstyne EL, Mitchell MI, Oconnor BJ. Effect of a leukotriene B$_4$ receptor antagonist, LY293111, on allergen induced responses in asthma. Thorax 1996; 51:1178–1184.

127. Roquet A, Dahlen B, Kumlin M, Ihre E, Anstren G, Binks S, Dahlen SE. Combined antagonism of leukotrienes and histamine produces predominant inhibition of allergen-induced early and late phase airway obstruction in asthmatics. Am J Respir Crit Care Med 1997; 155:1856–1863.

128. Gaddy JN, Margolskee DJ, Bush RK, Williams VC, Busse WW. Bronchodilation with a potent and selective leukotriene D4 (LTD4) antagonist (MK-571) in patients with asthma. Am Rev Respir Dis 1992; 146:358–363.

129. Hui KP, Barnes NC. Lung function improvement in asthma with a cysteinyl-leukotriene receptor antagonist. Lancet 1991; 337:1062–1063.

130. Impens N, Reiss TF, Teahan JA, Desmet M, Rossing TH, Shingo S, Ji Z, Schandevyl W, Verbesselt R, Dupont AG. Acute bronchodilation with an intravenously administered leukotriene-D(4) antagonist, MK-679. Am Rev Respir Dis 1993; 147:1442–1446.

131. Israel E, Rubin P, Kemp JP, Grossman J, Pierson WE, Siegel SC, Tinkelman D, Murray JJ, Busse W, Segal AT, Fish J, Kaiser HB, Ledford D, Wenzel S, Rosenthal R, Cohn J, Lanni C, Pearlman H, Karahalios P, Drazen JM. The effect of inhibition of 5-lipoxygenase by zileuton in mild to moderate asthma. Ann Intern Med 1993; 119:1059–1066.

132. Fujimura M, Sakamoto S, Kamio Y, Matsuda T. Effect of a leukotriene antagonist, ONO-1078, on bronchial hyperresponsiveness in patients with asthma. Respir Med 1993; 87:133–138.

133. Barnes NC, Pujet JC. Pranlukast, a novel leukotriene receptor antagonist: results of the first European placebo controlled, multicentre clinical study in asthma. Thorax 1997; 52:523–527.

134. Reiss TF, Altman LC, Chervinsky P, Bewtra A, Stricker WE, Noonan GP, Kundu S, Zhang J. Effects of montelukast (MK-0476), a new potent cysteinyl leukotriene (LDT(4)) receptor antagonist, in patients with chronic asthma. J Allergy Clin Immunol 1996; 98:528–634.

135. Israel E, Cohn J, Dube L, Drazen JM. Effect of treatment with zileuton, a 5-

lipoxygenase inhibitor, in patients with asthma: a randomized controlled trial. JAMA 1996; 275:931–936.

136. Liu MC, Dube LM, Lancaster J. Acute and chronic effects of a 5-lipoxygenase inhibitor in asthma: a 6-month randomized multicenter trial. J Allergy Clin Immunol 1996; 98:859–871.

137. Kemp JP, Dockhorn RJ, Shapiro GG, Nguyen HH, Reiss TF, Seidenberg BC, Knorr B. Montelukast once daily inhibits exercise-induced bronchoconstriction in 6- to 14-year-old children: a randomized double-blind trial. J Pediatr 1998; 33:424–428.

138. Noonan MJ, Chervinsky P, Brandon M. Montelukast, a potent leukotriene receptor antagonist, causes dose-related improvements in chronic asthma. Eur Respir J 1998; 11:1232–1239.

139. Cloud ML, Enas GC, Kemp J, Platts-Mills T, Altman LC, Townley R, Tinkelman D, King T Jr, Middleton E, Sheffer AL, et al. A specific LTD4/LTE4-receptor antagonist improves pulmonary function in patients with mild, chronic asthma. Am Rev Respir Dis 1989; 140:1336–1339.

140. Tamaoki J, Kondo M, Sakai N, Nakata J, Takemura H, Nagai A, Takizawa T, Kunno K. Leukotriene antagonist prevents exacerbation of asthma during reduction of high dose inhaled corticosteroids. Am J Respir Crit Care Med 1997; 155:1235–1240.

141. Suissa S, Dennis R, Ernst P, Sheehy O, Wooddauphinee S. Effectiveness of the leukotriene receptor antagonist zafirlukast for mild-to-moderate asthma—a randomized, double-blind, placebo-controlled trial. Ann Intern Med 1997; 126:177–177.

142. Fish JE, Kemp JP, Lockey RF, Glass M, Hanby LA. Zafirlukast for symptomatic mild-to-moderate asthma: a 13-week multicenter study. Clin Ther 1997; 19:675–690.

143. Knorr B, Matz J, Bernstein JA, Nguyen H, Seidenberg BC, Reiss TF, Becker A. Montelukast for chronic asthma in 6- to 14-year-old-children: a randomized, double-blind trial. JAMA 1998; 279:1181–1186.

144. Montelukast package insert. Rahway, NJ: Merck, 1998.

145. Chapman KR, Friedman BS, Shingo S, Heyse S, Reiss T, Spector R. The efficacy of an oral inhibitor of leukotriene synthesis (MK-0591) in asthmatics treated with inhaled steroids (abstr). Am J Respir Crit Care Med 1994; 149: A215.

146. Virchow JC, Noller PS, Wiessman KJ, Buhl R, Thalhofer S, Dorow G, Kunkel G, Ukena D, Ulbrich E, Sybrecht G, Matthys H. Multicenter trial of BAY x 1005, a new 5-lipoxygenase activating protein inhibitor in the treatment of chronic asthma (abstr). Am J Respir Crit Care Med 1995; 151:A377.

147. Wenzel S, Chervinsky P, Kerwin E, Silvers W, Faiferman I, Dubb J, Study Group Altair. Oral pranlukast (Ultair) versus inhaled beclomethasone: results of a 12-week trial in patients with asthma (abstr). Am J Respir Crit Care Med 1997; 155:A203.

148. Laitinen LA, Naya IP, Binks S, Harris A. Comparative efficacy of of zafirlukast and low dose steroids in asthmatics on prn β-agonists. Eur Resp J 1997; 10: 419S.

149. Kelloway JS, Wyatt RA, Adlis SA. Comparison of patients' compliance with prescribed oral and inhaled asthma medications. Arch Intern Med 1994; 154: 1349–1352.

150. Schwartz HJ, Petty, T, Dube LM, Swanson LJ, Lancaster JF. A randomized controlled trial comparing zileuton with theophylline in moderate asthma. Arch Intern Med 1998; 158:141–148.

151. Rickard KA, Wolfe JD, LaForce CF, Anderson WH, Kalberg CJ. A comparison of salmeterol and zafirlukast in patients with persistent asthma (abstr). Chest 1998; 114:297S.

152. Nathan RA, Glass M, Snader L. Effects of 13 weeks of treatment with ICI 204,219 (Accolate) or cromolyn sodium (Intal) in patients with mild to moderate asthma (abstr). J Allergy Clin Immunol 1995; 95:388.

153. Holgate ST, Anderson KD, Rodgers EM. Comparison of Accolate (zafirlukast) with sodium cromoglycate in mild to moderate asthmatic patients (abstr). Allergy 1995; 50:319–320.

154. Physicians' Desk Reference, 53d ed. Montvale, NJ: Medical Economics, 1999.

155. Lazarus SC, Lee T, Kemp JP, Wenzel S, Dube LM, Ochs RF, Carpentier PJ, Lancaster JF. Safety and clinical efficacy of zileuton in patients with chronic asthma. Am J Mgd Care 1998; 4:841–848.

156. Wechsler ME, Garpestad E, Flier SR, Kocher O, Weiland DA, Polito AJ, Klinek MM, Bigby TD, Wong GA, Helmers RA, Drazen JM. Pulmonary infiltrates, eosinophilia, and cardiomyopathy following corticosteroid withdrawal in patients with asthma receiving zafirlukast. JAMA 1998; 279:455–457.

157. Katz RS, Papernik M. Zafirlukast and Churg-Strauss syndrome. JAMA 1998; 279:1949 (letter).

158. Knoell DL, Lucas J, Allen JN. Churg-Strauss syndrome associated with zafirlukast. Chest 1998; 114:332–334.

159. Green RL, Vayonis AG. Churg-Strauss syndrome after zafirlukast in two patients not receiving steroid treatment. Lancet 1999; 353:725–726.

160. Franco J, Artes MJ. Pulmonary eosinophilia associated with montelukast. Thorax 1999; 54:558–560.

161. Haranath SP, Freston C, Fucci M, Lee E, Anwar MS. Montelukast-associated Churg-Strauss syndrome. Am J Resp Crit Care Med 1999; 159(3):A646.

162. Wechsler ME, Finn D, Jordan M, Gunawardena D, Drazen JM. Montelukast and the Churg-Strauss syndrome. (abstr.) Am J Resp Crit Care Med 1999; 159(3):A646.

163. Honsinger RW. Zafirlukast and Churg-Strauss syndrome. JAMA 1998; 279: 1949 (letter).

164. Churg A, Brallas M, Cronin SR, Churg J. Formes frustes of Churg-Strauss syndrome. Chest 1995; 108:320–323.

165. Martin RM, Wilton LV, Mann RD. Prevalence of Churg-Strauss syndrome, vasculitis, eosinophilia and associated conditions: retrospective analysis of 58 prescription-event monitoring cohort studies. Pharmacoepidemiol Drug Safety 1999; 8:179–189.

166. Finkel TH, Hunter DJ, Paisley JE, Finkel RS, Larsen GL. Drug-induced lupus in a child after treatment with zafirlukast (Accolate). J Allergy Clin Immunol 1999; 103:533–534.

167. United States Food and Drug Administration. Freedom of information act—zileuton file. 1998.

168. Kinoshita M, Shiraishi T, Ayabe M, Rikimaru T, Oizumi K. Churg-Strauss syndrome after corticosteroid withdrawal in an asthmatic patient treated with pranlukast. J Allergy Clin Immunol 1999; 103:534–535.

169. Schurman SJ, Alderman JM, Massanari M, Cacson AG, Perlman SA. Tubulointerstitial nephritis induced by the leukotriene receptor antagonist pranlukast. Chest 1998; 114:1220–1223.

170. Van Hecken A, Depre M, Verbesselt R, Wynants K, De Lepeleire I, Arnout J, Wong PH, Freeman A, Holland S, Gertz B, De Schepper PJ. Effect of montelukast on the pharmacokinetics and pharmacodynamics of warfarin in healthy volunteers. J Clin Pharmacol 1999; 39(5):495–500.

171. Garey KW, Peloquin CA, Godo PG, Nafziger AN, Amsden GW. Lack of effect of zafirlukast on the pharmacokinetics of azithromycin, clarithromycin and 14-hydroxyclarithromycin in healthy volunteers. Antimicrob Agents Chemother 1999; 43(5):1152–1155.

172. Deykin A, Israel E. Newer therapeutic agents for asthma. In: Schrier RW, Baxter JD, Dzau V, Fauci A, eds. Advances in Internal Medicine. 44th ed. St Louis: Mosby, 1999:209–236.

5

Anticholinergic Bronchodilators
Historical Perspective, Basic Pharmacology, and Overview of Clinical Use

STEPHEN I. RENNARD

University of Nebraska Medical Center
Omaha, Nebraska

I. Historical Perspective

Acetylcholine is an important neurotransmitter in both the central and peripheral nervous systems. It acts through two distinct classes of receptors: nicotinic cholinergic receptors and muscarinic cholinergic receptors initially characterized by their differential response to plant alkaloids. The nicotinic receptors are activated by nicotine and the muscarinic receptors are activated by muscarine. It is now recognized that these classes of receptors are themselves heterogeneous (see below).

Plants synthesize a variety of alkaloids that are active on cholinergic receptors, presumably because interference with cholinergic transmission provides a means of chemical defense against insect predators (1,2). That these alkaloids have pharmacological effects has been known since antiquity. Nicotine has been used since antiquity for its psychoactive effects (3). Atropine and related compounds function as antagonists on the muscarinic receptors. The pharmacological effects of these agents have also been known since antiquity and have found a number of varied uses (4,5). Preparations made from the deadly nightshade were used as poisons. The mydriatic response was used cosmetically, since dilated pupils were popular among Italian women. It is reported that these two uses led Linnaeus to select the name *Atropos bella-donna* for the deadly nightshade, after Atropos, the oldest of the three fates, responsible for cutting and thus ending the thread of life, and *belladonna* from the Italian for "beautiful woman." Interestingly, fashion photographers are reported still to use muscarinic antagonists for the same purpose (4).

Medicinal benefits of muscarinic antagonists have also been known since antiquity (4,5). These agents can slow gastrointestinal motility and, through these actions, may have a number of potentially beneficial effects. In addition, antagonism of muscarinic receptors can reduce airway tone. In India, smoking of *Datura stramonium* was widely used to treat respiratory disorders. Similar uses were discovered by Native Americans and residents of the Middle East (6). The use of *D. stramonium* for the treatment of respiratory disease was brought to western Europe from India by the British about 1800. Atropine was identified as the active agent in *D. stramonium* in the early nineteenth century. Physiological effects of atropine mediated by blockade of the para-sympathetic nervous system were studied in detail in the last half of the nine-teenth century. By the turn of the century, muscarinic antagonists administered via inhalation through the burning of *D. stramonium* or similar plants was common practice to relieve bronchospasm. Because these agents are readily absorbed from the lungs, however, they had considerable systemic parasympa-tholytic effect. As a result, when theophylline and epinephrine became avail-able in the 1920s, the use of anticholinergic bronchodilators declined (6,7).

The renewal of interest in anticholinergics, particularly for the treatment of bronchospasm, stems from the development of ipratropium bromide (6,7). Because this agent is a quaternary amine, it is poorly absorbed when adminis-tered via inhalation. As a result, it can function as a bronchodilator without the systemic side effects caused by atropine and other readily absorbable mus-carinic antagonists (4). These agents have, therefore, once again become an important tool in the therapeutic armamentarium for the management of air-way disease.

II. Pharmacological Mechanisms

The vagus nerve provides parasympathetic innervation to the lung (7,8). A branch of the vagus enters the lung at the hilum, and the preganglionic fibers synapse in ganglia within the lung. The postganglionic neurons then provide innervation to airway smooth muscle, airway glands, the airway epithelium, and blood vessels within the lung. In addition to acetylcholine, these neurons release a variety of other mediators, including nitric oxide and peptidergic mediators (9). Cholinergic receptors are also present on epithelial cells within the alveolar parenchyma. Acetylcholine released by parasympathetic nerves decrease airflow by stimulating airway smooth muscle contraction, can stimulate the production of secretions both by airway glands and airway epithelium, and stimulate mucociliary clearance. While the alveolar structures are not believed to be innervated, cholinergic receptors are present in the alveoli, and acetylcholine may stimulate secretion by alveolar type II cells as well.

It is likely that normal airways have a certain degree of ''cholinergic tone,'' leading to some smooth muscle contraction. Consistent with this, muscarinic cholinergic antagonists can increase airflow even in normal individuals (10,11). Cholinergically mediated increases in bronchial tone can be initiated by several mechanisms. Central activation of parasympathetic pathways may play an important role in the bronchospasm related to psychological stress (12,13). Irritant receptors throughout the respiratory tract can be activated by dusts, cold air, ozone, and other irritants as well as allergens and inflammatory mediators, leading to reflex activation (14–17). These pathways, which require synaptic transmission, may contribute to bronchospasm, increased secretions, and cough not only from irritant exposures within the lungs but also the nares, esophagus, and potentially other sites. Interestingly, activation of these receptors in the lung may lead to gastrointestinal symptoms (18). In addition, afferent fibers contained in the vagus can, through retrograde activation, lead to neurotransmitter discharge within the lung (8). This ''axonal reflex'' need not involve synaptic transmission and could serve to activate responses within a region of the lung.

As noted above, cholinergic receptors fall into two major classes. Nicotinic receptors are pentamers comprising transmembrane proteins, which together form an ion channel activated by acetylcholine (19,20). Muscarinic receptors, in contrast, are seven-membrane-spanning receptors that act through G-proteins (4,21–23). Five muscarinic receptor subtypes have been identified by molecular cloning methods. Three are believed to be active in the human lung.

The M1 and the M3 receptor activate a Gs protein, leading to activation of phospholipase C and the generation of inositol-1,4,5-triphosphate (IP3) and diacylglycerol (DAG). (See Ref. 21 for a detailed review of muscarinic receptor signal transduction.) IP3 induces calcium release from intracellular stores and initiates smooth muscle contraction. DAG activates protein kinase C (Fig. 1).

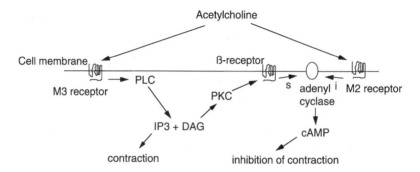

Figure 1 Cholinergic signal transduction: interactions with beta agonists. Acetylcholine can interact with several receptors. Many cells will express more than one receptor. Acetylcholine interaction with the M3 receptor leads, through G-proteins, to activation of phospholipase C. This enzyme then generates inositol-triphosphate (IP3) and diacylglycerol (DAG). IP3 leads to smooth muscle contraction. DAG can activate protein kinase C (PKC), which can, among other activities, phosphorylate and downregulate the beta receptor. Acetylcholine can also interact with the M2 receptor, which, through G-proteins, can inhibit (i) adenyl cyclase. This activity is the opposite of that of the β-receptor, which, through G-proteins, stimulates(s) adenylcyclase. The product of adenyl cyclase, cyclic AMP, can inhibit smooth muscle contraction. See text and Ref. 21 for details.

In contrast, the M2 (and probably M4) receptor activates Gi proteins that downregulate the activity of adenylcyclase. By this mechanism, M2 receptors can mediate a decrease in β-agonists' responsiveness in the presence of acetylcholine. A decrease in β-agonist responsiveness can also be induced by the activation of protein kinase C (PKC) through the M1 or M3 receptor, through phosphorylation of the β-receptor (24,25). These mechanisms of "cross talk" between cholinergic receptors and the β-receptor provide for at least two types of functional antagonism. That is, cholinergic agonists, by altering the function of the β-receptor, may decrease the potency of β-agonists. This cross talk thus provides an important rationale by which combination therapy may have selected benefits. That is, maximal bronchodilation achievable by β-agonist bronchodilators may be reduced by the functional antagonism of cholinergic agonists. Anticholinergics, therefore, could potentiate the action of β-agonists.

Transmission in the parasympathetic ganglia is mediated predominately by nicotinic receptors (8). M1 muscarinic receptors, however, are also located within the ganglia and likely serve to facilitate transmission (22,23,26). Whether antagonism of M1 muscarinic receptor modulation of ganglionic transmission has clinically relevant effects is unknown.

M2 muscarinic receptors are located on the postganglionic parasympathetic nerves, where they serve to downregulate acetylcholine release (21–23). In this capacity, the M2 receptor functions as a negative feedback modulating cholinergic transmission. Interestingly, M2 muscarinic receptors may have a similar function on sympathetic nerves (27). M2 receptors are also present in airway smooth muscle, where, as noted above, they may serve to decrease sympathetic responsiveness (21). There are species differences in M2 receptor expression. However, while early autoradiographic studies failed to demonstrate M2 receptor mRNA in human lung (28) and M2 receptors mRNA is present in human lung (29), cultured human airway smooth muscle cells express functional M2 receptors (30).

The M2 cholinergic receptor is subject to injury by a variety of stimuli. Cationic proteins released from eosinophils, for example, can bind to the receptor, leading to its dysfunction (31,32). Viral infections can damage the receptor (33,34) and neuraminidase induced by influenza virus can alter the structure of the receptor, also leading to its dysfunction. M2 receptor expression, moreover, may be downregulated by a variety of stimuli (35,36). All these mechanisms that lead to a decrease in M2 receptor function can lead to loss of a modulatory effect on cholinergic transmission and, as a result, to increased acetylcholine release by the postganglionic parasympathetic nerves. This is thought to contribute to increased smooth muscle contraction and therefore to bronchospasm in asthma, where viral infections and eosinophilic inflammation are frequently associated with clinical worsening. Loss of M2 downregulation of cholinergically mediated reflex bronchoconstriction may also contribute to the exaggerated response seen in asthmatics to noxious stimuli such as sulfur dioxide (37).

M3 muscarinic receptors are present on both airway smooth muscle and in gland cells (21–23). Acetylcholine, acting through these receptors, can lead to smooth muscle contraction and glandular secretion. It is likely that muscarinic anticholinergic drugs have their main bronchodilator effects as well as their main effects in inhibiting airway secretions through blockade of the M3 receptor.

A number of muscarinic anticholinergic compounds are available (4) (Table 1). Some are approved for a variety of uses, including the treatment of

Table 1 Types of Anticholinergic Agents

Tertiary amines
  Atropine
  Scopolamine
  Homatropine hydrobromide
  Cyclopentolate hydrochloride
  Tropicamide
  Benztropine mesylate
  Trihexyphenidyl hydrochloride
  Dicyclomine hydrochloride
  Oxyphencyclimine hydrochloride
  Flavoxate hydrochloride
  Oxybutynin chloride
Quaternary amines
  Ipratropium bromide
  Atropine methonitrate
  Oxitropium bromide
  Glycopyrrolate
  Tiotropium
  Flutropium bromide
  Methscopolamine
  Homatropine methylbromide
  Methantheline bromide
  Probantheline bromide
  Anisotropine methylbromide
  Clidinium bromide
  Iospropamide iodide
  Tridihexethyl chloride
  Mepenzolate bromide
  Hexocyclium methylsulfate

ophthalmological and gastrointestinal disorders. Atropine and similar tertiary amines are readily absorbable across mucosal surfaces. As a result, they have considerable systemic effects and are not generally used as bronchodilators. Synthetic quaternary amines, in contrast, do not cross mucosal surfaces readily. Several of these compounds are used for their effects on the gastrointestinal tract. Ipratropium and oxitropium have been approved (in various countries) as bronchodilators. In addition, other anticholinergics have been evaluated in this regard.

The available compounds are similar in that all appear to bind non-specifically to all three classes of muscarinic receptors believed to be important in the human lung. Tiotropium differs in that its duration of action is markedly longer (38). In addition, it dissociates more slowly from the M1 and M3 receptor than it does from the M2 receptor (38). As a result, tiotropium shows a temporal selectivity, inhibiting the M1 and M3 receptors after the M2 receptor has regained function. As the M2 receptor may serve as a downregulatory feedback control mechanism, this may have some potential clinical benefits.

III. Clinical Use

A. General Considerations

See Refs. 4, 6, and 7 for general reviews of the clinical pharmacology of anticholinergics. Anticholinergics are used in lung diseases primarily to improve airflow. As noted above, anticholinergics can reduce cholinergiallis mediated airway tone. The resulting decrease in smooth muscle tone is believed to be associated with an increase in airway diameter and therefore with increased airflow. Clinical benefits from anticholinergics, however, may derive from other effects. For example, anticholinergic agents may affect lung volumes more than β-agonist bronchodilators (39,40). Anticholinergics can affect airway secretions, although the effect of the anticholinergics used in clinical practice on airway secretions has not been regarded as physiologically important (41–44). A recent report, however, suggests that ipratropium may be associated with reduced exacerbation frequency in chronic obstructive pulmonary disease (COPD) (45), although the mechanism for such a benefit is undetermined.

Tertiary amine anticholinergics such as atropine are active on the airway when administered either topically or systemically. As atropine is readily absorbed from the mucosal surface, however, significant blood levels are achieved and systemic effects result when the drug is administered to the lung via inhalation. The quaternary amine anticholinergics such as ipratropium are also active when administered either topically or systemically. If they are administered intravenously, systemic effects will be similar to those of atropine (46). As these agents are poorly absorbed across mucosal surfaces, however, very low blood levels and minimal systemic effects result from administration to the lung via inhalation. Topical administration to the airways via inhalation is, therefore, the preferred route of administration. The bronchodilator response after administration via inhalation is similar to that after intravenous use, although the effect may be greater in the larger airways, where deposition via inhalation is likely greater (47).

Two types of inhalation devices are currently used to administer anticholinergics. A solution containing the drug can be nebulized and then inhaled. With conventional nebulizers, much of the nebulized drug is lost from the nebulizer during exhalation (48,49). Devices that are coordinated with the respiratory cycle may reduce such losses. In addition, much of the drug is deposited in the device, in the mouth, and in the pharynx. As a result, the nominal dose delivered by the device is much greater than the dose delivered to the airways. Metered dose inhalers (MDIs) generally deliver much more of the inhaled dose to the lung. These devices, however, still result in considerable deposition of drug to the mouth and pharynx (49,50), although the use of a spacer can reduce this deposition as a result of deposition in the spacer. Even though an MDI may be 5–10 times more efficient than a nebulizer at delivering drug to the airway, it will still deliver only 10–20% of the nominal dose to the airway. Dry powder inhalers deliver drug more efficiently to the airways but are not currently available for use with anticholinergics.

The delivery of drug to the airway by inhalation devices can vary tremendously with technique. One of the most common reasons for the lack of clinical efficacy of bronchodilators administered by these routes is poor inhaler technique. This is often much more of a problem with MDIs owing to the complexity of their use (51). This may also account for the reported low compliance with these devices (52,53). The variable delivery also has confounded dose-response relationships, particularly when the results of different studies are being compared. Current convention is to report the nominally delivered dose, recognizing that the active dose delivered to the lung is a fraction of the dose that exits the device.

Ipratropium has an onset of action of 15–30 min, reaching a peak effect after 1–2 h (7,54,55). Initial studies with ipratropium in asthmatics with relatively mild airflow limitation suggested a maximal bronchodilator effect with a nominal inhaled dose (by MDI) of 20–40 μg (56), although other studies suggested an increasing bronchodilator effect with increasing dose (57–59). A dose of 40 μg administered by inhalation of two inhalations of 20 μg from an MDI was selected for development as a commercial product and is the FDA-approved dose. This dosage has been evaluated in numerous clinical trials. In patients with increasing airflow limitation, an increased nominal dose may be required in order to assure adequate delivery to the airways (60,61). In patients with COPD, a dose response with nebulized solution suggested that a maximal effect was observed with a delivered dose of 400 µg (54) (Fig. 2). By way of comparison, 40 µg delivered by MDI was approximately equivalent to 100 µg administered by nebulizer. This would suggest that a fourfold increase, compared to the conventional 40-µg MDI dose, could still be beneficial.

The variable delivery of inhaled medications to the airways, the need for an increased dose in more severe disease, and the likelihood that the FDA-approved dose of ipratropium is not the peak of the dose response has resulted in the recommendation that doses above those indicated in the product labeling be used (62,63). This recommendation is reasonable, as the poor absorption of ipratropium assures a very high therapeutic index when the drug is adminis-

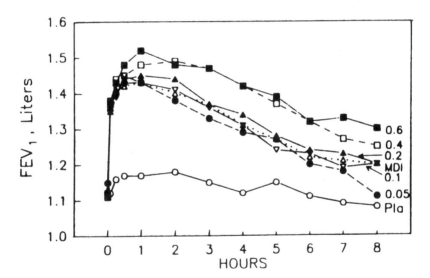

Figure 2 Bronchodilator response to ipratropium in COPD. Patients with COPD were exposed to varying doses of ipratropium administered via nebulizer or to two puffs from a conventional metered dose inhaler. (Vertical axis, FEV_1 in liters; horizontal axis, time following inhalation in hours.) Ipratropium at all doses used caused significant bronchodilatation, in contrast to the placebo (Pla). A maximal response was observed at approximately 0.4–0.6 mg administered via nebulizer. A metered dose inhaler resulted in a bronchodilator response comparable to 0.1 mg administered via nebulizer. Note that the duration of action, assessed as bronchodilation greater than an arbitrary level, increases with increasing dose. (From Ref. 54.)

tered topically. Systemic effects with inhaled ipratropium, therefore, are almost nonexistent, although caution should be used in men with bladder outlet obstruction. Side effects due to inadvertent topical administration—e.g., by direct spray into the eye—do represent a hazard, however. The major limitation to administration of higher than recommended doses is the inconvenience and expense of administering eight or more inhalations. It is difficult to imagine that many patients will be able to adhere to such a regimen.

Oxitropium and flutropium, which are not available in the United States, are quaternary amine anticholinergics with actions similar to those of ipratropium. Bronchodilator effect has been directly compared among these agents in a blinded crossover study (64). Maximal effect was observed at 280 µg (14 puffs) of ipratropium, 420 µg (14 puffs) of flutropium and 600 µg (6 puffs) of oxitropium. This study supports the notion that doses greater than those recommended in the package labeling may be of benefit. In countries where formulations that can achieve the maximal bronchodilatory effect with fewer puffs are available, there may be advantages to their use.

The duration of bronchodilator response is usually determined by the time at which FEV_1 falls to an arbitrary cutoff, usually 15% above the predrug baseline. This time depends on the maximal bronchodilation achieved. As a result, the duration of action of an anticholinergic such as ipratropium depends on the dose administered (54) (Fig. 2). The conventional 40-µg dose (two puffs administered by MDI) is regarded as lasting 4–6 h. A "maximal" dose of 600 µg, administered by nebulizer, however, can result in a duration of at least 8 h (54). For patients who need continual bronchodilation, this may represent a significant clinical advantage. It is likely that the longer duration of action reported for oxitropium is due to its relatively higher dosing compared to ipratropium (65).

Tiotropium is an anticholinergic agent currently (1999) in clinical trials. It associates rapidly with cholinergic receptors but dissociates much more slowly than ipratropium. Its dissociation constant from the M3 receptor, for example, is 133-fold slower than that of ipratropium (38). As a result, tiotropium has a markedly prolonged duration of action compared to that of ipratropium. Bronchodilation in COPD patients lasts at least 24 h (66). An effect lasting 48 h has been reported in asthma (67). This prolonged duration has suggested the appropriateness of once-daily dosing (68). Interestingly, tiotropium dissociates somewhat faster from the M2 receptor than from the M3 receptor, raising the possibility that it can function at least some of the time as a selective antagonist. Whether this will have any clinical advantages remains to be determined.

B. Asthma

Ipratropium is an effective bronchodilator in both acute and chronic asthma. In general, as compared with commonly used, rapidly acting β-agonist bronchodilators, ipratropium is regarded as less potent. The onset of the bronchodilator action of ipratropium is also considerably slower than that of rapid-acting β-agonists such as albuterol. As a result, ipratropium is not generally used as rescue medication for asthmatics needing acute bronchodilation (69). Ipratropium is most often used in combination with other agents when maximal therapy is required. Other anticholinergic agents have also been found to have similar effects when added to β-agonists (70,71). Ipratropium added to inhaled glucocorticoids has not been compared to an increased dose of glucocorticoids, as have salmeterol, formoterol, and theophylline. Ipratropium has no known anti-inflammatory actions of relevance to asthma.

Ipratropium is particularly effective, however, in asthmatics with bronchospasm in the face of β-blocking agents (72,73). In this situation, β-agonists are relatively less effective owing to the presence of the receptor blocking agent, although they may still be of some benefit. Anticholinergics, therefore, may be particularly important in this situation. Psychogenic bronchospasm may be completely relieved by anticholinergics, consistent with the concept of vagally mediated smooth muscle contraction (12,13). In contrast, anticholinergics are generally of partial benefit following exposure to noxious stimuli and are less effective than β-agonists (14–17). This is consistent with intact β-agonist–mediated smooth muscle relaxation in individuals exposed to noxious stimuli (in contrast to those exposed to β-blockers). Moreover, these observations suggest that noxious stimuli can lead to bronchospasm through both vagal reflex mechanisms, which are sensitive to anticholinergic interruption, and through other effects, such as local inflammatory mechanisms, that are not affected by anticholinergic drugs.

C. COPD

In COPD, ipratropium is generally regarded as at least as effective as a bronchodilator, as are rapidly acting β-agonists (62,63,74,75). As in asthma, the onset of action of ipratropium is somewhat slower than that of rapidly acting β-agonists. The duration of bronchodilator effect, however, is generally regarded as being longer, 4–6 h for ipratropium compared to 3–4 h for albuterol. As noted above, the effective duration of action is increased with increasing doses and increasing bronchodilator response.

Because patients with COPD, by definition, always have some degree of fixed airflow limitation, most symptomatic individuals are on continuous bronchodilator therapy. In this setting, ipratropium's slow onset of action is a less important disadvantage. In contrast, the increased duration of action is a potentially important clinical advantage. Ipratropium may have a further advantage in this setting, as the effectiveness of β-agonists diminishes slightly with continuous use (76). In contrast, ipratropium does not manifest tachyphylaxis and may become slightly more effective with chronic use (see below).

Ipratropium not only improves airflow in COPD but may also have a beneficial effect on lung volumes (39). In this context, many patients with COPD are hyperinflated (77,78). In addition, because of expiratory airflow limitation, hyperinflation worsens with increasing minute ventilation (79,80). The hyperinflation has an advantage in that airflows are generally greater at higher volumes, and a greater minute ventilation can be accommodated. This mechanism to increase expiratory airflow, however, comes with a price, as inspiration at higher volumes (and hence higher pressures) results in increased work of breathing and is associated with dyspnea (81–83). By decreasing hyperinflation, ipratropium may have beneficial effects in reducing dyspnea. These effects may be most important during exercise and may not be accurately reflected in routine spirometry measures obtained at rest (84–86). As a result, the FEV_1 correlates relatively poorly with clinical symptoms in patients with severe COPD. While not yet in wide use, measurement of inspiratory capacity may serve as a surrogate for the functional residual capacity or, more correctly, end-expiratory lung volume (86,87) (Fig. 3). Other measures of airflow limitation are being developed but remain research tools (88).

In the current setting, the use of ipratropium in clinical practice is best guided by careful observation of the response of an individual patient—what has been termed "a clinical trial of one." Patient response may be variable based on the dose, the magnitude of the response, and the type of response. Clearly, subjective patient responses—e.g., reduced dyspnea and increased ability to perform daily activities—should be the main guide of therapeutic response. Participation in an active program of pulmonary rehabilitation, however, may be required to maximize these latter effects (89). Many specialists, therefore, would also use spirometric measures of airflow to guide therapy. On the other hand, just as the FEV_1 correlates poorly with symptoms in severe COPD, improvement in symptoms may result from therapy with little change in FEV_1, presumably because of the effects on lung volumes noted above.

One issue that sometimes confuses the use of bronchodilator therapy in COPD is the expected clinical response. The magnitude of the clinical re-

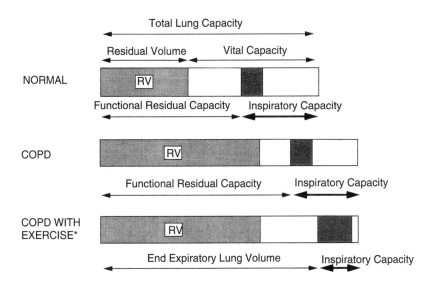

Figure 3 Lung volumes in normal and COPD patients. Schematic lung volumes are shown for normal and COPD individuals with and without exercise. Asterisk (∗) indicates the presence of dynamic hyperinflation. In normal individuals, residual volume (light stipple, RV) plus the vital capacity (open bar) comprises the total lung capacity. Tidal breathing (dark stipple) occurs near the middle of the vital capacity. Tidal breathing begins at a volume defined as the functional residual capacity. The maximal inspiratory effort from this volume is indicated by the inspiratory capacity (heavy arrow). In COPD, there is an increase in the residual volume which exceeds a decrease in vital capacity. As a result, total lung capacity. Tidal breathing occurs at a larger volume, hence an increase in functional residual capacity is present and the inspiratory capacity is decreased. With exercise, dynamic hyperinflation occurs, so that tidal breathing begins at a yet higher volume, here termed *end-expiratory lung volume*. The inspiratory capacity is, therefore, further reduced. Tidal breathing with exercise may also be associated with an increased breath volume and may require a large fraction of the inspiratory capacity.

sponse, assessed by milliliters of FEV_1 is often similar in both mild and severe disease. The relative importance of the response, however, is much greater in the presence of severe disease (90). Consider a patient with mild COPD with a baseline FEV_1 of 2.5 L who improves by 200 mL—an 8% increase that is unlikely to be of much clinical importance. In contrast, a patient with severe COPD with a baseline FEV_1 of 1.0 L who improves by 150 mL will have a 15% increase. More importantly, at the lower range of lung function, even small increases may have great effect on a patient's ability to engage in the activities of daily living. Therefore, it is important to use bronchodilators more aggressively as disease worsens. A clinical trial of bronchodilators in a mildly symptomatic patient may not be of much benefit. However, several years later, when the disease worsens, the same medications may offer important clinical benefits. Repeat clinical trials with ipratropium and trials with increasing dosages are reasonable as disease progresses. In addition, the therapeutic goals for the use of anticholinergics increase as the disease progresses (Table 2).

Table 2 Therapeutic Goals for Use of Anticholinergics in COPD

Stage I: $FEV_1 > 50\%$ predicted; asymptomatic
Grade A[a]: Bronchodilation during exacerbations as needed
Stage II: FEV_1 35–50%; symptomatic
Grade A: Bronchodilation
Consider PRN if symptoms are episodic
Consider regular anticholinergics if symptoms are common
May be combined with other agents
Use is empiric and guided by symptom relief
Stage III: FEV_1 <35%; symptomatic; functionally limited
Grade A: Bronchodilation
Consider PRN if symptoms are episodic
Consider regular anticholinergics if symptoms are common
May be combined with other agents
Use is empiric and guided by symptom relief
(repeat clinical trials indicated as disease progresses)
Grade C: Consider use to facilitated participation in rehabilitation programs
Grade B: May consider use to prevent exacerbations

[a] Grade indicates evidence-based support. (Grade A indicates multiple placebo-controlled trials; grade B indicates limited controlled trials; grade C indicates consistent with available data and clinical practice.)

The Lung Health Study evaluated the effectiveness of ipratropium in slowing the rate of decline of lung function in COPD (91). To accomplish this, nearly 6000 subjects were randomized into three groups. One received usual care and the other two received an aggressive smoking cessation intervention. These two groups were then further randomized to receive placebo or ipratropium 40 μg tid. After the first year, ipratropium was associated with a small increase in lung function. Thereafter, however, lung function declined at precisely the same rate in the placebo and the ipratropium groups. While this very large and well-done study has not been confirmed, it is generally well accepted that ipratropium does not alter the rate of decline of lung function in COPD.

A follow-up of Lung Health Study subjects after the discontinuation of treatment demonstrated that the small increment in baseline lung function observed with ipratropium required continuous administration of drug (91). Interestingly, a retrospective analysis of seven bronchodilator trials comparing ipratropium with a short-acting β-agonist also observed this increase in baseline lung function with extended ipratropium use (76). The small increment in lung function noted with ipratropium use remains incompletely understood. It is unlikely, though possible, that the bronchodilator effect of the doses of ipratropium used in these trials was persistent enough to account for this effect. An as yet poorly understood effect of ipratropium remains possible.

A recent report evaluated exacerbation frequency in subjects treated with ipratropium (45). This study observed both a reduced number and severity, and hence a reduced total cost, of exacerbations in patients treated with ipratropium when compared to those treated with albuterol. If this post hoc analysis is confirmed, it would represent an important therapeutic goal for ipratropium in addition to increasing lung function. As noted above, ipratropium, unlike atropine, is not believed to have clinically important effects on airway secretions. Mechanisms to account for reduced exacerbations with ipratropium therapy, therefore, remain speculative. However, a recent report that ipratropium may decrease reflex-induced esophageal spasm raises a number of interesting questions in this regard (18).

IV. Summary

Anticholinergic agents have been used since antiquity for a variety of purposes including the treatment of respiratory disorders. The development, over the last few decades, of poorly absorbable quaternary amine anticholinergics has permitted the topical use of these agents in the lung when administered via inhalation. This has provided local benefits without systemic side effects. In the United States, only ipratropium, is currently available, it is effective in both asthma and COPD. In asthma, anticholinergic therapy is generally regarded as less effective than other forms of treatment, although it is often added to these treatments for refractory patients. In COPD, anticholinergic therapy may have significant advantages over rapidly acting bronchodilators, and ipratropium is used as a mainstay of treatment for many patients. As new formulations of anticholinergics are developed, and, in particular, as clinical trials explore additional therapeutic outcomes, it is likely that the uses for these agents in respiratory diseases will expand.

Acknowledgment

This work was supported in part by the Larson Endowment of the University of Nebraska Medical Center, Omaha, Nebraska.

References

1. Soloway SB. Naturally occurring insecticides. Environ Health Perspect 1976; 14:109–117.
2. Eldefrawi ME, Eldefrawi AT. Neurotransmitter receptors as targets for pesticides. J Environ Sci Health B 1983; 18:65–88.
3. Slade J. Historical notes on tobacco. In: Bolliger CT, Fagerstrom KO, eds. The Tobacco Epidemic. Basel: Karger, 1997; 28:1–11.
4. Brown JH, Taylor P. Muscarinic receptor agonists and antagonists, In: Goodman LS, Gilman A, eds. The Pharmacological Basis of Therapeutics. New York: McGraw-Hill, 1996:141–160.
5. Gandevia B. Historical review of the use of parasympatholytic agents in the treatment of respiratory disorders. Postgrad Med J 1975; 51:13–20.
6. Gross NJ, Skorodin MS. Anticholinergic, antimuscarinic bronchodilators. Am Rev Respir Dis 1984; 129:856–870.
7. Gross NJ. Anticholinergic drugs. In: Barnes PJ, Grunstein MM, Leff AR, Woolcock AJ, eds. Asthma. Philadelphia: Lippincott-Raven. 1997:1555–1568.
8. Laitinen LA, Laitinen A. Neural system. In: Crystal RG, West JB, eds. The Lung: Scientific Foundations. Philadelphia: Lippincott-Raven, 1997.
9. Uddman R, Sundler F, Cardell L-O, Luts A. Neuropeptides in the lung. In: Crystal RG, West JB, eds. The Lung: Scientific Foundations. Philadelphia: Lippincott-Raven, 1997:103–115.

10. Ingram RH Jr, Wellman JJ, McFadden ER Jr, Mead J. Relative contributions of large and small airways to flow limitation in normal subjects before and after atropine and isoproterenol. J Clin Invest 1977; 59:696–703.

11. Hensley MJ, O'Cain CF, McFadden ER Jr, Ingram RH Jr. Distribution of bronchodilatation in normal subjects: beta-agonist versus atropine. J Appl Physiol 1978; 45:778–782.

12. Neild JE, Cameron IR. Bronchoconstriction in response to suggestion: its prevention by an inhaled anticholinergic agent. BMJ 1985; 290:674.

13. Rebuck AS, Marcus HI. SCH 1000 in psychogenic asthma. Scand J Respir Dis Suppl 1979; 103:186–191.

14. Groot CA, Lammers JW, Festen J, van Herwaarden CL. The protective effects of ipratropium bromide and terbutaline on distilled water-induced bronchoconstriction. Pulm Pharmacol 1994; 7:59–63.

15. McManus MS, Koenig JQ, Altman LC, Pierson WE. Pulmonary effects of sulfur dioxide exposure and ipratropium bromide pretreatment in adults with nonallergic asthma. J Allergy Clin Immunol 1989; 83:619–626.

16. Clarke PS, Jarrett RG, Hall GJ. The protective effect of ipratropium bromide aerosol against bronchospasm induced by hyperventilation and the inhalation of allergen, methacholine and histamine. Ann Allergy 1982; 48:180–183.

17. Santing RE, Pasman Y, Olymulder CG, Roffel AF, Meurs H, Zaagsma J. Contribution of a cholinergic reflex mechanism to allergen-induced bronchial hyperreactivity in permanently instrumented, unrestrained guinea-pigs. Br J Pharmacol 1995; 114:414–418.

18. Triadafilopoulos G, Tsang HP. Olfactory stimuli provoke diffuse esophageal spasm: reversal by ipratropium bromide. Am J Gastroenterol 1996; 91:2224–2227.

19. Conti-Tronconi BM, McLane KE, Raftery MA, Grando SA, Protti MP. The nicotinic acetylcholine receptor: structure and autoimmune pathology. Crit Rev Biochem Mol Biol 1994; 29:69–123.

20. Conti-Fine BM, Lei S, McLane KE. Antibodies as tools to study the structure of membrane proteins: the case of the nicotinic acetylcholine receptor. Annu Rev Biophys Biomol Struct 1996; 25:197–229.

21. Roffel AF, Meurs H, Zaagsma J. Muscarinic receptors and the lung: relevance to chronic obstructive pulmonary disease and asthma. In: Barnes PJ, Buist AS, eds. The Role of Anticholinergics in Chronic Obstructive Pulmonary Disease and Chronic Asthma. Cheshire, UK: Gardiner-Caldwell, 1997:92–125.

22. Hulme EC, Birdsall NJ, Buckley NJ. Muscarinic receptor subtypes. Annu Rev Pharmacol Toxicol 1990; 30:633–673.

23. Caulfield MP. Muscarinic receptors—characterization, coupling and function. Pharmacol Ther 1993; 58:319–379.

24. Abdel-Latif AA. Cross talk between cyclic AMP and the polyphosphoinositide signaling cascade in iris sphincter and other nonvascular smooth muscle. Proc Soc Exp Biol Med 1996; 211:163–177.

25. Houslay MD. "Crosstalk": a pivotal role for protein kinase C in modulating relationships between signal transduction pathways. Eur J Biochem 1991; 195: 9–27.
26. Levey AI. Immunological localization of m1-m5 muscarinic acetylcholine receptors in peripheral tissues and brain. Life Sci 1993; 52:441–448.
27. Racke K, Hey C, Wessler I. Endogenous noradrenaline release from guinea-pig isolated trachea is inhibited by activation of M2 receptors. Br J Pharmacol 1992; 107:3–4.
28. Mak JCW, Barnes PJ. Autoradiographic visualization of muscarinic receptor subtypes in human and guinea pig lung. Am Rev Respir Dis 1990; 141:1559–1568.
29. Mak JC, Baraniuk JN, Barnes PJ. Localization of muscarinic receptor subtype mRNAs in human lung. Am J Respir Cell Mol Biol 1992; 7:344–348.
30. Widdop S, Daykin K, Hall IP. Expression of muscarinic M2 receptors in cultured human airway smooth muscle cells. Am J Respir Cell Mol Biol 1993; 9:541–546.
31. Fryer AD, Adamko DJ, Yost BL, Jacoby DB. Effects of inflammatory cells on neuronal M2 muscarinic receptor function in the lung. Life Sci 1999; 64:449–455.
32. Jacoby DB, Gleich GJ, Fryer AD. Human eosinophil major basic protein is an endogenous allosteric antagonist at the inhibitory muscarinic M2 receptor. J Clin Invest 1993; 91:1314–1318.
33. Fryer AD, Jacoby DB. Parainfluenza virus infection damages inhibitory M2 muscarinic receptors on pulmonary parasympathetic nerves in the guinea-pig. Br J Pharmacol 1991; 102:267–271.
34. Costello RW, Schofield BH, Kephart GM, Gleich GJ, Jacoby DB, Fryer AD. Localization of eosinophils to airway nerves and effect on neuronal M2 muscarinic receptor function. Am J Physiol 1997; 273:L93–L103.
35. Jacoby DB, Xiao HQ, Lee NH, Chan-Li Y, Fryer AD. Virus- and interferon-induced loss of inhibitory M2 muscarinic receptor function and gene expression in cultured airway parasympathetic neurons. J Clin Invest 1998; 102:242–248.
36. Rousell J, Haddad EB, Mak JC, Barnes PJ. Transcriptional down-regulation of m2 muscarinic receptor gene expression in human embryonic lung (HEL 299) cells by protein kinase C. J Biol Chem 1995; 270:7213–7218.
37. Minette PA, Lammers JW, Dixon CM, McCusker MT, Barnes PJ. A muscarinic agonist inhibits reflex bronchoconstriction in normal but not in asthmatic subjects. J Appl Physiol 1989; 67:2461–2465.
38. Disse B, Reichl R, Speck G, Traunecker W, Ludwig Rominger KL, Hammer R. Ba 679 BR, a novel long-acting anticholinergic bronchodilator. Life Sci 1993; 52:537–544.
39. Gross NJ, Skorodin MS. Role of the parasympathetic system in airway obstruction due to emphysema. N Engl J Med 1984; 311:421–425.
40. Braun SR, Levy SF. Comparison of ipratropium bromide and albuterol in chronic

obstructive pulmonary disease: a three-center study. Am J Med 1991; 21:28S–32S.

41. Matthys H. Quantitative and selective bronchial clearance studies using 99mtc-sulfate particles. Scand J Respir Dis 1974; 55(suppl 85):337.
42. Ghafouri MA, Patil K, Kass I. Sputum changes associated with the use of ipratropium bromide. Chest 1984; 86:387–393.
43. Taylor RG, Pavia D, Agnew JE, Lopez-Vidriero MT, Newman SP, Lennard-Jones T, Clarke SW. Effect of four weeks' high dose ipratropium bromide treatment on lung mucociliary clearance. Thorax 1986; 41:295–300.
44. Taylor SM, Pare PD, Armour CL. Airway reactivity in chronic obstructive pulmonary disease. Am Rev Respir Dis 1985; 132:30–35.
45. Friedman M, Serby CW, Menjoge SS, Wilson JD, Hilleman DE, Witek TJ Jr. Pharmacoeconomic evaluation of a combination of ipratropium plus albuterol compared with ipratropium alone and albuterol alone in COPD. Chest 1999; 115:635–641.
46. Kikis D, Esser H, Heinrich K. Influence of ipratropium bromide on heart rate and hemodynamics in patients with sinus bradycardia. Clin Cardiol 1982; 5:441–445.
47. Weiss JW, McFadden ER Jr, Ingram RH Jr. Parenteral vs inhaled atropine: density dependence of maximal expiratory flow. J Appl Physiol 1982; 53:392–396.
48. Johnson MA, Newman SP, Bloom R, Talaee N, Clarke SW. Delivery of albuterol and ipratropium bromide from two nebulizer systems in chronic stable asthma: efficacy and pulmonary deposition. Chest 1989; 96:6–10.
49. Melchor R, Biddiscombe MF, Mak VH, Short MD, Spiro SG. Lung deposition patterns of directly labelled salbutamol in normal subjects and in patients with reversible airflow obstruction. Thorax 1993; 48:506–511.
50. Kim CS, Eldridge MA, Sackner MA. Oropharyngeal deposition and delivery aspects of metered-dose inhaler aerosols. Am Rev Respir Dis 1987; 135:157–164.
51. van Beerendonk I, Mesters I, Mudde AN, Tan TD. Assessment of the inhalation technique in outpatients with asthma or chronic obstructive pulmonary disease using a metered-dose inhaler or dry powder device. J Asthma 1998; 35:273–279.
52. Simmons MS, Nides MA, Rand CS, Wise RA, Tashkin DP. Trends in compliance with bronchodilator inhaler use between follow-up visits in a clinical trial. Chest 1996; 109:963–968.
53. Rand CS, Wise RA, Nides M, Simmons MS, Bleecker ER, Kusek JW, Li VC, Tashkin DP. Metered-dose inhaler adherence in a clinical trial [see comments]. Am Rev Respir Dis 1992; 146:1559–1564.
54. Gross NJ, Petty TL, Friedman M, Skorodin MS, Silvers GW, Donohue JF. Dose response to ipratropium as a nebulized solution in patients with chronic obstructive pulmonary disease. Am Rev Respir Dis 1989; 139:1188–1191.

55. Marlin GE. Studies of ipratropium bromide and fenoterol administered by metered-dose inhaler and aerosolized solution. Respiration 1986; 50:290–293.
56. Gross MJ. Sch 1000: a new anticholinergic bronchodilator. Am Rev Respir Dis 1975; 112:823–828.
57. Baigelman W, Chodosh S. Bronchodilator action of the anticholinergic drug, ipratropium bromide (Sch 1000), as an aerosol in chronic bronchitis and asthma. Chest 1977; 71:324–328.
58. Gomm SA, Keaney NP, Hunt LP, Allen SC, Stretton TB. Dose-response comparison of ipratropium bromide from a metered-dose inhaler and by jet nebulisation. Thorax 1983; 38:297–301.
59. Yeager H Jr, Weinberg RM, Kaufman LV, Katz S. Asthma: comparative bronchodilator effects of ipratropium bromide and isoproterenol. J Clin Pharmacol 1976; 16:198–204.
60. Dolovich MB, Sanchis J, Rossman C, Newhouse MT. Aerosol penetrance: a sensitive index of peripheral airways obstruction. J Appl Physiol 1976; 40:468–471.
61. Pavia D, Thomson M, Shannon HS. Aerosol inhalation and depth of deposition in the human lung. The effect of airway obstruction and tidal volume inhaled. Arch Environ Health 1977; 32:131–137.
62. Celli BR, Snider GL, Heffner J, Tiep B, Ziment I, Make B, Braman S, Olsen G, Phillips Y. Standards for the diagnosis and care of patients with chronic obstructive pulmonary disease. Am J Respir Crit Care Med 1995; 152:S77–S120.
63. Ferguson GT, Cherniack RM. Management of chronic obstructive pulmonary disease. N Engl J Med 1993; 328:1017–1022.
64. Ikeda A, Nishimura K, Koyama H, Izumi T. Comparative dose-response study of three anticholinergic agents and fenoterol using a metered dose inhaler in patients with chronic obstructive pulmonary disease. Thorax 1995; 50:62–66.
65. Skorodin MS, Gross NJ, Moritz T, King FW, Armstrong W, Wells D, Galavan E, Slutsky L. Oxitropium bromide, a new anticholinergic bronchodilator. Ann Allergy 1986; 56:229–232.
66. Maesen FPV, Smeets JJ, Sledsens TJH, Wald FDM, Cornelissen PJ. Tiotropium bromide, a new long-acting antimuscarinic bronchodilator: a pharmacodynamic study in patients with chronic obstructive pulmonary disease (COPD). Eur Respir J 1995; 8: 1506–1513.
67. O'Connor BJ, Towse LJ, Barnes PJ. Prolonged effect of tiotropium bromide on methacholine-induced bronchoconstriction in asthma. Am J Respir Crit Care Med 1996; 154:876–880.
68. Disse B, Speck GA, Rominger KL, Witek TJ Jr, Hammer R. Tiotropium (Spiriva): mechanistical considerations and clinical profile in obstructive lung disease. Life Sci 1999; 64:457–464.
69. Expert Panel: Guidelines for the Diagnosis and Management of Asthma. NIH Report 97-4051A. Bethesda, MD: National Institutes of Health, 1997:1–50.
70. Vichyanond P, Sladek WA, Sur S, Hill MR, Szefler SJ, Nelson HS. Efficacy of

atropine methylnitrate alone and in combination with albuterol in children with asthma. Chest 1990; 98:637–642.

71. Sur S, Mohiuddin AA, Vichyanond P, Nelson HS. A random double-blind trial of the combination of nebulized atropine methylnitrate and albuterol in nocturnal asthma. Ann Allergy 1990; 65:384–388.

72. Ind PW, Dixon CM, Fuller RW, Barnes PJ. Anticholinergic blockade of beta-blocker-induced bronchoconstriction. Am Rev Respir Dis 1989; 139:1390–1394.

73. Grieco MH, Pierson RN Jr. Mechanism of bronchoconstriction due to beta adrenergic blockade: studies with practolol, propranolol, and atropine. J Allergy Clin Immunol 1971; 48:143–152.

74. Siafakas NM, Vermeire P, Pride NB, Paoletti P, Gibson J, Howard P, Yernault JC, Decramer M, Higgenbottom T, Potsma DS, Rees J. Optimal assessment and management of chronic obstructive pulmonary disease (COPD). Eur Respir J 1995; 8:1398–1420.

75. Nisar M, Earis JE, Pearson MG, Calverley PMA. Acute bronchodilator trials in chronic obstructive pulmonary disease. Am Rev Respir Dis 1992; 146:555–559.

76. Rennard SI, Serby CW, Ghafouri M, Johnson PA, Friedman M. Extended therapy with ipratropium is associated with improved lung function in COPD: a retrospective analysis of data from seven clinical trials. Chest 1996; 110:62–70.

77. Snider GL, Faling LJ, Rennard SI. Chronic bronchitis and emphysema. In: Murray JF, Nadel JA, eds. Textbook of Respiratory Medicine. Philadelphia: Saunders, 1994:1331–1397.

78. Gibson GJ. Pulmonary hyperinflation a clinical overview. Eur Respir J 1996; 9: 2640–2649.

79. Niewoehner DE, Sobonya RE. Structure-function correlations in chronic obstructive pulmonary disease. In: Baum GL, Wolinsky E, eds. Textbook of Pulmonary Diseases. Boston: Little, Brown, 1994:973–993.

80. Solway J, Rossing TH, Saari AF, Drazen JM. Expiratory flow limitation and dynamic pulmonary hyperinflation during high-frequency ventilation. J Appl Physiol 1986; 60:2071–2078.

81. Wijkstra PJ, TenVergert EM, van der Mark TW, Postma DS, Van Altena R, Kraan J, Koeter GH. Relation of lung function, maximal inspiratory pressure, dyspnoea, and quality of life with exercise capacity in patients with chronic obstructive pulmonary disease. Thorax 1994; 49:468–472.

82. Gorini M, Misuri G, Corrado A, Duranti R, Iandelli I, De Paola E, Scano E. Breathing pattern and carbon dioxide retention in severe chronic obstructive pulmonary disease. Thorax 1996; 51:677–683.

83. Collett PW, Engel LA. Influence of lung volume on oxygen cost of resistive breathing. J Appl Physiol 1986; 61:16–24.

84. Belman MJ, Botnick WC, Shin JW. Inhaled bronchodilators reduce dynamic hyperinflation during exercise in patients with chronic obstructive pulmonary disease. Am J Respir Crit Care Med 1996; 153:967–975.

85. Ikeda A, Nishimura K, Koyama H, Tsukino M, Mishima M, Izumi T. Dose re-

sponse study of ipratropium bromide aerosol on maximum exercise performance in stable patients with chronic obstructive pulmonary disease. Thorax 1996; 51: 48–53.

86. Pellegrino R, Brusasco V. Lung hyperinflation and flow limitation in chronic airway obstruction. Eur Respir J 1997; 10:543–549.

87. Yan S, Kaminski D, Sliwinski P. Reliability of inspiratory capacity for estimating end-expiratory lung volume changes during exercise in patients with chronic obstructive pulmonary disease. Am J Respir Crit Care Med 1997; 156:55–59.

88. Tantucci C, Duguet A, Similowski T, Zelter M, Derenne JP, Milic-Emili J. Effect of salbutamol on dynamic hyperinflation in chronic obstructive pulmonary disease patients. Eur Respir J 1998; 12:799–804.

89. Pulmonary rehabilitation: joint ACCP/AACVPR evidence-based guidelines. ACCP/AACVPR Pulmonary Rehabilitation Guidelines Panel: American College of Chest Physicians. American Association of Cardiovascular and Pulmonary Rehabilitation (see comments). Chest 1997; 112:1363–1396.

90. Anthonisen NR, Wright E. Bronchodilator response in chronic obstructive pulmonary disease. Am Rev Respir Dis 1986; 133:814–819.

91. Anthonisen NR, Connett JE, Kiley JP, Altose MD, Bailey WC, Buist AS, Conway WA, Enright PL, Kanner RE, O'Hara P, Owens GR, Scanlon PD, Tashkin DP, Wise RA. Effects of smoking intervention and the use of an inhaled anticholinergic bronchodilator on the rate of decline of FEV_1. JAMA 1994; 272:1497–1505.

6

Circadian Rhythm Dependencies of Asthma Medications and Their Chronotherapy

MICHAEL H. SMOLENSKY

University of Texas Health Science
    Center
Houston, Texas

GILBERT E. D'ALONZO

Temple University School of Medicine
Philadelphia, Pennsylvania

ALAIN E. REINBERG

Fondation Adolph de Rothschild
Paris, France

I. Introduction

Nocturnal symptoms are a clinical feature of most asthma patients. Nonetheless, the contents of published consensus reports (1–3) have largely neglected this fact in formulating treatment plans. Although the consensus reports recognize the need to reduce the 24-h variability in airflow and prevent nocturnal exacerbations, treatment strategies recommended for achieving these goals are imprecise. Moreover, the guidelines convey the impression all of the various long-acting aerosol and tablet bronchodilator medications are of equal efficiency in controlling asthma during the day and night and that medicines within the different classes—like sustained-release (SR) β_2-agonists, theophyllines, or corticosteroids—are interchangeable. Furthermore, the there is no mention of the potential role of drug dosing time on the kinetics and effects of asthma medications. This article reviews the manner in which circadian rhythms in gastrointestinal and organ functions affect the pharmacokinetics and pharmacodynamics of commonly prescribed asthma medications. It also focuses on progress in the chronotherapy of asthma—that is, treatment strategies aimed at optimizing the effects of medicines by timing conventional or special dosage forms to circadian rhythms of disease activity.

II. β₂-Adrenergic Therapies

SR terbutaline and albuterol tablet medications are popular asthma treatments (4–8). Sometimes they are dosed in unequal morning and evening doses to optimize their effect on nocturnal asthma (9–11). Short-acting β-agonist medications are useful in managing acute episodic attacks of asthma but not in the long-term management of the disease. The duration of action of short-acting β-agonist therapies is generally no longer than 4 to 6 h. The consequence of this is clearly shown by the results of a study in which albuterol was used on a regular qid basis; patients continued to experience asthma attacks most frequently between 4 and 8 A.M. (12) (Fig. 1). In contrast, the incidence of nighttime symptoms was moderated with a medication having a greater duration of effect, SR theophylline, dosed twice daily.

Short-acting β-agonist aerosol therapies have been used by several investigators to explore circadian rhythm–dependent differences in bronchodilator effect. In day-active persons, infused or inhaled epinephrine achieved best bronchodilation and highest peak expiratory flows (PEF) when dosed at 4 P.M. (13,14). Administration of the same dose at 4 A.M. produced considerably less bronchodilation and lower PEFs (Fig. 2). At all times of treatment, the airflow response to epinephrine was dose-dependent. However, the percentage increase in PEF from the respective clock-time placebo-control baseline was greatest when epinephrine was dosed at 4 A.M. Similar findings have been documented in studies with orciprenaline in asthmatic children and with isoproterenol in healthy persons (15–17).

SR albuterol and terbutaline tablets are commonly prescribed therapies for asthma; generally, they are ingested at 12-h intervals in equal doses (4–8). Nonetheless, significant overnight declines in airflow rates and exacerbations of nocturnal asthma remain problematic, particularly in patients with severe asthma. An unequal morning-evening dosing regimen of terbutaline tablets with one-third of the daily dose taken at 8 A.M. and the remaining two-thirds at 8 P.M. has been explored as a chronotherapy of nocturnal asthma (11). This treatment strategy significantly improved the mean 24-h PEF and FEV₁ and markedly attenuated the nocturnal decline in airflow (Fig. 3).

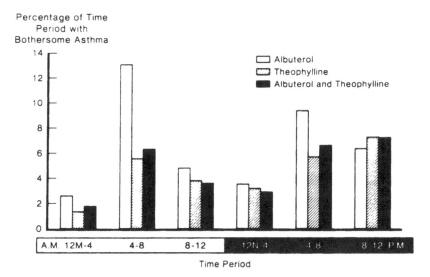

Figure 1   The timing of acute exacerbation of asthma during the 24 h in 18 patients studied during a month-long period of treatment by inhaled albuterol or SR theophylline tablet therapy. Asthma was two times more frequent between 04:00 (4 A.M.) and 08:00 (8 A.M.) during albuterol-only than with SR theophylline treatment. These findings show the effect-duration of albuterol is too short to be protective against nocturnal asthma. (From Ref. 12.)

A tablet form of albuterol (Proventil Repetabs, Schering, USA) has also been assessed as a chronotherapy of nocturnal asthma. This formulation releases medication in a pulse-like fashion, working as a tablet within a tablet. An outer coat of albuterol surrounds an inner coat. A third insoluble antacid coat that degrades in an alkaline environment protects an inner core of albuterol until the medication reaches the small intestine. Thus, one-half of the 4-mg dose is released from the outer coat within the initial 6 h of ingestion and the remaining 2 mg is released from the inner core during the subsequent 6 h. Therapeutic levels of albuterol are thus sustained over the 12-h dosing interval (4,18–20).

Storms and coworkers (21) studied the chronotherapy of Proventil Repetabs in 98 presumably diurnally active patients exhibiting nighttime declines in FEV_1 of at least 15% and who had a medical history of asthma-induced sleep disruptions of 3 nights per week or more. In a placebo-controlled study, patients received a fixed 4-mg dose of albuterol in the morning and varying

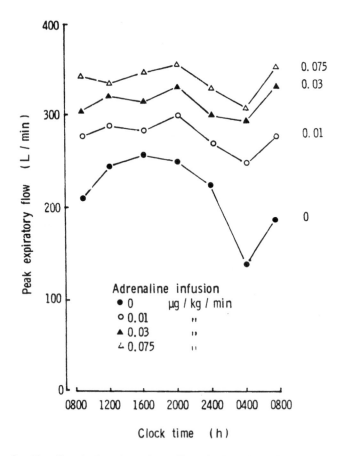

Figure 2 Circadian rhythm–dependent effect of adrenaline infusion on airway patency in presumably diurnally active asthmatic persons. The airway response to adrenaline is dose-dependent; the greater the dose, the greater the increase in peak expiratory flow (PEF) over the clock-time reference value determined under placebo infusion. Daytime in comparison to nighttime adrenaline infusions result in greatest PEF values. However, the percent increase in PEF from baseline is greatest with drug infusion at 04:00 (4 A.M.). Day-night differences in adrenaline effect on pulmonary function result from circadian rhythmicity in β-adrenergic tone. (From Ref. 14.)

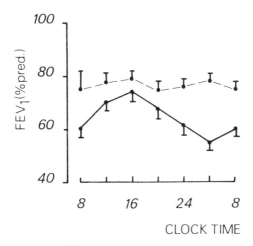

Figure 3 Chronotherapy of SR terbutaline achieved by an unequal morning (5 mg)–evening (10 mg) dosing regimen in diurnally active patients with reversible airway disease. The upper curve shows the circadian pattern in FEV_1 when one-third the daily dose of terbutaline is taken at 08:00 (8 A.M.) and the remaining two-thirds at 20:00 (8 P.M.). The 24-h mean FEV_1 is significantly increased over placebo conditions (lower curve) and the nocturnal decline in airway caliber averted. (From Ref. 11.)

doses, from 4 to 16 mg, at bedtime. The unequal morning-evening Proventil Repetabs dosing regimens reduced the number of nights when PEF declined by more than 15% and, most importantly, the number of nights disturbed by asthma.

Another SR albuterol tablet therapy that makes use of a different drug-delivery system (Volmax, Glaxo, UK; Muro, USA) has also been assessed as a chronotherapy for nocturnal asthma. Volmax relies on osmotic pump tablet technology to achieve the controlled and steady release of albuterol over 12- to 24-h dosing intervals (7,22–24). Moore-Gillon (25) studied 34 patients experiencing asthma at least 5 nights per week. In comparison with placebo, 8 mg of Volmax administered as a single evening dose resulted in higher morning PEF and better overnight asthma control. Van Keimpema and associates (26) studied 35 patients who had a medical history of nocturnal asthma attacks or significant overnight decline in PEF. Of these patients, 32 used inhaler corticosteroids. An equal-dose, equal-interval, twice-daily Volmax regimen was compared with a once-daily evening regimen and with placebo. Although the twice-daily albuterol treatment group improved slightly, this investigation failed to demonstrate that a dose of 8 mg of albuterol, as Volmax, whether ingested all at once in the evening or twice daily at 12-h intervals, significantly alleviates the risk of nocturnal asthma. Finally, Creemers (27) compared the efficacy of a once-a-day evening dose of either 8 mg of Volmax or 300 mg of SR theophylline (Theo-Dur, Key-Schering, USA; Astra Draco, Sweden) in a study of 55 patients complaining of asthma-induced sleep disruption at least 5 nights per week. Compared to the run-in control period, both medications were equally effective in reducing asthma-induced sleep disruption. Evening Volmax treatment, however, better enhanced the stability of pulmonary function during the 24 h and better controlled daytime asthma symptoms than the evening SR theophylline therapy.

A prodrug of terbutaline marketed in Europe, bambuterol (Bambec, Astra Draco, Sweden), exerts a bronchodilator effect for as long as 24 h with less adverse effects than albuterol and terbutaline. Bambuterol is the carbamate prodrug of terbutaline, which possesses high affinity for lung tissue and substantial presystemic metabolic stability. Hydrolysis and oxidation of the parent compound are controlled by plasma cholinesterase and cytochrome P-450 enzymes. Because plasma cholinesterase is reversibly inhibited by bambuterol in a dose-dependent manner, its metabolism takes place in a slow and controlled fashion throughout the 24 h (28,29). D'Alonzo and colleagues (30) compared the effect of a once-a-day 7 A.M. versus 10 P.M. 20-mg regimen of bambuterol in 22 diurnally active patients with a history of nocturnal asthma. This double-blind, placebo-controlled study evaluated the kinetics and dynamics of bambuterol under rigidly controlled experimental conditions, including around-the-clock subject sequestration and control of meal composition and timing. Inpatient studies assessed airway function and adverse drug effects at 3-h intervals during a series of 36-h inpatient investigations. Associated outpatient 7-day diary studies further surveyed drug efficacy and safety. The inpatient bambuterol investigations documented a substantial increase in the mean 24-h FEV_1 relative to placebo no matter the dosing time (Fig. 4). Both the morning and evening treatment regimens improved pulmonary function overnight to a comparable and substantial extent relative to the placebo condition. However, evening in comparison to morning dosing was better, since it improved the PEF and FEV_1 at 7 A.M., the commencement of the daily activity span, in a statistically significant greater amount. Neither bambuterol treatment regimen was associated with significant cardiovascular or central nervous system side effects, including tachycardia and tremor.

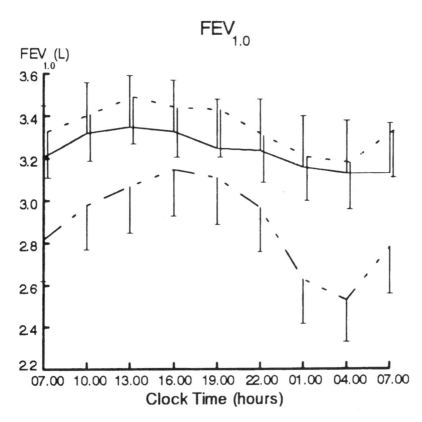

Figure 4 Mean FEV₁ measured every 3 h throughout the day and night during three steady-state conditions of treatment—20 mg bambuterol in the morning and 20 mg bambuterol in the evening versus placebo in 22 asthmatic patients. The lower plot shows the circadian rhythm in FEV₁ under placebo treatment and the upper solid and dashed lines indicate bambuterol treatment in the morning and evening, respectively. The 24-h mean FEV₁ and, in particular, the 04:00 (4 A.M.) FEV₁ are significantly greater for bambuterol versus placebo. Evening bambuterol treatment is superior to either one of the other two treatments since it increases the awakening (07:00 or 7 A.M.) FEV₁ to the greatest extent. (From Ref. 30.)

Other studies demonstrate the substantial efficacy of bambuterol in controlling nocturnal asthma. Petrie and coworkers (31) compared evening bambuterol and placebo treatment in 28 apparently diurnally active patients with nocturnal asthma. All were symptomatic despite the use of inhaled β-agonists, inhaled corticosteroids (mean daily dose 1500 μg), and oral corticosteroids by eight patients (mean daily dose, 10 mg). This randomized double-blind, crossover study involved patients who exhibited a 20% or greater overnight decline in PEF during 7 of the 14 days of run-in. The 20-mg evening dose of bambuterol produced a mean improvement of 16% in the morning PEF and mean improvement of 10% in the evening PEF measured 24 h after the previous drug administration. Evening bambuterol significantly reduced the frequency and intensity of nocturnal asthma as well as use of inhaled β_2-agonist rescue medicine.

Gunn and colleagues (32) compared the efficacy and safety of once-daily evening bambuterol versus twice-daily albuterol (Volmax) as therapies of nocturnal asthma. A total of 152 adult patients with nocturnal asthma who were concomitantly treated with a regimen of inhaled corticosteroid therapy received one of the β-agonists for 3 weeks and then the other for the same duration in an unblinded crossover investigation. Both therapies significantly increased lung function parameters and, more importantly, decreased the severity of nocturnal asthma symptoms by 63% relative to the baseline situation. Compared to the albuterol medication, bambuterol reduced the severity of tremor—considered in terms of both the number of days it occurred and its intensity when experienced—as a side effect. Moreover, patient preference was greater for the evening once-a-day bambuterol than twice-a-day albuterol (Volmax) treatment. The authors concluded that both bambuterol and albuterol were effective; however, patients preferred bambuterol, since it had to be taken only once a day and caused less adverse effects.

The long-acting inhaled β-agonists salmeterol (Glaxo-UK and Glaxo-USA) and formoterol (Ciba Geigy, Europe) are also popular asthma treatments. Each has a duration of action of approximately 12 h (33–35), although one study suggests that salmeterol exerts its effect for as long as 18 h (33). The action exerted by formoterol is similar to that of salmeterol, although it is claimed to have a more rapid onset of action (27,36).

So far, salmeterol has been studied more extensively than formoterol. Salmeterol xinafoate, a unique chemical analogue of albuterol, is 10 times more potent and about 750-fold more selective for β_2- versus β_1-adrenoceptors than albuterol. Differing from albuterol by an elongated side chain, salmeterol binds to the β_2-receptor in an area termed *the exocite*, with the remainder of the molecule repetitively exciting the receptor by rocking on and off it (38,39). Results of large-scale multicenter clinical investigations on diurnally active patients with mild to moderately severe asthma demonstrate that 12-h interval 50-μg salmeterol aerosol dosing better improves overnight asthma symptoms—as well as morning PEF and FEV_1—than 180–200 μg of albuterol aerosol medication inhaled four times daily (40–48). Attenuation of the frequency of nighttime asthma resulted in a concomitant decreased reliance upon aerosol rescue $β_2$-agonist medication and improved nighttime sleep plus enhanced daytime performance (43). A recent study by Weersink and associates (49) evaluated the effect of combined salmeterol and inhaled fluticasone corticosteroid therapy, both administered twice-daily in the morning and evening. The FEV_1 at 4 A.M. and 4 P.M. was normalized, and the bronchial hyperresponsiveness to adenosine-5′-monophosphate was markedly reduced when the two aerosol medications were used in combination.

Faurschou and coworkers (50) compared the safety and efficacy of a regimen of 50 μg salmeterol dosed twice daily and 100 μg dosed only at night relative to placebo treatment in 41 adult patients with poorly controlled asthma. This double-blind, randomized crossover study, with each treatment period lasting 3 weeks, demonstrated that both the twice-daily and evening-only salmeterol dosing schedules improved the morning and evening PEF in a comparable manner. However, the diurnal variation in PEF was greater with the evening-only regimen, suggesting less stability of airway function over the 24 h. Nonetheless, both salmeterol dosing strategies controlled asthma during the day and night with equal effectiveness, and apparently because of this there was no differential preference by patients for one treatment regimen over the other. Compared to placebo, salmeterol exerted little effect on blood pressure or heart rate. This investigation, albeit a single one, suggests that once-nightly dosing of 100 μg of salmeterol is an effective means of improving the control of asthma in unstable patients treated with a combination of medications that includes oral or inhaled corticosteroids and/or SR theophylline therapy.

Selby and associates (51) compared the effectiveness of 50 μg of salmeterol inhaled at 12-h intervals with dose-titrated SR oral theophylline therapy on sleep quality and cognitive performance in 15 sufferers of nocturnal asthma. Cognitive testing and polysomnography were performed on every patient. The overnight decline in PEF was similar with both treatments, but salmeterol was more protective against nighttime asthma; there were fewer nights of nocturnal awakenings and arousals plus a better quality of life and higher level of cognitive performance and visual vigilance in the daytime. Nonetheless, there was no difference in patient preference for one therapy over the other. The authors concluded that there is no major clinical advantage of salmeterol over theophylline in patients with nocturnal asthma. Nonetheless, the better quality of sleep and life plus higher daytime cognitive functioning favor salmeterol.

Finally, Martin and colleagues (52) compared the effect of 84 μg of salmeterol inhaled every 12 h versus albuterol as Volmax (Muro) taken in tablet doses of 4 mg in the morning and 8 mg in the evening in 46 patients with a medical history of nocturnal asthma. Relative to the run-in baseline, both treatments significantly improved PEFR and FEV_1. However, nighttime asthma was somewhat better controlled by the twice-a-day equal-interval, equal-dose salmeterol regimen. Even though there was no difference in the percentage of patients who were not awoken by nocturnal symptoms, there was greater use of beta-agonist rescue medicine by those treated with Volmax in the evening. Overall, the several studies indicate that the asymmetrical morning-evening dosing regimen of tablet β_2-agonist therapy is advantageous in the control of nocturnal asthma; however, it has not been demonstrated whether it is better than long-acting aerosol therapy taken twice a day.

III. Anticholinergic Therapies

Cholinergic tone is thought to play a role in precipitating asthma. It is speculated that the circadian rhythm in vagal tone is amplified in asthma patients, and in this regard there seems to be a relationship between the worsening of airway inflammation and the upregulation of muscarinic receptors at night. Nonetheless, the impact of anticholinergic medications on improving airflow and controlling nocturnal asthma is quite variable between patients. Overall, the therapeutic effectiveness of anticholinergic medications has been disappointing. Some investigations show these agents improve asthma and moderate the nighttime decline in airflow, while others do not (53,54). Differences in the findings between studies may be related to problems of dosing strategy— poor choice of dosing time or inappropriate distribution of doses during the 24 h—and/or disparities in the duration of therapeutic activity of the various medicines plus differences between patients in their responsiveness to them.

Administration time–dependent differences in the effect of anticholinergic medications have been little investigated. Gaultier and coworkers (15) assessed the effect of two dose levels of inhaled ipratropium bromide at different clock times on airflow resistance in a group of diurnally active children. The low dose reduced airflow resistance when administered at 7 A.M. but not at 10 P.M. The high one, in contrast, was effective when administered at both times. Coe and Barnes (53) studied the effect of 0.2 and 0.4 mg of oxitropium administered at bedtime to 18 asthma patients for a 2-week period. The low dose was not effective in attenuating the nocturnal fall in airflow; however, the high one was. It reduced the decline in PEF by 40% compared to placebo. Individual differences were identified between patients in their response to the vagolytic agent. Some showed a marked improvement in airflow, while others did not. In the responsive patients, approximately half of the study group, a dose-dependent effect was documented. The greater the bedtime dose, the greater the moderation of the overnight decline in PEF. Other investigators also found that late-night or early-morning dosing of anticholinergic medications reduces the nocturnal fall in PEF (15,53–56). The collective results of these studies imply that (1) there are individual differences between patients in their responsiveness to anticholinergic agents, (2) the effect of at least some vagolytic medications varies with the time of their administration, and (3) high doses of medications may be required, especially at night even by responsive patients, to be effective against nocturnal asthma.

Morrison and colleagues (56) compared the effect of atropine versus placebo on PEF when dosed intravenously at 4 P.M. and 4 A.M. in patients who exhibited a 20% or greater overnight fall in PEF. In comparison to placebo, the 4 A.M. atropine infusion significantly improved the nighttime PEF, from an average value of 260 L/min with placebo to 390 L/min with atropine. The 4 P.M. atropine infusion also had a significant although tempered effect on PEF. The PEF was 400 L/min with placebo and 440 L/min with atropine (Fig. 5).

Long-acting inhaled anticholinergic agents are now under investigation. Tiotropium bromide, a novel anticholinergic agent, has a long duration of action and kinetic receptor selectivity for the M_1 and M_3 subtypes of muscarinic receptors. O'Connor and coworkers (57) used this medication to treat a group of adult asthmatic patients not necessarily prone to nocturnal exacerbations. Once-a-day morning administration resulted in prolonged bronchodilator response and protection against methacholine challenge. Cazzola and associates (58) investigated telenzepin, a M_1-selective muscarinic receptor antagonist, administered orally at bedtime to nocturnal asthma patients. Although the 1.5-, 3-, and 5-mg doses increased the PEF at 6 A.M. and midnight relative to placebo baselines, it was ineffective in preventing breakthrough asthma overnight. Further studies are required to fully assess the value of anticholinergic medications in the management of nocturnal asthma, particularly in regard to dose and timing.

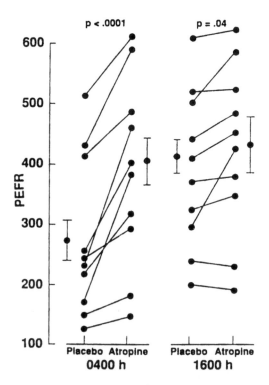

Figure 5 Effect of vagal blockade induced by i.v. infusion of atropine at 16:00 (4 P.M.) or 04:00 (4 A.M.) on peak expiratory flow rate (PEFR) in 10 asthmatic subjects. Vagal blockade results in significant bronchodilation at both treatment times; however, the magnitude of improvement in PEFR from the pretreatment baseline level is greatest with the 4 A.M. atropine treatment. (From Ref. 56.)

IV. Theophylline Therapies

Theophylline is a weak bronchodilator that exerts anti-inflammatory action (59–62). The exact manner in which theophylline exerts this action remains to be clearly elucidated. It inhibits the late-phase bronchospastic reaction triggered by inhaled allergen, increases the titer of CD8 cells in peripheral blood, and decreases the quantity of T lymphocytes in the airways (59–61,63). Some feel that the attenuation of airway inflammation by theophylline during the night involves leukotriene B_4-mediated mechanisms (64–66).

The kinetics of certain oral SR theophylline formulations can differ dramatically following morning versus evening dosing (67–69). Some SR theophyllines that have been studied under steady-state conditions exhibit shorter T_{max} and greater C_{max} when ingested in the morning than evening; this is particularly true in children and adolescents (Fig. 6). These administration time–dependent differences are not the result of meal timings and contents, since these influences were controlled. Rather, differences in theophylline kinetics arise from circadian rhythms in gastrointestinal function, although alteration in posture during the day and night likely plays a role as well (67,69). Day-night differences in drug absorption rather than elimination seem to be responsible for the difference in theophylline pharmacokinetic behavior.

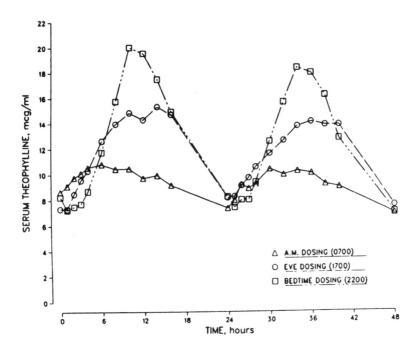

Figure 6 Example of extreme circadian rhythm–dependent differences in the pharmacokinetics of theophylline. Mean steady-state serum theophylline concentrations (STC) during 48-h study spans in healthy subjects administered 900 mg Theo-24 (Whitby, USA) once daily either at 07:00 (7 A.M.), 15:00 (3 P.M.), or 22:00 (10 P.M.) on different occasions. The area under the theophylline-time concentration curve (AUC) differs significantly according to treatment time; it is about threefold greater with once-daily 22:00 (10 P.M.) than 07:00 (7 A.M.) treatment. (From Ref. 68.)

The precipitation and intensity of theophylline-induced side effects may also be circadian rhythm–dependent. Laboratory animal studies clearly demonstrate a greater degree of tolerance to theophylline overdose between the middle and end of the daily rest span than at other times of the 24 h. Drug-induced mortality varied six- to sevenfold according to the timing of drug overdose (70). To date, however, there have been no follow-up studies of circadian rhythms in the tolerance of asthmatic patients to theophylline.

Certain SR theophyllines are specifically designed as asthma chronotherapies. Some are meant to be taken in the morning and evening in unequal doses, while others are intended for ingestion in the evening. The goal of theophylline chronotherapy is to achieve a higher drug level during the night than the day, since this is when airway patency is poorest and inflammation greatest and the risk of asthma highest. The German pharmaceutical company Byk Gulden appears to have been the first to embrace the concept of theophylline chronotherapy. In the early 1980s, it marketed Euphyllin; one-third of the daily dose of the medicine is ingested in the morning and the remaining two-thirds are taken before bedtime (71,72). This dosing strategy has a profound effect on nocturnal asthma, but the atypical dosing regimen is inconvenient.

Presently, once-a-day theophylline formulations are used to accomplish chronotherapy. Euphylong (Byk Gulden, Germany) and Uniphyl/Uniphyllin (Purdue Pharma, USA; Mundipharma, Germany) are the most popular theophylline chronotherapies in Asia, Europe, and United States (73,74). Figure 7 compares the pharmacokinetics and pharmacodynamics of a conventional theophylline ingested in equal doses at 12 h intervals with a chronotherapy ingested in the evening. The theophylline chronotherapy results in a greater level of medication overnight than the conventional treatment; as a consequence,

---

Figure 7 Comparison of day-night serum theophylline concentration (STC) and peak expiratory flow (PEF) with 20:00 (8 P.M.) once-daily chronotherapy of Uniphyllin (Munidpharma, Germany), a medication essentially identical to Uniphyl, shown as a solid line, versus bid SR theophylline (Phyllotemp) dosed at 08:00 (8 A.M.) and 20:00 (8 P.M.), shown as a dashed line in 9 asthmatic patients. Conventional 12-h SR theophylline dosing achieves a relatively stable STC; in contrast, evening chronotherapy results in large STC fluctuations characterized by intentionally elevated nighttime drug level. The nocturnal decline in PEF is excessive with the SR bid theophylline but significantly attenuated with the evening chronotherapy. Single arrows along the *x* axis indicate times of the twice-daily SR conventional treatment and double arrows indicate once-daily evening chronotherapy. (From Refs. 73 and 74.)

Theophylline
serum
concentration
(mg/L)

PEFR
(L/min)

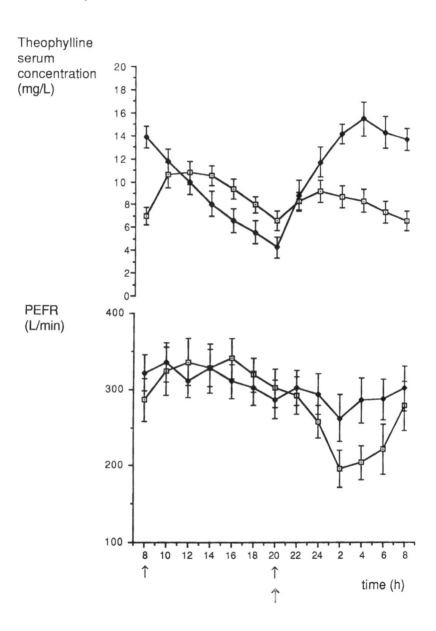

time (h)

it better attenuates the nocturnal dip in airflow and risk of asthma (75). Moreover, the increased nighttime protection against asthma is achieved without the elevated risk of daytime attacks. Reinberg and coworkers (76) reported similar results with another European SR theophylline formulation administered once a day in the evening. Collectively, the results of these well-controlled trials clearly support the conclusion that the airway response to theophylline at night depends on the serum concentration that is achieved then; the greater the nighttime drug level, the greater the improvement in PEF and FEV_1 (74). One study found that when Uniphyl was dosed in the evening to achieve an average serum theophylline concentration at 4 A.M. of 15.4 µg/mL, the neutrophil cell content and macrophage leukotriene B_4 concentration of bronchoalveolar lavage samples were significantly depressed in asthma patients studied at that hour (64–66). Moreover, drug-induced attenuation of the nocturnal fall in FEV_1 was correlated with the decrease of neutrophil cell count in bronchoalveolar lavage specimens ($r = 0.53$; $p < 0.01$). In addition, the change in the leukotriene B_4 concentration was significantly correlated with the theophylline-induced decrease in lavage granulocytes, neutrophils, and eosinophils. These findings further confirm that theophylline attenuates airway inflammation during the night, apparently involving a leukotriene B_4-mediated mechanism.

V. Glucocorticoid Therapy

Aerosol corticotherapy is recommended as a first-line of treatment for asthma (77–80). Glucocorticoids inhibit lung macrophages, T lymphocytes, and eosinophils as well as epithelial and other cells involved in airway inflammation (81,82). It decreases eosinophil cell numbers, especially low-density ones, by inducing apoptosis, and it reduces mast cell density in lung tissue. Glucocorticoids decrease mucus secretion and inhibit plasma exudation. Aerosol forms are preferred for the long-term management of asthma, in which chronic inflammation is characteristic, while tablet formulations are reserved for treating severe exacerbations and chronic severe, unstable asthma.

Administration-time differences in the pharmacokinetics of synthetic corticosteroid tablet medications have been little studied; nonetheless, several reports document them (83–86). For example, English et al. (84) assessed the kinetics of prednisolone tablets administered in a dosage of 2 mg/kg to a group of diurnally active healthy subjects. At 7-day intervals, separate administration-time studies were done at 6 A.M., noon, 6 P.M., and midnight under carefully controlled conditions to exclude effects of meal timing and contents. C_{max} and AUC were greatest and elimination half-life shortest with the noontime ingestion, while the T_{max} and apparent volume of distribution were greatest with the 6 P.M. one.

Circadian rhythm–dependent differences in the effects of corticosteroid medications have been investigated more in regard to adrenal suppression than pulmonary function. Ceresa et al. (87) infused methylprednisolone (MP) at rate of 660 µg/h or placebo at different spans of the day and night to a group of diurnally active healthy subjects. When MP was infused continuously between 8 A.M. and 4 P.M., cortisol secretion was unaffected. In contrast, when infused between 4 P.M. and 8 P.M., cortisol suppression was moderate. When MP was infused between midnight and 4 A.M., cortisol suppression was marked (Fig. 8). The dosing-time difference in MP effect on cortisol secretion results from the circadian rhythm in the susceptibility of the hypothalamic–pituitary–adrenocortical (HPA) axis to inhibition; inhibition is more likely and more severe when synthetic corticosteroids are infused late in the day and at night than in the morning or early afternoon. Additional clinical studies conducted primarily since the 1960s confirm this. Morning once-daily ingestion of small to moderate doses of corticosteroid medicines in tablet form causes little or no adrenocortical suppression. In contrast, when the same daily dose is split into several equal administrations that include an ingestion in the late afternoon or evening, significant HPA axis suppression is likely (88,89).

Investigation of circadian differences in the beneficial effect of MP on airway function began more than 20 years ago by Reinberg and colleagues (90). Twelve symptom-free, diurnally active, asthmatic boys between 7 and 12 years of age received single injections of 40 mg MP at 3 A.M., 7 A.M., 3 P.M., and 7 P.M. in random order during different study weeks. PEF was self-assessed five times daily 2 days before injection, the day of injection, and the day following each timed injection. MP improved the 24-h mean PEF at least to some extent after each timed treatment; however, improvement was best following the 3 P.M. one (Fig. 9).

Investigations by Beam and coworkers (91) confirm and extend the findings of Reinberg and associates (90). Seven diurnally active patients with a history of nighttime asthma and documented decline of PEF by at least 15% were studied. According to a double-blind, placebo-controlled crossover protocol, patients received either placebo or a 50-mg dose of prednisone as tablets at 8 A.M., 3 P.M., and 8 A.M. in different trials. The effect of the large dose of prednisone varied greatly with the time of treatment. Attenuation of the nocturnal decline in FEV_1 was best when the medicine was dosed at 3

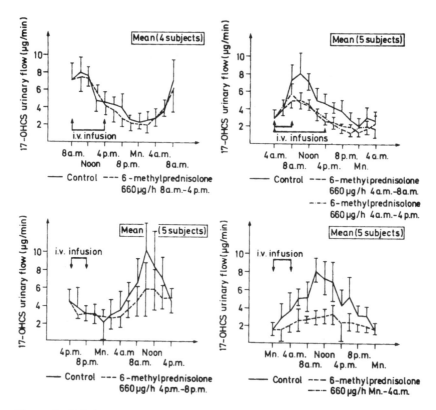

Figure 8 Infusion of 6-methylprednisolone (660 μg/h) during different 4, 8, or 12-h periods of the day or night resulted in differential suppression of the hypothalamic-adrenocortical-pituitary (HPA) axis as gauged by changes in the urinary excretion of 17-OHCS, the metabolic by-product of cortisol. When the methylprednisolone infusion coincided in time with the circadian stage of elevated cortisol concentration (8 A.M. to 4 P.M.), no suppression of 17-OHCS was induced. In contrast, moderate to severe adrenal suppression resulted from infusions done in the late afternoon and at night, respectively. (From Ref. 87.)

P.M. The average percentage decline in the overnight FEV$_1$ with the 3 P.M. placebo treatment amounted to 28.3%; with the 3 P.M. glucocorticoid dose, the decline was reduced to only 10.4%. Ingestion of high-dose prednisone at 8 A.M. and 8 P.M. was totally ineffective in moderating the overnight dip in FEV$_1$ (Fig. 10). Moreover, only with the 3 P.M. administration was a significant reduction in blood eosinophil count and pancellular BAL cytology achieved.

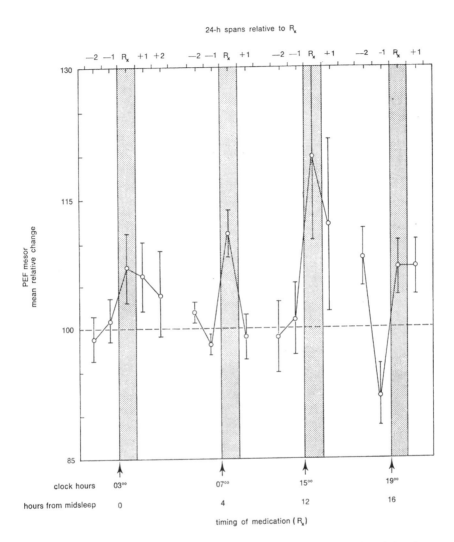

Figure 9 Circadian time-dependent effect of a single 40-mg injection of methylprednisolone on the peak expiratory flow (PEF) of a group of diurnally active asthmatic boys (7–15 years of age). PEF was assessed at five different clock times 2 days before, on the day of medication, and on the day after each of the timed treatments to derive 24-h average values. The data of each of the two pretreatment days were averaged and set equal to 100% as a baseline PEF value. Methylprednisolone only produced an 8% or so improvement in the 24-h mean PEF when injected at 03:00 (3 A.M.) or 19:00 (7 P.M.). The improvement averaged about 11% with (07:00) 7 A.M. treatment and nearly 20% with 15:00 (3 P.M.) treatment. (From Ref. 94.)

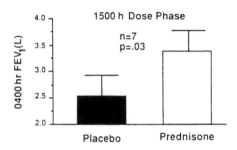

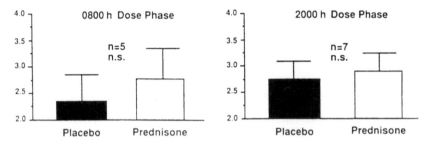

Figure 10 Effect of a single oral 50-mg dose of prednisone versus placebo on the nocturnal decline in FEV$_1$ in a group of diurnally active patients with a medical history of nighttime asthma. Prednisone dosing at 08:00 h (8 A.M.) or 20:00 h (8 P.M.) was no better than placebo in moderating the overnight decline in FEV$_1$. In contrast, oral dosing at 15:00 h (3 P.M.) resulted in a profound and statistically significant attenuation in its nocturnal decline. (From Ref. 91.)

This investigation implies that once-a-day early afternoon glucocorticoid dosing best attenuates the deterioration of nighttime pulmonary function and exacerbated airway inflammation. These findings are consistent with those of Reinberg and colleagues (90) discussed above. They are also consistent with the findings of an earlier study by Kowanko and associates (92) conducted on steroid-dependent arthritic patients. This group of investigators assessed the effect of low-dose (5–6 mg) prednisolone on the grip strength of arthritis sufferers as a function of its ingestion time. During different 1-week study periods, the medicine was taken either at 8 A.M., 1 P.M., or 11 P.M. In more than half the subjects, it was the 1 P.M. treatment that elevated grip strength the most.

The results of a number of investigations suggest that the therapeutic efficiency of synthetic corticosteroid tablet medicines is enhanced when a portion of the daily dose is taken in the early afternoon. However, additional study is yet required to explore whether afternoon-only glucocorticoid chronic dosing of diurnally active asthma patients constitutes the ideal chronotherapy. Under normal conditions, serum cortisol peaks at the commencement of the diurnal activity period. Since the circadian rhythm of cortisol clocks numerous metabolic, cognitive, physical, and other biological processes, the afternoon pulsing of corticotherapy, especially in large doses, for prolonged durations could conceivably alter the body's circadian time structure as a side effect. To date, this chronobiological concern has yet to be assessed.

The daily and alternate-day morning glucocorticoid tablet dosing regimen (Medrol; Upjohn, USA) was the first chronotherapy to be accepted into clinical medicine (93). Both of these morning treatment schedules successfully attenuate side effects, particularly adrenocortical suppression, since in diurnally active persons this is the time when the HPA axis best tolerates elevated steroid levels caused by the administration of exogenous glucocorticoid medication. A more elaborate tablet chronotherapy of corticosteroid medicines (Dutimelan; Hoechst, Italy) was introduced in the 1980s in selected European countries. Dutimelan is a corticosteroid formulation consisting of a different mix and concentration of synthetic glucocorticoids designated for morning (8 A.M.) and afternoon (3 P.M.) ingestion. The clock time, drug composition, and dose strength of the two daily administrations are intended to simulate the circadian rhythm of adrenocorticoid secretion of diurnally active persons to optimize the therapeutic potency and minimize the side effects of this type of treatment. The morning dose consists of 7 mg prednisolone acetate and 4 mg prednisolone alcohol, and the afternoon one consists of 3 mg prednisolone alcohol and 15 mg cortisone acetate. Dutimelan is marketed in two different strengths—''regular,'' as described above, and ''mite,'' which contains the same combination of corticosteroids but in half the dose. Trials by Reinberg and coworkers (94) have demonstrated the efficacy of this chronotherapy in patients with steroid-dependent asthma. A 1-month course of Dutimelan treatment improved PEF significantly without inducing adrenal inhibition or other side effects (Fig. 11). Comparable findings were published by Crepaldi and Muggeo (95) and Serafini and Bonini (96).

Since asthma is a nocturnal disease, many practitioners feel that glucocorticoids should be administered at night. The findings of Beam and colleagues (91) showed that the ingestion of a single large tablet dose of prednisone at 8 P.M. was totally ineffective in averting the overnight deterioration

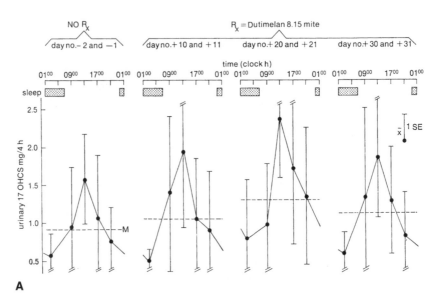

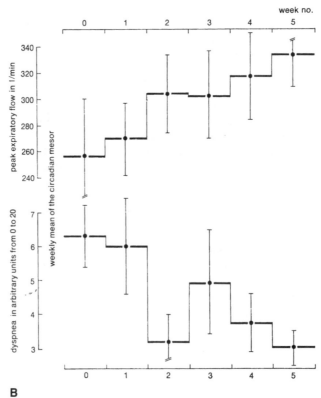

A

B

of airway patency. Reinberg and associates (90) also found that a large evening MP dose was only marginally effective in improving the PEF of asthmatic boys. The results of another investigation by Reinberg and associates (97) were the same. This group compared the effect of the twice-daily Dutimelan medication regimen given as intended—a strong dose in the morning, at 8 A.M., a weak dose at 3 P.M., and placebo at 8 P.M. (designated as DTM_{8-15})—versus a regimen in which the strong dose was given at 8 P.M., a weak one at 3 P.M., and placebo at 8 A.M. (designated as DTM_{15-20}). Eight asthmatic patients were studied using a double-blind, crossover protocol with each DTM treatment regimen administered for 8 days. DTM_{8-15} in comparison to DTM_{15-20} was more effective in improving and stabilizing pulmonary function throughout the entire 24 h (Fig. 12). These results are consistent with the conclusion that the dosing of synthetic corticosteroids in the evening has little beneficial effect on asthma control. Moreover, as discussed above, the ingestion of glucocorticoid medicines in the evening confers added risk of HPA axis suppression.

Inhaled glucocorticoids are routinely prescribed for the management of airway inflammation in asthma (77–80). Beclomethasone dipropionate, budesonide, flunisolide, fluticasone, and triamcinolone are the most common of the aerosol glucocorticoid preparations marketed presently, although not all of them are available in every country. Desired properties of inhaled glucocorticoids are high binding affinity, high topical potency, low systemic bioavailability, and rapid systemic clearance. Systemic absorption of inhaled glucocorticoids can be great, depending on the patient's skill level and drug-delivery technique. As much as 80–90% of the inhaled dose may be deposited in the oropharynx and swallowed. Only about 10% of the dose may reach the lung (98). Systemic drug exposure due to poor technique and absorption from the lung can be significant. Flunisolide and budesonide both undergo extensive first-pass liver metabolism; thus, relatively low amounts of these medications circulate systemically (99–100). Fluticasone possesses low oral availability,

Figure 11 Circadian rhythm of urinary 17-OHCS (top, panel A) plus weekly mean 24-h peak expiratory flow (PEF) and self-assessed dyspnea level (bottom, panel B) 2 days before (no medication) and at 10-day intervals during treatment of nine diurnally active asthmatics undergoing 1 month of chronocorticotherapy with low-dose (mite formulation) administration of Dutimelan 8-15 (Hoechst, Italy). The corticosteroid chronotherapy increased PEF and decreased dyspnea markedly without induction of adrenal suppression or alteration of the circadian rhythm in 17-OHCS excretion. (From Ref. 94.)

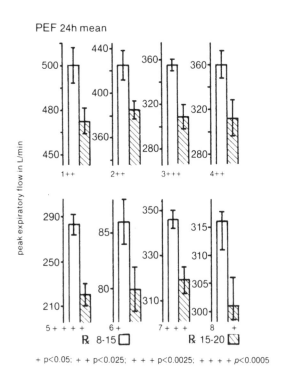

+ p<0.05; + + p<0.025; + + + p<0.0025; + + + + *p*<0.0005

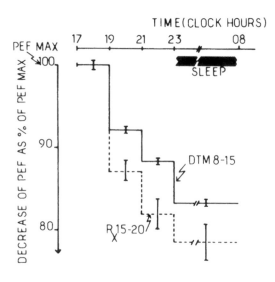

thereby minimizing its potential to induce systemic effects when used in low doses (101), although in higher dose it can cause HPA axis suppression (102,103). Beclomethasone dipropionate is administered as a prodrug and undergoes conversion in the lung to the active monopropionate form (104,105); nonetheless, it too can induce adrenal suppression when taken in higher doses.

Various types of side effects have been ascribed to the long-term use of beclomethasone diproprionate, budesonide, and triamcinolone aerosol medicines as reviewed elsewhere (98,103). In general, low-dose aerosol therapy is well tolerated with minimal risk of systemic effects; however, the risk of adverse effects increases with the long-term use of moderate- and especially high-dose regimens (103). Patients with severe asthma are occasionally treated with high-dose aerosol and tablet glucocorticoids. In these patients, it is not always possible to determine if systemic side effects result from the long-term use of aerosol, episodic tablet corticotherapy, or both (98,102).

As discussed above, the time of day when corticosteroid preparations are inhaled or ingested with reference to circadian rhythm of the HPA axis is a determinant of the risk of adrenal suppression and perhaps other unwanted effects. Based on studies done with tablet and parenteral corticosteroids, it is logical to expect that treatment regimens that entail the dosing of aerosol glucocorticoids having a low first-pass effect around supper and bedtime potentiate the risk of adrenal suppression. In this regard, Toogood and coworkers (106) assessed the effect of frequency (twice versus four-times daily administration), circadian (morning-only versus morning and evening) timings, and dose strength of budesonide on the PEF and HPA axis. A significant interaction between daily aerosol dose and administration schedule was detected. Morning doses best conserved endogenous cortisol secretion for budesonide doses greater than 800 µg/day. On the other hand, morning-only treatment schedules consisting of an 8 A.M. or noontime inhalation or a four-dose morning 7 A.M., 9 A.M., 10:30 A.M., and noontime regimen were less effective in improving pulmonary function, although not in a statistically significant manner, than the equal-interval, equal-dose schedule consisting of treatment times spread over the day. Shifting from a four-times-a-day (8 A.M., noon, 5:30 P.M.,

Figure 12 Effect of 8-day treatment with Dutimelan 8–15, versus Dutimelan 15–20 in the same total daily dose on the mean 24-h (top) and nocturnal decline in peak expiratory flow (PEF) (bottom) in eight steroid-dependent asthmatics. The 24-h mean was most improved and the nocturnal decline in PEF best attenuated when the largest of the bid corticosteroid doses was administered not at 8 P.M. but at 8 A.M., at the start of the activity period, that is with the Dutimelan 8–15 treatment. (From Ref. 97.)

and 10 P.M.) to a twice-a-day (8 A.M. and 10.00 P.M.) regimen reduced the effect on PEF.

Meibohm and colleagues (107) used mathematical simulation models based on the data of flunisolide and fluticasone pharmacokinetic and pharmacodynamic studies conducted at a single circadian time to predict their administration time–dependent risk of HPA axis suppression. Their simulations aimed at finding the safest time to take a 500- or 1000-µg dose of the medicines. According to the model, HPA axis suppression is significantly dependent on dosing time. For both flunisolide and fluticasone, induction of greatest HPA axis suppression is predicted from administration at 3 or 4 A.M. The model predicts that flunisolide should be dosed at 7 P.M. and fluticasone at 3 P.M. to minimize this side effect.

The findings of the simulation model are inconsistent with the literature regarding the vulnerability of the HPA axis to suppression. The literature suggests that administration of tablet and parenteral corticosteroids more than 9 h after the usual time of awakening from sleep, around 3 P.M., in persons adhering to a lifestyle of diurnal activity and nocturnal rest, increases the risk of HPA axis suppression. The later in the day they are administered, the greater the risk and extent of adrenal suppression (88,89). Moreover, the findings of the simulation are also at odds with the work of Toogood and colleagues (106), who found morning budesonide regimens to be most sparing of the HPA axis. Although unstated, two of the underlying assumptions of the simulation model are that (1) the pharmacokinetics of inhaled glucocorticoids and (2) the steroid dose–HPA axis suppression response relationship are invariable (are homeostatic) and independent of drug administration time. The vulnerability of the HPA axis to suppression by exogenous glucocorticoid medicines is strongly associated with circadian rhythms, as discussed earlier in this chapter. Moreover, it may not be true that the pharmacokinetics of aerosol glucocorticoids are invariable with the time of dosing, as suggested by the results of studies on tablet corticosteroids (88). Follow-up drug administration trials on asthmatic patients are required to substantiate the predictions of the simulations. Until then, we feel it is premature to recommend that flunisolide, fluticasone, or other aerosol corticosteroids be dosed preferentially in the late afternoon or evening to minimize the risk of HPA axis suppression.

Studies by Pincus and colleagues (108) addressed the often asked question of when is the best time to dose inhaled glucocorticoids to optimize their therapeutic effect. This group of investigators compared the effect of a regimen of 800 µg of triamcinolone acetate aerosol taken all at once 3 P.M. to one consisting of four daily doses, each of 200 µg, spread over the day. The choice of the afternoon dosing time was based on earlier findings showing that 3 P.M. MP and prednisone tablet dosing is best at improving airway flow rates and attenuating markers of airway inflammation (90,91). Aerosol treatment was taken as directed by two comparable groups of asthmatic patients daily for 4 months, during which PEF was self-assessed every morning and evening. Serum cortisol and urinary 17-OHCS studies were also done before and at the end of treatment. Improvement in the baseline FEV_1 level was comparable between treatments, as were the morning and evening PEFs. There was a trend ($p < 0.07$) toward greater improvement in the evening PEF with the 3 P.M. once-a-day versus the four times-a-day regimen. The systemic response to the two dosing regimens assessed by eosinophil count, morning serum cortisol concentration, and 24-h urinary cortisol studies was also comparable. Moreover, both groups experienced a comparable reduction in the requirement for supplemental β_2-agonist medication. In a follow-up study, the same investigators (109) assessed the effect of the 800-μg triamcinolone dose when administered to comparable groups of asthma patients either all at once at 8 A.M. or 5:30 P.M. or four times a day in 200-μg doses, as in the initial trial. The afternoon once-a-day and qid treatment groups displayed higher morning and evening PEFs than the 8 A.M. group, although the reduction in reliance on β_2-agonists was the same. Overall, the nature of the treatment responses favored, albeit it in a nonstatistically significant manner, the qid schedule. Nonetheless, based on the collective findings of the two triamcinolone studies, the investigators concluded that, in diurnally active subjects, a "window of opportunity" for optimizing the therapeutic efficiency of this medicine may exist in the afternoon.

The optimization of asthma corticotherapy is a complex task. Toogood and colleagues (106), Malo and associates (110), and Dahl and Johansson (111) found that dosing frequency was critical for achieving optimal therapeutic effect. In contrast, Pincus and coworkers (108) demonstrated that the circadian timing of once-a-day triamcinolone aerosol is a critical factor, perhaps of nearly equal importance as dosing frequency. The studies of Beam and associates (91) involving prednisone tablets indicate that morning and bedtime dosing is ineffective in controlling airway inflammation but that 3 P.M. dosing is. Reinberg and coworkers (90) also showed that once-a-day 3 P.M. MP dosing is more effective in improving the 24-h mean PEF than once-a-day 3 A.M., 7 A.M., or 7 P.M. dosing. Furthermore, Reinberg and associates (94) showed that 1 month treatment of asthma patients with Dutimelan, consisting of high-dose glucocorticoids, at 8 A.M. and a lesser yet substantial dose at 3 P.M. results in significant improvement in PEF without HPA axis suppression. Collectively, these studies imply that once-daily aerosol and tablet treatment timed in the afternoon, approximately 8–9 h following the commencement of the diurnal activity span, exerts a superior effect on airways patency and nighttime inflammation. The delivery of glucocorticoid medications at this time most likely interrupts the cascade of events that culminates in the exacerbation of airway inflammation nocturnally (112). However, further investigations involving other times of once-daily corticosteroid administration are required to better define the ideal treatment time.

VI. Mast-Cell Stabilizers

Cromolyn sodium (Intal; Fisons, UK) and nedocromil sodium (Tilade; Fisons, UK), a pyranoquinoline dicarboxylic acid derivative, exert an anti-inflammatory effect on the airways of asthmatic patients. Although the exact mechanism of their action is unknown, it is thought that they block the release of inflammatory mediators from pulmonary mast cells, thereby decreasing airways hyperresponsiveness (113,114). In clinical studies, both medicines have been shown to reduce the number of nights disturbed by asthma, although neither averted the nocturnal fall in spirometric measures (115–120).

Potential circadian rhythm dependencies of these medications have yet to be explored. Morgan et al. (117) assessed the impact of a single high 160-mg cromolyn sodium dose versus placebo at bedtime on nocturnal asthma. The high-dose cromolyn failed to attenuate the nocturnal dip in FEV_1. However, single-dose studies are unlikely to provide an appropriate assessment of this class of medications. Williams and Stableforth (120) demonstrated that four times daily dosing of nedocromil 4 mg delivered by metered-dose inhaler increased the 24-h mean and decreased the amplitude of the PEF circadian rhythm in a statistically significant manner during 12 weeks of treatment. Cessation of nedocromil treatment during an ensuing 12-week period resulted in a reversal of the improvement in pulmonary function to the pretreatment baseline level. Additional investigations are required to determine the circadian rhythm dependencies, if any, of these types of medicines.

VII. Discussion

Epidemiological and clinical studies clearly document that asthma is a nighttime disease in as many as 75% of patients. We feel strongly that the clinical approach to the successful management of asthma patients entails the attenuation of airway inflammation and stabilization of airway flow rates during the critical overnight hours. We feel that it is imperative to control asthma at night in order to control it during the day. One means of achieving this goal is to proportion the concentration of asthma medications to need during the 24 h in a chronotherapeutic manner. The concept of chronotherapeutics in clinical medicine is not new. The first chronotherapy of severe asthma was introduced in the 1960s as the morning daily and alternate-day methylprednisolone schedules. Both these schedules are aimed at averting or minimizing adrenal suppression by timing the glucocorticoid medicine to coincide with the peak of the circadian rhythm in cortisol (93). The morning is when the HPA axis is least vulnerable to suppression by exogenous steroids. During the early 1980s, theophylline chronotherapies were developed and popularized, first in Europe and then in the United States. Evening once-daily therapies that make use of special drug delivery systems produce an elevated theophylline drug level during the night, when the risk of asthma is greatest. Attainment of the highest medication levels then results in an optimization of the effects of theophylline therapy in patients prone to nocturnal bronchospasm. Similar strategies have been employed with SR tablet β_2-agonists medications, particularly in Europe. Today, long-acting inhaled β_2-agonist therapies are preferred. The contents of the package inserts of these medications recommend a twice-daily equal-interval, equal-dose regimen. The merit of an evening-only dosing schedule has been addressed in only one study thus far, and the results were encouraging (50). The findings of trials with anticholinergic medications are far from clear. Some suggest that their beneficial effect can be increased when medication is taken in high dose at night. Research regarding potential circadian rhythm dependencies of mast-cell stabilizer medications has yet to be initiated.

The amount of benefit derived as well as the occurrence and severity of adverse effects of some asthma medications can be significantly affected by the time during the day or night they are ingested, inhaled, or infused. Circadian rhythms in gastrointestinal function, blood flow to vital organs, liver enzyme activity, receptor site number or conformation, plus messenger activities of cells are capable of affecting the behavior of many types of medications (121–123). Based on the concept of homeostasis, it is assumed that the pharmacokinetics and dynamics of all medications are comparable no matter what the dosing time may be. Pharmacokinetic and pharmacodynamic trials are customarily conducted in the morning. In spite of the great number of persons who take at least a portion of their daily dose of medicine at night, we know surprisingly little about the therapeutic efficiency and safety of these drugs when used at any other time than in the morning. The pharmacokinetics of medications need not be the same when they are dosed in the morning and evening, even in fasted subjects. The current knowledge of circadian rhythm dependencies of asthma drugs and other medications is derived primarily from studies that have been conducted by academic scientists working in university rather than pharmaceutical company laboratories. Investigation of differences in the kinetics and effects of asthma medications according to dosing time is not currently required by regulatory agencies, nor is it routinely explored by pharmaceutical companies in Phase I–III studies aimed at documenting the safety and efficacy of new therapies. As a minimum, we feel the kinetics and effects of medicines should be studied at a minimum of two common dosing times, typically in the morning and evening. These recommendations are particularly germane to asthma. Since this is a nighttime disease in most patients, it is critical that medicines be at least as efficient in their effects following evening as after morning administration. Doctors require this information to make informed decisions about the medications they prescribe, and pharmacists require it to educate patients properly as to how and when they should take their medications.

In this chapter we reviewed the circadian rhythm dependencies of several classes of asthma medications. We discussed chronotherapeutic dosing strategies as an effective means of increasing the efficiency of asthma treatments to better avert nighttime attacks and reduce drug-induced side effects. The results of an impressive number of studies demonstrate the utility and merit of the chronotherapeutic approach for bronchodilator and anti-inflammatory medications. However, to date there have been no systematic study of circadian rhythm–adapted regimens of anticholinergic, mast-cell-stabilizing, or leukotriene-modifier or antagonist medicines. Moreover, to date there has been no systematic investigation of how to dose combination therapies consisting of β_2-agonist, theophylline, corticosteroid, or other commonly prescribed medications with reference to the circadian rhythms of asthma. Such investigations are eagerly awaited, especially on difficult-to-control patients, who seemingly are those most likely to benefit from the polychronotherapy of severe asthma.

References

1. National Asthma Education and Prevention Program. Expert Panel Report 2: Guidelines for the Diagnosis and Management of Asthma. NIH pub. no. 97-4051. Bethesda, MD: National Institutes of Health, 1997.

2. National Heart, Lung, and Blood Institute. International Consensus Report on Diagnosis and Management of Asthma. NIH pub. no. 92-3091. Bethesda, MD: National Institutes of Health, 1992.

3. National Heart, Lung, and Blood Institute and World Health Organization. Global Initiative for Asthma. NIH pub. no. 95-3659. Bethesda, MD: National Institutes of Health, 1995.

4. Bogin RM, Ballard RD. Treatment of nocturnal asthma with pulse-release albuterol. Chest 1992; 102:362–366.

5. Eriksson NE, Haglind K, Ljungholm K. A comparison of sustained-release terbutaline and ordinary terbutaline in bronchial asthma. Br J Dis Chest 1982; 76: 202–204.

6. Eriksson L, Jonson B, Eklundh G, et al. Nocturnal asthma: effects of slow-release terbutaline on spirometry and arterial blood gases. Eur Respir J 1988; 1:302–305.

7. Grossman J, Morris RJ, White KD, et al. Improved stability in oral delivery of albuterol provides less variability in bronchodilation in adults with asthma. Ann Allergy 1991; 66:324–327.

8. Maesen FPV, Smeets JJ. Comparison of a controlled-release tablet of salbutamol given twice daily with a standard tablet given four times daily in the management of chronic obstructive lung disease. Eur Respir J 1986; 31:431–436.

9. Postma DS, Koeter GH, Van der Mark TW, et al. The effects of oral slow-release terbutaline on the circadian variation in spirometry and arterial blood gas levels in patients with chronic airflow obstruction. Chest 1985; 87:653–657.

10. Postma DS, Koeter GH, Keyzer JJ. Influence of slow-release terbutaline on the circadian variation of catecholamines, histamine, and lung function in nonallergic patients with partly reversible airflow obstruction. J Allergy Clin Immunol 1986; 77:471–477.

11. Koeter GH, Postma DS, Keyzer JJ, et al. Effect of oral slow-release terbutaline on early morning dyspnea. Eur J Clin Pharmacol 1985; 28:159–162.

12. Joad JP, Ahrens RC, Lindgren SD, et al. Relative efficacy of maintenance therapy with theophylline, inhaled albuterol, and the combination for chronic asthma. J Allergy Clin Immunol 1987; 79:78–85.

13. Barnes PJ, Fitzgerald GA, Dollery CT. Circadian variation in adrenergic response in asthmatic subjects. Clin Sci 1982; 62:349–354.

14. Fitzgerald GA, Barnes P, Brown MN, Dollery CT. The circadian variability of circulating adrenaline and bronchomotor reactivity in asthma. In: Smolensky MH, Reinberg A, Labrecque G, eds. Recent Advances in Chronobiology of Allergy and Immunology. Oxford, UK: Pergamom Press, 1980:89–94.

15. Gaultier C, Reinberg A, Girard F. Circadian changes in lung resistance and dynamic compliance in healthy and asthmatic children: effects of two bronchodilators. Respir Physiol 1988; 31:169–182.

16. Gaultier C, Reinberg A, Motohashi Y. Circadian rhythm in total pulmonary

resistance of asthmatic children: effects of a β-agonist agent. Chronobiol Int 1988; 5:285–290.

17. Brown A, Smolensky M, D'Alonzo G, Frankhoff H, Gianotti L, Nilsetuen J. Circadian chronesthesy of the airways of healthy adults to the β-agonist bronchodilator isoproterenol. Annu Rev Chronopharmacol 1988; 5:163–166.

18. Bollinger AM, Young KYL, Gambertoglio JG, Newth CJL, Zureikat G, Powell M, Leung P, Affirme MB, Symchowicz S, et al. Influence of food on the absorption of albuterol Rapatabs. J Allergy Clin Immunol 1989; 83:123–126.

19. Hussey EK, Donn KH, Powell JR. Albuterol extended-release products: a comparison of steady-state pharmacokinetics. Pharmacotherapy 1991; 11:131–135.

20. Powell ML, Weisberger M, Dowdy Y, Gural R, Symchowicz S, Patrick JE. Comparative steady-state bioavailability of conventional and controlled-release formulation of albuterol. Biopharm Drug Disp 1987; 8:461–467.

21. Storms WW, Nathan RA, Bodman SF, Morris RJ, Selner JC, Greenstein SM, Zwillich CW. The effects of repeat action albuterol sulfate (Proventil Repetabs) in nocturnal symptoms of asthma. J Asthma 1992; 29:209–216.

22. Higenbottam MA, Khan A, Williams DO, Mikhail JR, Peake MD. Controlled release salbutamol tablets versus aminophylline in the control of reversible airways obstruction. J Intern Med Res 1989; 17:435–441.

23. Pierson WE, LaForce CF, Bell TD, MacCosbe PE, Sykes RS, Tinkelman D. Long-term, double blind comparisons of controlled-release albuterol versus sustained-release theophylline in adolescents and adults with asthma. J Allergy Clin Immunol 1990; 85:618–626.

24. Sykes RS, Reese ME, Meyer MC, Chubb JM. Relative bioavailability of a controlled-release albuterol formation for twice-daily use. Biopharm Drug Disp 1988; 9:551–556.

25. Moore-Gillon J. Volmax (salbutamol CR 8 mg) in the management of nocturnal asthma: a placebo-controlled study (abstr). Eur Respir J 1988; 1(suppl 2) 306s.

26. Van Keimpema AR, Ariaansz M, Raaijmakers JA, Nauta JJ, Postmus PE. Treatment of nocturnal asthma by addition of oral slow-release albuterol to standard treatment in stable asthma patients. J Asthma 1996; 33:119–124.

27. Creemers JD. A multicenter comparative study of salbuterol controlled release (Volmax) and sustained-release theophyllin (Theo-Dur) in the control of nocturnal asthma (abstr). Eur Respir J 1988; 1(suppl 2):333s.

28. Pedersen BK, Laursen LC, Gnosspelius Y, Faurschou P, Weeke B. Bambuterol: effects of a new anti-asthmatic drug. Eur J Clin Pharmacol 1985; 29:425–427.

29. Persson G, Gnosspelius Y, Anehus S. Comparison between a new once-daily, bronchodilating drug, bambuterol, and terbutaline sustained-release, twice-daily. Eur Respir J 1988; 1:223–226.

30. D'Alonzo GE, Smolensky MH, Feldman S, Gnosspelius Y, Karlson K. Bambuterol in the treatment of asthma: a placebo-controlled comparison of once-daily morning vs evening administration. Chest 1989; 107:406–412.

31. Petrie GR, Chookang JY, Hassan WU, Morrison JF, Pearson SB, Schneer-

son JM, Tang OT, Nig AC, Turbitt ML. Bambuterol: effective in nocturnal asthma. Respir Med 1993; 87:581–585.

32. Gunn SD, Ayres JG, McConchie SM. Comparison of the efficacy, tolerability and patient acceptability of once-daily bambuterol tablets against twice-daily controlled release salbutamol in nocturnal asthma: ACROBATICS Research Group. Eur J Clin Pharmacol 1995; 48:23–28.

33. Kemp JP, Bierman CW, Cocchetto DM. Dose-response study of inhaled salmeterol in asthmatic patients with 24-hour spirometry and holter monitoring. Ann Allergy 1993; 70:316–322.

34. Maesen FBV, Smeets JJ, Gubbelmans HLL, Zweers PG. Bronchodilator effect of inhaled formoterol vs salbutamol over 12 hours. Chest 1990; 97:590–594.

35. Maesen FBV, Smeets JJ, Gubbelmans HLL, Zweers PG. Formoterol in the treatment of nocturnal asthma. Chest 1990; 98:866–870.

36. Arvidsson P, Larsson S, Lofdahl CG, Melander B, Svedmyr N, Wahlender L. Inhaled formoterol during one year in asthma: a comparison with salbutamol. Eur Respir J 1991; 4:1168–1173.

37. Kesten S, Chapman KR, Broder I, Cartier A, Hyland RH, Knight A, Malo JL, Mazza JA, Moote DW, Small P. Sustained improvement in asthma with long-term use of formoterol fumarate. Ann Allergy 1992; 69:415–420.

38. Ball DI, Brittain RT, Coleman RA, Denyer LA, Jack D, Johnson M, Lunts LH, Nials AT. Salmeterol, a novel, long-acting beta$_2$-adrenergic agonist: characterization of pharmacological activity in vitro and in vivo. Br J Pharmacol 1991; 104:665–671.

39. Johnson M. The preclinical pharmacology of salmeterol: bronchodilator effects. Eur Respir Rev 1991; 1:253–256.

40. Brambilla C, Chastang C, Georges D, Bertin L. Salmeterol compared with slow-release terbutaline in nocturnal asthma. Allergy 1994; 49:421–426.

41. Britton MG, Earnshaw JS, Palmer JBD. A twelve month comparison of salmeterol and salbutamol in asthmatic patients. Eur Respir J 1992; 5:1062–1067.

42. D'Alonzo GE, Natim RA, Henochowicz S, Morris RJ, Ratner P, Rennard SI. Salmeterol xinafoate as maintenance therapy compared with albuterol in patients with asthma. JAMA 1994; 271:1412–1416.

43. Fitzpatrick MF, Mackay T, Driver H, Douglas NJ. Salmeterol in nocturnal asthma: a double-blind, placebo controlled trial of a long acting inhaled P2 agonist. BMJ 1990; 301:1365–1368.

44. Lundback B, Rawlinson DW, Palmer JBD. Twelve month comparison of salmeterol and salbutamol as dry powder formulations in asthmatic patients. Thorax 1993; 48:148–153.

45. Muir JF, Bertin L, Georges D. Salmeterol versus slow-release theophylline combined with ketotifen in nocturnal asthma: a multicentre trial. Eur Respir J 1992; 5:1197–1200.

46. Pearlman DS, Chervinsky P, LaForce C, et al. A comparison of salmeterol with

albuterol in the treatment of mild-to-moderate asthma. N Engl J Med 1992; 327:1420–1425.

47. Ullman A, Hednerj SN. Inhaled salmeterol and salbutamol in asthmatic patients. Am Rev Respir Dis 1990; 142:571–575.

48. Ullman A, Svedmyr N. Salmeterol, a new long acting inhaled beta$_2$-adrenorceptor agonist: comparison with salbutamol in adult asthmatic patients. Thorax 1998; 43:674–678.

49. Weersink EJ, Dourna RR, Postma DS, Koeter GH. Fluticasone propionate, salmeterol xinafoate, and their combination in the treatment of nocturnal asthma. Am J Respir Crit Care Med 1997; 155:1241–1246.

50. Faurschou P, Engel AM, Haanaes OC. Salmeterol in two different doses in the treatment of nocturnal bronchial asthma poorly controlled by other therapies. Allergy 1994; 49:827–832.

51. Selby C, Engleman HM, Fitzpatrick MF, Sime PM, Mackay TW, Douglas NJ. Inhaled salmeterol or oral theophylline in nocturnal asthma? Am J Respir Crit Care Med 1997; 155:104–108.

52. Martin RJ, Kraft M, Beaucher WN, Kiechel F, Sublett JL, LaVallee N, Shilstone J. A Comparative study of extended release albuterol sulfate and long acting inhaled salmeterol xinafoate in the treatment of nocturnal asthma. Ann Allergy Asthma Immunol 1999; 121–126.

53. Coe CI, Bames PJ. Reduction of nocturnal asthma by an inhaled anticholinergic drug. Chest 1986; 90:485–488.

54. Wolstenholme RJ, Shettan SP. Comparison of a combination of fenoterol with ipratropium bromide (Duovent) and salbutamol in young adults with nocturnal asthma. Respiration 1989; 55:152–157.

55. Catterall JL. Rhind GB, Whyte KF, Shapiro CM, Douglas NJ. Is nocturnal asthma caused by changes in airway cholinergic activity? Thorax 1988; 43: 720–724.

56. Morrison JFJ, Pearson SB, Dean HG. Parasympathetic nervous system in nocturnal asthma. BMJ 1988; 296:1427–1429.

57. O'Connor BJ, Towse LJ, Barnes PJ. Prolonged effect of tiotropium bromide on methacholine-induced bronchoconstriction in asthma. Am J Respir Crit Care Med 1996; 154(4, pt 1):876–880.

58. Cazzola M, Matera MG, Liccardi G. Effect of telenzepine, an MI-selective muscarinic receptor antagonist, in patients with nocturnal asthma. Pulm Pharmacol 1994; 7:91–97.

59. Barnes PJ, Pauwels RA. Theophylline in the management of asthma: time for reappraisal? Eur Respir J 1994; 7:579–591.

60. Sullivan P, Songul B, Jaffar Z, Page C, Jeffery P, Costello J. Anti-inflammatory effects of low dose oral theophylline in atopic asthma. Lancet 1994; 343:1006–1008.

61. Ward AJM, McKenniff M, Evans JM, Page CP, Costello JF. Theopylline: an immunomodulatory role in asthma? Am Rev Respir Dis 1993; 147:518–523.

62. Vassallo R, Lipsky JJ. Theophylline: recent advances in the understanding of its mode action and uses in clinical practice. Mayo Clin Proc 1998; 73:346–354.

63. Kidney JC, Dominguez M, Taylor P, Rose M, Aikman S, Chung KF, Barnes P. Withdrawing chronic theophylline treatment increases airway lymphocytes in asthma. Thorax 1994; 49:396.

64. Kraft M, Torvik JA, Trudeau J, et al. Theophylline potential anti-inflammatory effects in nocturnal asthma. J Allergy Clin Immunol 1996; 97:1242–1246.

65. Torvik JA, Borish LC, Beam WR, Kraft M, Wezel SE, Martin RJ. Does theophylline alter inflammation in nocturnal asthma (abstr)? Am J Respir Crit Care Med 1994; 149:A210.

66. Trudeau JB, Martin RJ, Kraft M, Torvik JA, Westcott JY, Wenzel SE. Theophylline decreases stimulated alveolar macrophage leukotriene B4 (LTB4) production in nocturnal asthmatics lavaged at 4 am (abstr). Am J Respir Crit Care Med 1994; 149:A941.

67. Smolensky MH, McGovern JP, Scott PH, et al. Chronobiology and asthma. II. Body-time–dependent differences in the kinetics and effects of bronchodilator medications. J Asthma 1987; 24:90–134.

68. Smolensky MH, Scott PH, Harrist RB, Hiatt PH, Wong TK, Baenziger JC, Klank BJ, Marbella A, Meltzer A. Administration-time dependency of the pharmacokinetic behavior and therapeutic effect of a once-a-day theophylline in asthmatic children. Chronobiol Int 1987; 4:435–448.

69. Smolensky MH. Chronopharmacology of theophylline and beta-sympathomimetics. In: Lemmer B, ed. Chronopharmacology: Cellular and Biochemical Interactions. New York: Marcel Dekker, 1989:65–113.

70. Kyle GM, Smolensky, MH, McGovern JP. Circadian variation in the susceptibility of rodents to the toxic effects of theophylline. In: Reinberg A, Halberg F, eds. Chronopharmacology. Oxford, UK: Pergamon Press, 1979:239–244.

71. Darow P, Steinijans VW. Therapeutic advantage of unequal dosing of theophylline in patients with nocturnal asthma. Chronobiol Int 1987; 4:439–357.

72. Schulz H-U, Frercks H-J, Hypa F. Vergleichende Theophyllin-Serum-Spiegel Messungen über 24 Stunden nach konventioneller Dosierung einer Theophyllin-retard-Präparation über 4 Tage. Ther Woche 1984; 34:536–543.

73. Neuenkirchen H, Wikens JH, Oellerich M, Sybrecht GW. Nocturnal asthma: effect of a once per evening dose of sustained-release theophylline. Eur J Respir Dis 1985; 66:196–204.

74. D'Alonzo GE, Smolensky MH, Feldman S, Gianotti LA, Emerson MB, Staudinger H, Steinjans VW. Twenty-four hour lung function in adult patients with asthma: chronoptimized theophylline therapy once-daily dosing in the evening versus conventional twice-daily dosing. Am Rev Respir Dis 1990; 142:84–90.

75. Helms S. Diurnal stabilization of asthma with once daily evening administration of controlled release theophylline. Immunol Allergy Pract 1987; 9:414–419.

76. Reinberg A, Pauchet F, Ruff F, Gervais A, Smolensky MH, Levi F, Ger-

vais P, Chaouat D, Abella ML, Zidani R. Comparison of once-daily evening versus morning sustained-release theophylline dosing for nocturnal asthma. Chronobiol Int 1987; 4:409–420.

77. British Thoracic Society. Guidelines on management of asthma. Thorax 1993; 48(suppl):1098–1111.

78. Sheffer AL. National Heart Lung and Blood Institute National Asthma Education Program Expert Panel Report: guidelines for the diagnosis and management of asthma. J Allergy Clin Immunol 1991; 88:425–534.

79. Sheffer AL. International consensus report on diagnosis and management of asthma. Eur Respir J 1992; 5:601–641.

80. Wettengel R, Berdel D, Cegla U, Fabel H, Geisler L, Hofmann D, Krause J, Kroidl RF, Lanser K, Leupold W. Empfehlungen der Deutschen Atemwegsliga zum Asthma Management bei Erwachsenen und bei Kindern. Med Klinik 1994; 89:57–67.

81. Barnes PJ. Effect of corticosteroids on airway hyperresponsiveness. Am Rev Respir Dis 1990; 141:S70–S76.

82. Barnes PJ. Current issues for establishing inhaled corticosteroids as the antiinflammatory agents of choice in asthma. J Allergy Clin Immunol 1998; 101: S427–S433.

83. English J, Marks V. Diurnal variations in methylprednisolone metabolism in the rat. IRCS Med Sci 1981; 9:721.

84. English J, Dunne M, Marks V. Diurnal variation in prednisone kinetics. Clin Pharmacol Ther 1983; 33:381–385.

85. McAllister WAC, Mitchell DM, Collins JV. Prednisolone pharmacokinetics compared between night and day in asthmatic and normal subjects. Br J Clin Pharmacol 1981; 11:303–304.

86. Morselli PL, Marc V, Garattini S, Zaccala M. Metabolism of exogenous cortisol in humans—diurnal variations in plasma disappearance rate. Biochem Pharmacol 1970; 19:1643–1647.

87. Ceresa F, Angeli A, Boccuzzi A, Molino G. Once-a-day neurally stimulated and basal ACTH secretion phases in man and their responses to corticoid inhibition. J Clin Endocrinol Metab 1969; 29:1074–1082.

88. Reinberg A. Chronopharmacology of corticosteroids and ACTH. In: Lemmer B, ed. Chronopharmacology: Cellular and Biochemical Interactions. New York: Marcel Dekker, 1989:137–178.

89. Reinberg A, Smolensky MH, D'Alonzo GE, McGovern JP. Chronobiology and asthma: III. Timing corticotherapy to biological rhythms to optimize treatment goals. J Asthma 1988; 25:219–248.

90. Reinberg A, Halberg F, Falliers C. Circadian timing of methylprednisolone effects in asthmatic boys. Chronobiologia 1974; 1:333–347.

91. Beam WR, Weiner DE, Martin RJ. Timing of prednisone and alteration of airways inflammation in nocturnal asthma. Am Rev Respir Dis 1992; 146:1524–1530.

92. Kowanko IC, Pownall R, Knapp MS, Swannell AJ, Mahoney PG. Time of day

of prednisolone administration in rheumatoid arthritis. Ann Rheum Dis 1982; 41:447–452.

93. Harter JG, Reddy WIJ, Thorn GW. Studies on an intermittent corticosteroid dosage regimen. N Engl Med 1963; 296:591–595.

94. Reinberg A, Guilet P, Gervais P, Ghata J, Vignaud D, Abuker C. One-month chronocorticotherapy (Dutimelan 8-15 mite): control of the asthmatic condition without adrenal suppression and circadian alteration. Chronobiologia 1977; 4: 295–312.

95. Crepaldi G, Muggeo M. Plurichronocorticoid treatment of bronchial asthma and chronic bronchitis. Clinical and endocrinometabolic evaluation. Chronobiologia 1974; 1(suppl 1):407–407.

96. Serafini U, Bonini S. Corticoid therapy in allergic disease. Clinical evaluation of a chronopharmacological attempt. Chronobiologia 1974; 1(suppl 1):339–406.

97. Reinberg AP, Gervais M, Chaussade G, Fraboulet G, Duburque B. Circadian changes in effectiveness of corticosteroids in eight patients with allergic asthma. J Allergy Clin Immunol 1983; 71:425–433.

98. Barnes PJ. Inhaled glucocorticods for asthma. N Engl J Med 1995; 332:868–875.

99. Chaplin MD, Rooks W II, Swenson EW, Cooper WC, Nerenberg C, Chu NI. Flunisolide metabolism and dynamics of a metabolite. Clin Pharmacol Ther 1980; 27:402–413.

100. Ryrfeldt A, Andersson P, Edsbacker S, Tonnesson M, Davies D, Pauwels R. Pharmacokinetics and metabolism of budesonide, a selective glucocorticoid. Eur J Respir Dis 1982; 63(suppl):86–95.

101. Holliday SM, Faulds D, Sorkin EM. Inhaled fluticasone propionate: a review of its pharmacodynamics and pharmacokinetic properties, and therapeutic use in asthma. Drugs 1994; 47:319–331.

102. Dluhy RG. Clinical relevance of inhaled corticosteroid and HPA axis suppression. J Allergy Clin Immunol 1988; 101(4, pt 2):S447–S450.

103. Smolensky MH, D'Alonzo GE. Medical chronobiology: concepts and applications. Am Rev Respir Dis 1993; 147:511–519.

104. Wurthwein G, Rohdewald P. Activation of beclomethasone dipropionate by hydrolysis to beclomethasone-17-monopropionate. Biopharm Drug Disp 1990; 11:381–394.

105. Derendorf H, Hochhaus G, Meibohm B, Mollmann H, Barth J. Pharmacokinetics and pharmacodynamics of inhaled corticosteroids. J Allergy Clin Immunol 1998; 101(4, pt 2):S440–S446.

106. Toogood JH, Baskerville JC, Jennings B, Lefco NM, Johansson SA. Influence of dosing frequency and schedule on the response of chronic asthmatics to the aerosol steroid, budesonide. J Allergy Clin Immunol 1982; 70:288–298.

107. Meibohm B, Hochhaus G, Rohatagi S, Mollmann H, Barth J, Wagner M, Krieg M, Stockman R, Derendorf H. Dependency of cortisol suppression on the administration time of inhaled corticosteroids. J Clin Pharmacol 1997; 37:704–710.

108. Pincus DJ, Szefler SJ, Ackerson LM, Martin RJ. Chronotherapy of asthma with

inhaled steroids: the effect of dosage timing on drug efficacy. J Allergy Clin Immunol 1995; 95:1171–1178.

109. Pincus DJ, Humeston TR, Martin RJ. Further studies on the chronotherapy of asthma with inhaled steroids: The effect of dosage timing on drug efficacy. J Allergy Clin Immunol 1997; 100:771–774.

110. Malo J-L, Cartier A, Merland N, Ghezzo H, Burek A, Morris J, Jennings BH. Four-times-a-day dosing frequency is better than twice-a-day regimen in subjects requiring a high-dose inhaled steroid, budesonide to control moderate to severe asthma. Am Rev Respir Dis 1989; 140:624–628.

111. Dahl R, Johansson SA. Clinical effect of bid and qid administration of inhaled budesonide, a double-blind controlled study. Eur J Respir Dis 1982; 63(suppl 122):268–269.

112. Labrecque G, Reinberg A. Chronopharmacology of nonsteroidal anti-inflammatory drugs. In: Lemmer B, ed. Chronopharmacology: Cellular and Biochemical Interactions. New York: Marcel Dekker, 1989:545–579.

113. Furukawa CT, Shapiro GG, Bierman CW, Kraemer MJ, Ward DJ, Pierson WE. A double-blind study comparing the effectiveness of cromolyn sodium and sustained-release theophylline in childhood asthma. Pediatrics 1984; 74:453–459.

114. Kay AM. The mode of action of anti-allergic drugs. Clin Allergy 1987; 17: 154–164.

115. Gonzalez JP, Brogden RH. Nedocromil sodium: a preliminary review of its pharmacodynamic and pharmacokinetic properties and therapeutic efficacy in the treatment of reversible airways disease. Drugs 1987; 34:560–577.

116. Hetzel MR, Clarke JH, Gilliam SJ, Isaac P, Perkins M. Is sodium cromoglycate effective in nocturnal asthma? Thorax 1985; 40:793–794.

117. Morgan AD, Connaughton JJ, Caterall JR, Shapiro CM, Douglas NJ, Flenley DC. Sodium cromoglycate in nocturnal asthma. Thorax 1986; 41:39–41.

118. Petty TL, Rollins DR, Christopher K, Good JT, and Oakley R. Cromolyn sodium is effective in adult chronic asthmatics. Am Rev Respir Dis 1989; 139: 694–701.

119. Ruffin R, Alpers JH, Kromer DK, Rubinfield AR, Pain MCF, Czarny D, Bowes G. A 4-week Australian multicentre study of nedocromil sodium in asthmatic patients. Eur J Respir Dis 1986; 69(suppl 147):336–339.

120. Williams AJ, Stableforth D. The addition of nedocromil sodium to maintenance therapy in the management of patients with bronchial asthma. Eur J Respir Dis 1986; 69(suppl 147):340–343.

121. Hrushesky WJM, Langer R, Theeuwes F, eds. Temporal control of drug delivery. Ann NY Acad Sci 1991; 618.

122. Lemmer B ed. Chronopharamcology. Cellular and Biochemical Interactions. New York: Marcel Dekker, 1989.

123. Redfern P, Lemmer B, eds. Physiology and Pharmacology of Biological Rhythms. Heidelberg: Springer-Verlag, 1997.

7

Combination Therapy in Asthma

Monica Kraft

National Jewish Medical and Research Center
Denver, Colorado

I. Introduction

In the treatment of asthma, the use of several medications with different mechanisms has become the mainstay of therapy. Combination therapy can result in improved asthma control at decreased doses of individual medications. Furthermore, the side-effect profile can also be improved. This later benefit is of particular interest in those patients who require long term anti-inflammatory therapy, such as inhaled or oral corticosteroids, where side effects are of concern (1,2). As corticosteroids are first-line therapy for asthma, the majority of this chapter focuses on the combination of medications with inhaled corticosteroids; however, a discussion of other combination therapies, particularly in acute and pediatric asthma, is also included.

II. Inhaled Corticosteroids in Combination with Other Agents

As inhaled corticosteroids are first-line therapy for asthma, many studies have focused on their efficacy. However, concern has been raised about steroid side effects occurring after long-term use (1,2). This issue, along with potentially complementary mechanisms of action appreciated with other pharmacological therapies, has led to many studies comparing inhaled steroids alone versus their combination with other agents. This section addresses such studies for the treatment of asthma, including nocturnal asthma, exercise-induced asthma, severe asthma, and pediatric asthma.

A. Inhaled Corticosteroids and Short-Acting β_2-Agonists

Combination therapy of inhaled corticosteroids with inhaled β_2-agonists has been evaluated for more than 10 years (3,4). Haahtela and colleagues reported in 1989 that patients using a combination inhaler of 100 µg beclomethasone and 200 µg salbutamol four times daily exhibited greater improvements in forced expiratory volume in 1s (FEV_1), peak expiratory flow rate (PEFR), and symptom scores than those patients using 400 µg of salbutamol alone four times daily (4). Studies in the 1990s have also demonstrated that the addition of inhaled corticosteroids to inhaled β_2-agonists improved many aspects of asthma control. A 4-year prospective study performed by Dompeling and colleagues (3) confirmed this issue. Twenty-nine general practices in the Netherlands participated in the study, resulting in a sample size of 56 patients with moderate asthma and 28 patients with chronic obstructive pulmonary disease (COPD). During the first 2 years of treatment, patients received only bronchodilator therapy (400 µg of salbutamol or 40 µg of ipratropium bromide) either four times daily or as needed. During years 3 and 4, subjects received 400 µg of beclomethasone twice daily in addition to salbutamol or ipratropium bromide. In the asthmatic subjects, the mean prebronchodilator FEV_1 improved by 562 mL and the mean postbronchodilator FEV_1 improved by 201 mL after 6 months of therapy. In addition, the mean residual volume decreased by 0.49 L (95% Cl 0.18–0.80 L). The provocative concentration of histamine producing a fall in FEV_1 of 20% (histamine PC_{20}) improved by three doubling doses per year. Exacerbations fell by 1.3 per year and severity of symptoms decreased by 17%. No significant adverse events were appreciated, although four patients used a spacer, as the severity of oral candidiasis had increased. These significant clinical improvements confirm the importance of inhaled steroids in the therapy of asthma.

The use of inhaled corticosteroids in combination with short-acting inhaled β_2-agonists in the treatment of nocturnal asthma specifically has not been extensively studied. Until recently, it was felt that they had little or no impact on nocturnal symptoms of asthma, as Turner-Warwick stated in her 1988 epidemiological analysis of nocturnal asthma (5). She stated that the "no drug or drug combination was associated with a significantly lower frequency of nocturnal awakenings" and suggested that the introduction of inhaled corticosteroids in the 1970s had not affected nighttime asthma control. McGivern and colleagues found that, at equivalent doses, once-daily inhaled beclomethasone resulted in lower morning and evening PEFRs and an increase in both daytime and nighttime symptoms compared to a three- or four-times-per-day dosing schedule (6). Malo and colleagues compared a twice-daily to a four-times-daily dosing regimen using variable doses of budesonide over 6 months (7). They demonstrated that the twice-daily regimen resulted in almost twice as many days with nocturnal asthma and cough and almost three times as many days with disability due to asthma. In addition, overnight variability in PEFR and relapse frequency were higher during the twice-daily schedule. These results are in agreement with those of Toogood and colleagues, who found a four-times-daily schedule superior to an equivalent dose used in a twice-daily schedule (8).

Although the four-times-daily schedule of dosing inhaled corticosteroids appears the most efficacious for the overall symptoms of asthma, nocturnal symptoms are still present 25% of the nights, as shown by Malo and colleagues (7). Furthermore, the maximum evening-to-morning variability in PEFR remained at 29% on the four-times-daily dosing schedule as compared to 33% during the twice-daily dosing schedule. Certainly the symptoms and signs are improved, but they are still clinically significant.

Other studies again support the limited ability of inhaled corticosteroids in combination with short-acting inhaled β_2-agonists to attenuate nocturnal worsening of asthma. Horn et al. evaluated nocturnal asthma symptoms and variability in PEFR in a group of asthmatics after use of beclomethasone at 400 µg qid inhaled (9). They demonstrated a variety of responses in which about one-half of the subjects significantly reduced their overnight fall in PEFR and the other half showed no significant improvement in their overnight PEFR compared to baseline. In a subsequent study, Horn and colleagues evaluated the overnight variability in PEFR in a group of asthmatics using inhaled beclomethasone at variable doses up to 2000 µg/day for 36 weeks (10). At the end of the study, one-half of the subjects continued to experience nocturnal awakenings due to asthma. Despite high doses, which can also lead to systemic absorption and clinically important side effects, frequent dosing regimens have demonstrated limited effectiveness in improving nocturnal symptoms and/or overnight spirometry (8–11).

As the timing of medication is an important issue in the treatment of nocturnal asthma, Pincus and colleagues found that a single daily 800 μg dose of triamcinolone at 3 P.M. did not increase systemic effects and produced a similar improvement in morning FEV_1, morning and evening PEFR, and inhaled β_2-agonist use as compared to 200 μg four times daily (12). The authors concluded that a dosing strategy based on once-daily dosing can increase compliance.

In the treatment of asthma in the pediatric population, inhaled corticosteroids in combination with short-acting β_2-agonists have been evaluated. Waalkens and colleagues evaluated the combination of budesonide, 200 μg twice daily, and terbutaline, 500 μg twice daily, as compared to terbutaline alone (13). After 8 weeks of therapy, the budesonide/terbutaline group demonstrated a decrease in bronchial hyperresponsiveness, with mean differences of 2.1 versus 1.3 doubling doses of histamine within the budesonide/terbutaline and terbutaline groups, respectively. The mean FEV_1 did not change in either group. Afternoon and nocturnal PEFR improved significantly in the group receiving budesonide, as did symptoms of wheezing. Van Essen-Zandvliet and colleagues also studied the use of budesonide in pediatric asthma. In the group receiving budesonide and a short-acting β_2-agonist, 32% were symptom-free in the 2-week period before each visit at the end of 12 months, and this increased to 47% at 22 months (14). As discussed in the next section, the addition of a long-acting β_2-agonist may allow for a reduction in the inhaled steroid dosage. This is an attractive option given the concerns over the effects of inhaled steroids on growth in children (15–19).

The question of whether short-acting inhaled β_2-agonists can be used intermittently or regularly in conjunction with inhaled corticosteroids has also been addressed. Ganassini et al. demonstrated that inhaled β_2-agonists can be used regularly by persons with mild asthma while taking low doses of inhaled corticosteroid (beclomethasone 250 μg three times daily) (20). Tormey and colleagues showed that either regular or intermittent use of β_2-agonists can be used in conjunction with inhaled corticosteroids (beclomethasone 500 μg daily) without significant differences in lung function, histamine PC_{20}, or symptom scores (21).

Several mechanisms may contribute to the many clinical benefits seen with the combinations of inhaled corticosteroids and inhaled β_2-agonists. Certainly, the anti-inflammatory action of corticosteroids alone exerts a very powerful effect on airway inflammation and airway hyperresponsiveness (22–32). However, steroids have been shown to potentiate the relaxing effect of β_2-agonists in a number of animal studies and *in vitro* studies of human bronchial smooth muscle (33). The direct influence on β_2 receptors appears to be mediated by lipocortin through the synthesis of new β_2 receptors, increased coupling between receptors and their functional unit, increased synthesis of catecholamine, and reversal of β_2 receptor dysfunction due to repeated β_2 stimulation (tachyphylaxis). However, there are data to suggest that high-dose β_2-agonists may exhibit antiglucocorticold activity (34,35). In addition, Cockcroft and colleagues demonstrated that budesonide did not prevent tolerance to the bronchoprotective effect of salbutamol or the increased airway responsiveness to allergen seen after regular salbutamol use (36). Further studies are needed to determine the clinical relevance of these data.

B. Inhaled Corticosteroids and Long-Acting β_2-Agonists

It appears that the addition of a long acting β_2-agonist to inhaled corticosteroids confers additional symptomatic and physiological benefit. International guidelines have recommended the use of long-acting β_2-agonists such as salmeterol, either as an addition to conventional doses of inhaled steroids or as additive treatment in patients on higher doses of inhaled steroids (37–39). Van der Molen et al. demonstrated that the addition of formoterol to a stable dose of inhaled corticosteroids (100–3200 µg/day) resulted in improved morning PEFR and symptoms and decreased short-acting β_2-agonist use (40).

In a double-blind, randomized, placebo-controlled trial of salmeterol over 1 year in 87 asthmatic adults, Wilding et al. reported that there was a 17% reduction in the dose of inhaled corticosteroid on salmeterol as compared with placebo and even accompanied by improved pulmonary function, reduced symptom scores, and bronchodilator use (41). Greening and colleagues demonstrated that in patients still symptomatic on 400 µg of beclomethasone or budesonide daily, 50 µg of salmeterol twice daily together with 200 µg of beclomethasone twice daily was more effective than 500 µg of beclomethasone twice daily (42). The patients exhibited better PEFR, less diurnal variation in PEFR, and fewer symptoms after 21 weeks of treatment (Fig. 1). Similar results were shown by Woolcock et al. where the addition of 50 µg of salmeterol and 100 µg salmeterol twice daily to 500 µg beclomethasone twice daily was compared to 1000 µg of beclomethasone twice daily without salmeterol (43). In contrast, Sears and colleagues observed that increasing the dose of inhaled corticosteroid was more effective than adding more bronchodilator in patients with moderate asthma (44).

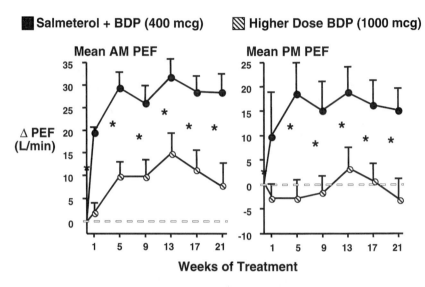

Figure 1 The mean change in A.M. and P.M. peak expiratory flow (PEF) over 21 weeks with salmeterol plus 400 μg beclomethasone (BDP) (closed circles) and 1000 μg beclomethasone (striped circles). (Adapted from Ref. 42.)

The addition of a long-acting β_2-agonist may also decrease exacerbations of asthma, as shown by Pauwels et al. (45). They randomized patients with moderate asthma to one of four treatment groups: low-dose budesonide (100 μg twice daily) plus placebo, low-dose budesonide plus formoterol (12 μg twice daily), high-dose budesonide (400 μg twice daily) plus placebo, and high-dose budesonide plus formoterol. Treatment was continued for 1 year. The rates of severe and mild exacerbations in the group as a whole decreased by 26 and 40%, respectively. Patients treated with formoterol and the higher dose of budesonide experienced the greatest reductions (63 and 62%, respectively). The addition of formoterol to budesonide did not cause any long-term loss of asthma control. There were no signs of worsening of disease or tolerance to the effects of medication with regard to any clinical or functional variable examined except for a decrease in the effect of formoterol on PEFR in the morning after the first 2 days of treatment. Despite this change, the PEFR remained significantly higher than in the budesonide-only groups for the rest of the 1-year study period. One possible explanation is the development of limited tolerance to the bronchodilating effect of formoterol during the early phase of regular treatment, as demonstrated in other studies (36,46–52). The findings from this study suggest that tolerance has little or no clinical significance.

In the treatment of nocturnal asthma, the use of long acting β_2-agonists has been evaluated in several trials. One such study by Fitzpatrick and colleagues, using a randomized, double-blind crossover design, involved 20 patients with nocturnal asthma (53). It demonstrated that salmeterol, as compared to a short-acting β_2-agonist along, improved the overnight PEFR using both 50- and 100-µg doses twice daily (53). These improvements were associated with a reduction in the mean 24-h "rescue" use of albuterol by both doses of salmeterol (Fig. 2). Furthermore, an objective improvement in sleep quality was found while the patients were taking salmeterol 50 µg twice daily. It was noted that the subjects spent less time awake or in light sleep and more time in stage 4 sleep. Dahl and colleagues also demonstrated that salmeterol, 50 µg twice daily, decreased diurnal variation in PEFR and the number of nocturnal awakenings, as compared to 200 mg qid of salbutamol, in a parallel study of 692 asthmatic patients (54). Similarly, Dahl and colleagues also demonstrated that the combination of inhaled corticosteroids plus the long-acting oral β_2-agonist sustained-release terbutaline (Bricanyl) improved nocturnal worsening of asthma better than each drug did separately (55). The studies by Greening

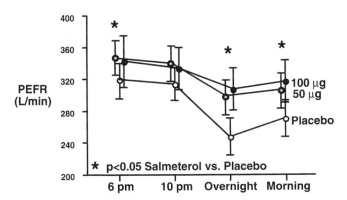

Figure 2 The peak expiratory flow rate (PEFR) measured from 6 P.M. to morning in placebo (open circles), 50 µg salmeterol (gray circles), and 100 µg salmeterol (closed circles). (Adapted from Ref. 53.)

(42) and Woolcock (43) discussed above also showed improvement in several aspects of nocturnal asthma. These improvements included decreased nocturnal awakenings and improved morning PEFR.

Recently, Selby and coworkers compared inhaled corticosteroids plus salmeterol or theophylline in the treatment of nocturnal asthma (56). Although the overnight falls in PEFR were similar in both groups, subjects experienced fewer nocturnal awakenings while using salmeterol. The authors concluded that there is no major clinical advantage in patients with nocturnal asthma, but a small benefit in sleep quality, quality of life, and daytime cognitive function was appreciated with salmeterol.

In contrast, Weersink and colleagues evaluated the combination of salmeterol (50 µg twice daily) and fluticasone (250 µg twice daily) and the two medications separately in the treatment of nocturnal asthma (57). Interestingly, the combination of the two did not offer any advantage as compared to fluticasone alone when circadian changes in PEFR and bronchial hyperresponsiveness were evaluated. The combination did offer an advantage when adenosine 5′ monophosphate (AMP), not methacholine or histamine, was used to measure bronchial hyperresponsiveness. AMP is an indirect bronchoconstrictor through activation of mast cells, suggesting that the anti-inflammatory actions of fluticasone and possibly salmeterol may offer greater protection than fluticasone alone. Note that although salmeterol has been shown to inhibit mast cells in vitro (58), a significant anti-inflammatory effect is not consistently shown in vivo (59).

Although these improvements in nocturnal awakenings may seem minor at first glance, they are probably significant from the standpoint of cognitive performance. Investigators have shown that even small amounts of sleep deprivation can lead to appreciable impairments of cognitive performance (60,61). It has also been shown that patients with nocturnal asthma who had minor problems with sleep quality do have impaired daytime cognitive performance to a degree that could affect work performance (62). Weersink and colleagues demonstrated that treatment of nocturnal airway obstruction improves daytime cognitive performance (63).

In the pediatric population, long-acting β_2-agonists have also been used in conjunction with inhaled corticosteroids. Verberne et al. evaluated 177 children who were using inhaled corticosteroids and randomized them in a double-blind parallel study to either 200 µg of beclomethasone twice daily plus salmeterol 50 µg twice daily, 800 µg beclomethasone alone, or 200 µg beclomethasone twice daily plus placebo (64). The primary outcome variables were FEV_1 and methacholine PC_{20}. In this population, there were no significant differences between the three groups in airway caliber, airway responsiveness, symptom scores, or exacerbation rates. These results differed from those of the studies in adults described above (42,43). The authors proposed that the differences may be due to differences in selection criteria for the adult studies as compared to their pediatric study. They hypothesized that the adult populations may have been more symptomatic, as the baseline FEV_1 was 72% in the Woolcock study and the baseline PEFR was 74% in the Greening study. This is in contrast to the baseline FEV_1 of 86% in the Verberne study (64). Therefore, there may have been more room for improvement with a bronchodilator in the adult studies, given the lower lung function exhibited at baseline.

However, Meijer and coworkers studied the effect of adding salmeterol, 50 µg twice daily, to beclomethasone (either 200 µg or 400 µg twice daily) in a pediatric population (mean age 11.4 years) (65). After 16 weeks of therapy, the mean FEV_1 was $4.9 \pm 2.0\%$ higher in the salmeterol group ($p = 0.01$). The methacholine PC_{20} did not differ between the groups. Salmeterol was discontinued, and bronchial hyperresponsiveness was assessed 1 week later. There was no rebound increase in methacholine PC_{20} or worsening in FEV_1. These authors concluded that the addition of salmeterol to inhaled corticosteroids in this pediatric population led to a sustained bronchodilator effect.

The combination of salmeterol with inhaled corticosteroids has also been evaluated in exercise-induced asthma. In a study by Simons et al. in a pediatric population aged 12–16 years, patients received salmeterol 50 µg once daily in addition to their usual dose of beclomethasone 100–200 µg twice daily (66). The salmeterol group exhibited a significant protective effect against exercise-induced asthma at 1 and 9 h after salmeterol dosing. After 28 days of treatment, the bronchoprotective effect was significantly greater than placebo at 1 h but not 9 h. In this study, subjects lost the protective effect of salmeterol despite the use of inhaled corticosteroids. A similar result was shown in adults, where subjects received salmeterol, 50 µg twice daily (67). The initial protection in the fall in FEV_1 by salmeterol was $5 \pm 2\%$ on day 1, $10 \pm 3\%$ on day 14, and $9 \pm 3\%$ on day 28 (Fig. 3). The duration of action of the drug, however, shortened with long-term use. By the end of the second week, the extent of protection recorded in the evening was less than that on day 1 (decrease in FEV_1 from morning to evening on day 1, $6 \pm 2\%$; on day 14, $15 \pm 3\%$, $p = 0.003$). These changes remained constant, as the decrease in FEV_1 from morning to evening on day 29 was $14 \pm 3\%$. Finally, the number of patients for whom salmeterol did not offer protection against exercise-induced asthma later in the day (those with more than a 10% fall in FEV_1 after exercise) increased from 2 on study day 1 to 11 on study day 29 ($p = 0.02$).

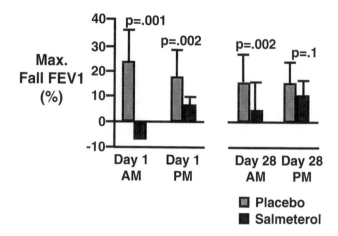

Figure 3 The protective effect of salmeterol initially and after 28 days is shown. The initial dose of salmeterol (dark squares) exhibited a protective effect that waned (nonsignificantly) after 28 days as compared to placebo (gray squares). (Adapted from Ref. 66.)

Despite these changes, the benefit afforded by salmeterol was still better than placebo. As stated above, the clinical significance of these observations is currently unclear and requires further study.

It is important to note that when salmeterol was first available, its use was associated with increased exacerbations of asthma and respiratory arrests (68). The mechanisms resulting in these adverse events are unclear. A postulated mechanism includes the use of salmeterol alone, as it provides no clinically significant anti-inflammatory effects (69). Second, patients did not always have shorter-acting β_2-agonist such as albuterol available as "rescue" medication. Just as glucocorticoids and short-acting β_2-agonists exhibit significant interactions, so, apparently, do glucocorticoids and long-acting β_2-agonists, as discussed in a review by Chung (70). Therefore, salmeterol is probably best used concomitantly with inhaled corticosteroids and albuterol, the latter as needed.

In addition to the use of inhaled corticosteroids and salmeterol separately, a combination inhaler containing fluticasone and salmeterol (Seretide®) has been approved in Europe. Its counterpart, Advair®, is soon to be approved in the United States (70a, 70b). The combination inhaler has been studied by Chapman and colleagues in a randomized, double-blind, double-dummy parallel study in 43 centers in five countries. During the initial 2-week run-in period, patients with moderate asthma (FEV_1 approximately 75% predicted) continued to take inhaled beclomethasone or budesonide, 800–1200 µg/day or fluticasone 400–600 µg/day and salbutamol. Patients qualified for the study if, at the end of the run-in period, they demonstrated via symptoms score and PEFR that their asthma was not adequately controlled.

During the 28-week treatment period, patients received either Seretide (salmeterol/fluticasone at 50 µg/250 µg) twice daily via a single Diskus inhaler and placebo twice daily via another Diskus inhaler, or the same dosages of the active components via separate Diskus inhalers (concurrent therapy). Patients were allowed to use salbutamol as needed.

The primary outcome variable was morning PEFR. In both groups, the mean morning PEFR improved, with mean changes of 43 and 36 L/min for the combination and concurrent therapy, respectively. Thiry-five percent of patients receiving combination inhaler and 31% of those receiving concurrent therapy had a mean daytime symptom score of zero over weeks 1 to 12 compared with 1 and 2%, respectively, at baseline. There were no differences in adverse events between the two treatment groups. Thus, the combination appeared to be as efficacious as both inhalers separately. Further studies are required to determine whether compliance is improved with the combination inhaler.

C. Inhaled Corticosteroids and Theophylline

Recently, attention has been focused on the use of theophylline preparations as steroid-sparing agents (71,72). However, studies dating back to 1979 suggest that the combination of inhaled corticosteroids and theophylline is more effective than corticosteroids alone (73,74). Evans and colleagues treated 62 patients with moderate asthma by adding theophylline (250 or 375 mg, depending on weight) to inhaled corticosteroids (400 or 800 µg budesonide) over a 3-month treatment period (71). The group receiving the low-dose budesonide plus theophylline exhibited greater improvements in FEV_1 (2.48 ± 0.18 L to a peak of 2.76 ± 0.18 L, $p = 0.002$) as compared to the group receiving high-dose budesonide (2.50 ± 0.14 L to a peak of 2.62 ± 0.15 L, $p = 0.37$) (Fig. 4). Improvements of similar magnitude were appreciated for the forced vital capacity (FVC). A similar study was performed first by Ukena and colleagues (72). In this study, 133 patients received theophylline 250 mg twice daily plus either 400 or 800 µg of budesonide for 6 weeks. In this study, PEFR and FEV_1 were the main outcome variables, which improved by 30% in both groups. There were no significant differences between the two treatment groups. Inter-

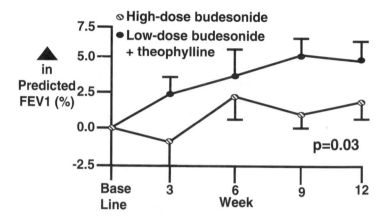

Figure 4 The mean changes in percentage predicted FEV₁ over 12 weeks using high-dose (800 μg) budesonide (striped circles) and low-dose (400 μg) budesonide plus theophylline (closed circles). (Adapted from Ref. 71.)

estingly, Evans and colleagues also evaluated PEFR and found no differences between the groups, but the theophylline/budesonide group experienced a greater improvement in peak flow variability (71). Perhaps the greater sample size evaluated in the Ukena study resulted in equivalence between the two treatment regimens, as compared to superiority of one regimen over the other.

Theophylline and inhaled corticosteroids have also been evaluated in the treatment of nocturnal asthma. Youngchaiyud and colleagues studied the effects of theophylline (Theodur) 200 mg twice daily taken at 8 A.M. and 8 P.M., budesonide 200 μg twice daily, and their combination in 61 patients with nocturnal asthma (75). Morning and evening PEFRs were significantly higher when the patients used either budesonide alone or combination therapy. There were also significantly fewer nocturnal awakenings and less nocturnal β_2-agonist use when the patients used either budesonide or the combination of budesonide and theophylline. There were no significant differences in efficacy between the budesonide and combination regimens; however, the authors did not measure theophylline levels, so it is unclear if they were in the therapeutic window for the majority of patients.

In pediatric asthma, three combinations of albuterol, theophylline, and beclomethasone were compared by Meltzer and colleagues (76). In this double-blind, parallel, multicenter study, children aged 6–16 years with moderately severe asthma (percent predicted FEV₁, 67–71%) were randomized to one of three regimens: theophylline (oral Theobid Jr.) twice daily in addition to albuterol two puffs (180 µg) four times daily; beclomethasone, two puffs (84 µg) four times daily after albuterol; and beclomethasone plus theophylline plus albuterol. Theophylline levels were measured during the 1- to 2-week run-in until the levels were between 8 and 18 µg/mL. After 12 weeks of treatment, all three treatment regimens resulted in significant improvements in the FEV_1 and FVC. The FEV_1 improvement ranged from 20–26% and the FVC improvement from 18–28%. There were no significant differences in lung function between the three regimens. However, the group that received beclomethasone had lower symptom scores, fewer exacerbations, fewer requirements for prednisone bursts, and reduced rescue medication use. Therefore, beclomethasone appeared to exert the greatest effect on asthma control.

D. Inhaled Corticosteroids and Cromolyn/Nedocromil

Although most studies in this area have compared cromolyn or nedocromil directly to inhaled corticosteroids, there have been studies evaluating the combination of nedocromil with other agents. Rebuck and coworkers evaluated the efficacy of nedocromil sodium in patients who had persistent asthma symptoms despite inhaled or oral corticosteroids (77). Nedocromil, 2 mg four times daily or placebo was given to 188 patients for 12 weeks. A total of 43% of the nedocromil group and 47% of the placebo group used beclomethasone 400 µg/day. Both groups contained similar proportions of patients taking 800 µg/day or more of inhaled corticosteroid. In the nedocromil group, 33% of patients took oral corticosteroids, as compared to 22% in the placebo group. Pulmonary function tests (FEV_1, FVC) showed no significant differences between the two groups. Morning and evening PEFRs were significantly higher in the nedocromil group during the first 6–8 weeks, but these differences diminished by 12 weeks (Fig. 5). Symptoms decreased significantly within 4 weeks after starting nedocromil; there were no differences in symptom scores within the placebo-treated group. The authors concluded that the addition of nedocromil may offer small but important improvements in asthma therapy.

High-dose nedocromil was studied in combination with inhaled corticosteroids by adding 8 mg of nedocromil four times daily or placebo to the treatment of 29 asthmatic patients for 6 weeks (78). All patients were taking inhaled corticosteroids in a dose of up to 1000 µg/day. Morning PEFR increased slightly in the nedocromil group, approaching statistical significance ($p = 0.06$). Daytime asthma symptoms were significantly reduced in the nedocromil group, but nighttime symptoms and bronchodilator use were not differ-

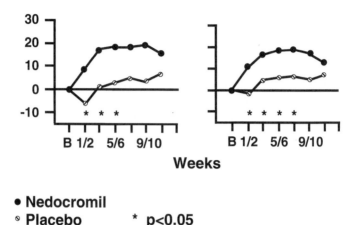

Weeks

- **Nedocromil**
- ⊘ **Placebo**   * **p<0.05**

Figure 5   The change in morning and evening peak expiratory flow rate (PEFR) over 12 weeks from baseline (B) with nedocromil (2 mg four times daily) (closed circles) and placebo (striped circles). (Adapted from Ref. 77.)

ent. There was also no difference in the side-effect profile. Again, these changes are small, but they suggest that the addition of nedocromil may further improve asthma therapy.

Furthermore, a study by Svendson et al. also suggested that adding nedocromil to high-dose inhaled corticosteroids may improve symptoms and morning PEFR (79). Acute administration of cromolyn has also been found to reduce the fall in lung function after challenge with 4.5% saline in patients treated for 3 months with budesonide (80).

In the treatment of asthma in the pediatric population, cromolyn and nedocromil are critical aspects (81). The expert panel guidelines from the National Institutes of Health suggest that cromolyn or nedocromil can be used as first-line therapy in milder asthma. The response should be monitored for 4–6 weeks (81). If symptoms persist or pulmonary function remains impaired, an inhaled corticosteroid should be given at a medium dose and then gradually reduced to the lowest dose that maintains good control of symptoms. Thus, the combination of inhaled corticosteroids and cromolyn/nedocromil is a mainstay of asthma therapy in this population.

E.   Inhaled Corticosteroids and Leukotriene Modifiers

Cysteinyl leukotrienes (leukotriene C4, D4, and E4) are released by inflammatory cells present in the airways of asthmatic patients. Considerable evidence, including evidence from clinical trials using orally and intravenously administered cysteinyl leukotriene receptor antagonists, suggests that these agents are important mediators of asthma (82–86). Two classes of leukotriene modifiers are currently used in the treatment of asthma: zileuton, which is a 5-lipoxygenase enzyme inhibitor, and the leukotriene D4 (LTD4) receptor antagonists zafirlukast and montelukast. The third LTD4 receptor antagonist, pranlukast, has been studied but is not currently approved for use in the United States. Both classes of leukotriene modifiers have been studied in combination with inhaled corticosteroids in the treatment of asthma.

Zileuton has been studied in combination with inhaled corticosteroids by Dahlen and colleagues (87). These patients had asthma that was exacerbated by aspirin, therefore referred to as aspirin-intolerant asthma (AIA). These patients experience chronic rhinosinusitis, nasal polyposis, and acute bronchospasm when they ingest aspirin (88). In recent years, observations have accumulated to suggest that leukotrienes may have a central role in AIA (89–93). In these patients, zileuton at 600 mg four times daily was added to existing therapy, which included medium- to high-dose inhaled (average dose 1030 µg beclomethasone or budesonide) or oral corticosteroids (4–25 mg/day). There was an acute (within 4 h of ingestion) and chronic improvement in pulmonary function, expressed as both an acute and chronic increased FEV_1 from baseline compared with placebo (acute: 12.7% increase with zileuton vs. 6.8% with placebo, $p < 0.01$; chronic: 7% improvement over placebo at the end of 6 weeks, $p < 0.01$). These improvements occurred despite reduced rescue bronchodilator use in the zileuton group. Other improvements included higher morning and evening PEFR measurements. Zileuton also diminished nasal dysfunction, one of the cardinal signs of AIA. There was a return of smell, less rhinorrhea, and a trend toward less congestion. This study suggests that in AIA, the addition of zileuton may bring about greater control of asthma than that achieved by treatment with medium to high doses of corticosteroids.

Montelukast, an LTD4 receptor antagonist, has also been shown to be efficacious in combination with inhaled corticosteroids. Reiss and colleagues randomized 22 asthmatic patients with moderate asthma to receive montelukast at 100 or 250 mg or placebo in a three-period crossover trial (94). Ten of these patients were using inhaled corticosteroids at doses ranging from 200–1200 µg/day. FEV_1 was measured hourly for 10 h after each dose. Both doses of montelukast increased the FEV_1 acutely (within 2–6 h) by 8.6% and 8.5% for the 100- and 250-mg dosages, respectively ($p < 0.05$). These improvements occurred regardless of whether patients used inhaled corticosteroids.

Zafirlukast has been studied in patients whose asthma was not well controlled despite high-dose corticosteroids (mean dose 1600 µg/day) (95). Patients were randomized to receive zafirlukast (80 mg twice daily) or placebo in addition to their usual therapy. After 6 weeks of treatment, patients who received zafirlukast exhibited significantly higher morning PEFR than did patients who received placebo (18.7 vs. 1.5 L/min, respectively, $p = 0.001$). There was evidence of incremental improvement each week of the trial in the zafirlukast arm. There was no evidence of any increases in adverse events in the zafirlukast group, and only about half as many patients in the zafirlukast group experienced worsening asthma over the course of the trial that necessitated a change in therapy.

A recent study evaluated pranlukast (ONO-1078) and its effect on asthma control in the face of a reduced dose of inhaled corticosteroid (96). Seventy-nine patients requiring high doses (>1500 µg/day) of beclomethasone were treated with either pranlukast, 450 mg twice daily, or placebo. At the end of 2 weeks, the doses of inhaled corticosteroid in each group were halved. After 6 weeks, the FEV_1 in the placebo group decreased by 0.33 ± 0.2 L and the morning and evening PEFR decreased by 46 ± 7 and 18 ± 6 L/min, respectively. In contrast, these variables were sustained above baseline in the pranlukast group. Use of inhaled β_2-agonist and nighttime asthma symptoms increased in the placebo group and remained at baseline in the pranlukast group. The authors concluded that pranlukast prevented the asthma deterioration provoked by a 6-week reduction of inhaled corticosteroid.

Montelukast has also been used in the treatment of asthma in the pediatric population (97). In this double-blind, multicenter, placebo-controlled trial, 336 patients were given 5 mg of montelukast or placebo for 8 weeks. Approximately one-third of the patients used inhaled corticosteroids. Mean morning FEV_1 increased from 1.85 to 2.01 L in the montelukast group and from 1.85 to 1.93 L in the placebo group. This represents a change of 8.23%, with $p <$ 0.01 (Fig. 6). Although these changes are modest, they are consistent with those reported in other pediatric trials using currently available therapies (98–101).

F. Inhaled Corticosteroids and Other Miscellaneous Agents

Inhaled corticosteroids have been evaluated by Guttman and colleagues with intravenous corticosteroids for the treatment of acute asthma (102). In a double-blind, placebo-controlled, randomized trial, 60 patients who presented to the emergency department with acute asthma received 80 mg of intravenous methylprednisolone, inhaled salbutamol, and either inhaled beclomethasone 7 mg or placebo. The inhaled medications (beclomethasone and placebo) were

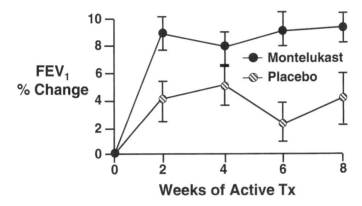

Figure 6 The effect of montelukast (closed circles) and placebo (striped circles) on the mean percent change from baseline in FEV_1 over the 8-week treatment period. The FEV_1 was measured at every visit (2-week intervals). (Adapted from Ref. 97.)

administered with a holding chamber over 8 h. Patients were treated and observed for 12 h, with FEV_1 as the primary outcome variable. FEV_1 and dyspnea, the latter measured by the Borg scale, improved significantly from baseline in both groups. However, there were no differences between the groups over this 12-h period.

Inhaled corticosteroids as the main treatment for acute asthma have also been studied. Rodrigo et al. evaluated the efficacy of inhaled flunisolide or placebo administered at a dose of four puffs (400 μg flunisolide) every 10 min for 3 h in patients whose FEV_1 was less than 50% of that predicted (103). Approximately 25% of subjects in both the flunisolide and placebo groups had used corticosteroids within the previous week and approximately 45% used theophylline preparations. FEV_1 and PEFR were significantly higher in the flunisolide group at 90, 120, 150, and 180 min. The admission rate in the flunisolide group was approximately half that of the placebo group. The studies by Guttman et al. and Rodrigo et al. reveal different results, suggesting that there may be efficacy in using inhaled corticosteroids during an acute exacerbation, but the response is not uniform among all patients. This issue has been further illustrated in several other studies where inhaled corticosteroids appeared to provide benefit in acute asthma in some but not in others (104–106).

Inhaled furosemide has also been used in conjunction with inhaled corticosteroids and other agents in the treatment of exacerbations of acute asthma

(107). Forty subjects presenting with acute asthma were randomized to either 20 mg of furosemide or placebo; 25% of the furosemide group and 19% of the placebo group used inhaled or oral corticosteroids. All patients also received 250 mg of intravenous aminophylline and 100 mg intravenous hydrocortisone upon presentation. The baseline FEV_1 or serum theophylline concentrations did not differ significantly between the two groups. At 60 min, the mean FEV_1 of the group that received furosemide increased by 28 ± 5.9%, a significantly higher figure than that in the control group. The mechanism is unclear, but previous studies suggest that furosemide may inhibit sodium, potassium, and chloride transport or may block the release of substance P (108,109).

III. Oral Corticosteroids in Combination with Other Agents

Oral corticosteroids have been used in combination with other agents in hopes of reducing the oral corticosteroid requirement. Several studies have employed high-dose nedocromil as a potential steroid-sparing agent (110–113). Boulet et al. (110) studied 37 oral corticosteroid–dependent patients with reverse asthma who were receiving daily or alternate-day oral corticosteroids who had participated in a 12-week double-blind study where they received either nedocromil, 16 mg daily, or placebo. Boulet and colleagues describe a continuation of this study, where therapy was continued for an additional 12 weeks. During the 12-week period, patients were evaluated every 2 weeks. The nedocromil group was able to achieve a greater percentage reduction in oral steroid dose, although it was only statistically significant when the percentage change in dose was calculated (nedocromil group: decrease of 4.6 mg/day, placebo group: decrease of 2.0 mg/day, p = 0.054). The percentage change in steroid dose was −61% in the nedocromil group and −28% in the placebo group, p = 0.03. There were 9 withdrawals in the nedocromil group; 1 subject was lost to follow-up, and 8 withdrew for worsening asthma; 7 patients withdrew in the placebo group, 1 patient was lost to follow-up, and 6 experienced a worsening of their asthma. In general, there were trends in favor of nedocromil as an oral steroid–sparing agent, but the differences between the groups were not statistically significant except for the percentage change in corticosteroid dose discussed above.

   In acute asthma, inhaled corticosteroids have been studied as an adjunct to oral corticosteroids (114). In this study, nebulized budesonide was compared with placebo in acute pediatric asthma in a randomized, double-blind trial. Children aged 6 months to 18 years with a moderate to severe exacerbation of asthma and a pulmonary index score > 5 or < 11 after nebulized salbutamol were eligible. The pulmonary index score is a previously published scale of severity that correlated significantly with FEV_1 and hospitalization rates in a prior study of asthmatic children aged > 6 years who presented to an emergency department (115). All 38 patients received prednisone 1 mg/ kg orally and nebulized salbutamol 0.15 mg/kg every 30 min for three doses and then every hour for 4 hours. Patients were then given 2 mg of nebulized budesonide or 4 mL of nebulized saline. Of note, 15 of 38 patients used inhaled corticosteroids, and the data were analyzed in a stratified fashion to take this into account. The group that received budesonide was discharged sooner, but there were no significant differences in the pulmonary index score, although there was trend toward a lower score in the budesonide group ($p = 0.07$). These results are preliminary and the approach cannot be widely recommended until it is further validated in future studies.

Oral corticosteroids have also been compared with intramuscular corticosteroids in acute asthma (116–121). Schuckman and colleagues studied 154 patients in a randomized, double-blind, placebo-controlled trial (116). Patients were eligible if they exhibited a PEFR < 350 L/min and were to be discharged from the emergency department after taking oral corticosteroids. Patients were randomized to receive either triamcinalone (40 mg i.m.) or placebo injection plus prednisone (40 mg/day orally for 5 days). Patients were instructed to use an inhaled β_2-agonist and to continue other routine medications. The main outcome measure was relapse of asthma. Mean PEFRs were 244 ± 64 L/min for the triamcinalone group and 245 ± 83 L/min in the prednisone group. Fifty percent of patients were smokers, but the pack-years were not described. Inhaled corticosteroids were used by 17% of the triamcinalone group and 23% of the prednisone group ($p = 0.35$). The relapse rate was 9% in the triamcinalone group and 14.5% in the prednisone group ($p = 0.29$). The study was powered to detect a relapse difference of 15%. Therefore, this study reveals that in the face of some inhaled corticosteroid use, intramuscular triamcinalone resulted in a relapse rate similar to that of oral prednisone in the treatment of acute asthma.

The treatment of the corticosteroid-dependent patient with asthma can be very challenging, as standard therapies will not often result in a significant reduction in oral corticosteroid usage. Thus, many studies have been published adding "alternative" therapies to a treatment regimen. These alternative therapies involve agents not commonly used in asthma, such as cyclosporine (122–124), methotrexate (125–130), gold (131–134), and troleandomycin (135–139).

Lock and colleagues evaluated the use of cyclosporine in the treatment of corticosteroid-dependent asthma (124). In a year-long trial with a 36-week treatment period, patients received cyclosporine at 5 mg/kg per day or placebo. The primary outcome was a decrease in oral prednisolone dosage, which ranged from 5 to 22.5 mg/day.

Nineteen subjects received cyclosporine, but three withdrew during the first 12 weeks of treatment—one due to an asthma exacerbation, and one because of hypertrichosis; one subject died suddenly after exertion, which was felt to be secondary to a cardiac dysrhythmia and not cyclosporine use. The cyclosporine group reduced their prednisolone use by 62% (from 10 to 3.5 mg) as compared to 25% in the placebo group (from 10 to 7.5 mg) ($p = 0.043$). Although morning PEFR improved in the cyclosporine group, FEV_1, FVC, PEFR variability, and symptoms did not change significantly in either group. Thus, cyclosporine allowed a reduction in corticosteroid dosage, but side effects (gastrointestinal disturbance, hypertrichosis, headache, gum hypertrophy, and hypertension) were frequent and patients required close monitoring.

Shiner and colleagues evaluated the use of methotrexate 15 mg by mouth weekly or placebo in the treatment of corticosteroid-dependent asthma (128). The methotrexate-treated group were able to decrease their daily prednisolone dose by 50%, as compared to a 14% reduction in the placebo group ($p = 0.005$). As in the study by Lock and colleagues described above, lung function and symptoms did not change significantly in either group. Liver function abnormalities were the most common serious side effect (in 12 of 38 patients) and resulted in discontinuation of treatment in 5.

In contrast, the study by Erzurum and colleagues did not show a benefit when patients were given 15 mg of methotrexate or placebo intramuscularly (129). Both the methotrexate and placebo groups were able to reduce their prednisone use significantly (39.6 and 40.2% in the methotrexate and placebo groups, respectively). The authors concluded that improved compliance and frequent physician visits allowed both groups to undergo significant reductions in steroid use.

High-dose intramuscular triamcinalone has been studied in acute asthma, as discussed above, but also in corticosteroid-dependent asthma (121,130,137,140). In a study by Ogirala and coworkers, 19 patients with corticosteroid-dependent asthma were randomized to receive 360 mg of intramus-

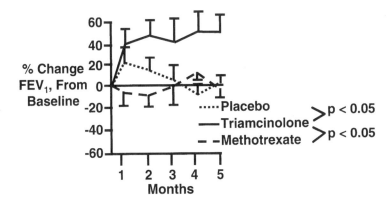

Figure 7 Comparison of mean FEV_1 in the three treatment groups, placebo (dotted line), triamcinalone (unbroken line), and methotrexate (dashed line) expressed as percent change from baseline. Only the triamcinolone-treated patients showed a significant and sustained increase in FEV_1. (Adapted from Ref. 130.)

cular triamcinalone plus methotrexate placebo, placebo triamcinalone plus low-dose methotrexate (7.5 mg followed by 15 mg weekly), or placebo triamcinalone and placebo methotrexate. The mean corticosteroid use was similar in the three groups: 6.0 ± 8.3 mg, 5.0 ± 4.5 mg, and 7.1 ± 6.9 mg in the placebo, triamcinalone, and methotrexate groups, respectively. The baseline FEV_1 was also similar in the three groups, ranging from 67–75% predicted. Methacholine challenge was performed every 6 weeks, pulmonary function tests were done every 4 weeks, and PEFRs were recorded at home twice daily. The study duration was 6 months.

The patients in the triamcinalone group showed a significant and sustained increase in home PEFR, and their FEV_1 persistently improved by a mean of 40%, whereas the methotrexate and placebo groups' FEV_1 did not change significantly from baseline ($p < 0.05$) (Fig. 7). Steroid side effects were worse in the triamcinalone group and included cushingoid appearance in 4 patients, muscle cramps in 5, transient hypertension requiring therapy in 2, mild diabetes requiring an oral hypoglycemic agent in 1, and polyuria and polydipsia in 3. In the methotrexate group, side effects included increases in transaminases in 3 patients, a rash in 1 patient, and nausea and abdominal pain in 1. The placebo group experienced milder chronic steroid side effects. According to the analysis, the overall differences in the side-effect profiles among the three groups were not statistically significant. As this study evalu-

Table 1 Therapeutic Success in All Patients Randomized to Treatment Classified by Baseline Oral Corticosteroid Dose Pretreatment

Treatment Group	Dose at Randomization (mg)	Total Randomized (n)	Therapeutic Success			
			Completed		Compliant + Noncompliant	
			n	%	n	%
Placebo	<10	3	2	66.7	2	66.7
	10–19	92	26	28.3	31	33.7
	≥20	44	9	20.5	12	27.3
Auranofin	<10	4	1	25.0	2	50.0
	10–19	92	45	48.9[a]	55	59.8[b]
	≥20	40	10	25.0	19	47.5

% of patients receiving 10–19 mg prednisone per day who were successful at reducing their dose by at least 50%—$p < 0.05$ as compared to placebo.
[a] % of patients who completed study.
[b] % includes patients who enrolled, regardless of compliance.

ated only one injection of high-dose triamcinalone, repeat injections have not been studied, and these results must be extrapolated with caution.

Gold (auranofin) as a steroid-sparing agent has been studied by Bernstein and colleagues (131,133) and others (134). Patients were eligible if they required at least 10 mg of prednisone per day for the control and prevention of asthma exacerbations (131). A total of 279 patients were randomized to receive auranofin 3 mg twice daily or placebo during an 8-month clinical trial, which was divided into three phases, including a 4-week baseline period (Phase I), a 6-month double-blind treatment and steroid-reduction phase (Phase II), and a 4-week posttreatment observation period (termed Phase III) during which steroid and auranofin doses or placebo doses were maintained at levels achieved by the end of Phase II. The primary outcome variable was a reduction in daily corticosteroid by 50% or more.

Baseline FEV_1 was similar in both groups (64 and 63% in placebo and auranofin groups, respectively). The majority of patients in each group used between 10 and 19 mg of oral prednisone per day (66.2 and 67.7% in the placebo and auranofin groups, respectively). The proportion of patients achieving a > 50% reduction in oral corticosteroid dose was significantly higher in the auranofin group as compared to the placebo group (41 vs. 27%, $p = 0.01$) (Table 1). This effect was greatest in the group requiring 10–19 mg of oral prednisone per day ($p < 0.001$). This was not appreciated in the group receiving > 20 mg of prednisone per day, although the difference trended toward significance (47.5 vs. 27.3%, $p = 0.06$). There were no significant differences between the groups in symptoms, concomitant medication use, or lung function. However, gastrointestinal and cutaneous adverse events (abdominal pain, diarrhea, dyspepsia, rash, and pruritus) were greater in the auranofin group ($p < 0.001$ and $p < 0.015$ for the gastrointestinal and skin adverse event comparisons, respectively). Thus, auranofin did exhibit a steroid-sparing effect in this study, but mainly in patients using 10–19 mg of prednisone per day. As with all alternative therapies, the side-effect profiles are significant, and patients require close follow-up.

Troleandomycin (TAO) was introduced in 1957, and as early as 1959 it was reported that TAO appeared to be effective in patients with severe asthma (138). It was felt to have a steroid-sparing effect and the mechanism is thought to occur through alterations in steroid metabolism, as described by Spector and colleagues (139). However, its steroid-sparing effect is most consistent when it is used with methylprednisolone rather than prednisone. Nelson and colleagues performed a randomized, double-blind, placebo-controlled trial in 75 patients with asthma requiring daily corticosteroids (135). The primary outcomes were determination of the lowest stable methylprednisolone dose and assessment of corticosteroid side effects. A total of 30 patients receiving TAO and 27 patients receiving placebo completed 1 year of the 2-year study; 17 on TAO and 8 on placebo completed the 2-year study. The vast majority of patients in both groups achieved alternate-day dosing (29 of 30 on TAO and 23 of 27 on placebo in the first year). The lowest stable doses of methylprednisolone achieved were 10.4 mg/day on placebo and 6.3 mg/day on TAO. However, the baseline dose of methylprednisolone was higher in the placebo group; thus the reductions were not statistically significant. Differences between the groups were appreciated in fasting blood sugar, serum cholesterol, and progression toward osteoporosis. In each of these adverse events, the more unfavorable response occurred in the TAO group. Thus the addition of TAO did not result in a significant reduction of methylprednisolone dosage but did result in increased side effects.

IV. Theophylline in Combination with Other Agents

A. Theophylline with Intravenous and/or Oral Corticosteroids

Theophylline has been studied in acute asthma to determine whether its addition to conventional therapy (which includes intravenous or oral corticosteroids) adds any benefit. Huang and colleagues studied 21 adult asthmatics presenting to the emergency department with acute exacerbations of asthma (141). Subjects received intravenous aminophylline or placebo in addition to nebulized albuterol given every 0.5–4 h and intravenous methylprednisolone 60 mg every 4 h. Treatment with this regimen was continued for 48 h. Upon admission from the emergency department, the baseline percent predicted FEV_1 was 49 ± 19% in the aminophylline group versus 43 ± 13% in the placebo group. The improvement in FEV_1 at 3 h was greater in the aminophylline group (29 ± 23% vs. 10 ± 10% in the aminophylline and placebo groups, respectively; $p = 0.023$). At 48 h, the percent predicted FEV_1 was 75 ± 19% in the aminophylline group and 58 ±15% in the placebo group, $p= 0.048$. Finally, the aminophylline group required fewer doses of nebulized albuterol. Thus, the authors concluded that the addition of aminophylline to intravenous corticosteroids appeared to benefit adults presenting with acute asthma.

In contrast, Self and colleagues showed that intravenous aminophylline in addition to oral prednisone (0.5 mg/kg every 6 h) and albuterol did not improve FEV_1 or duration of hospitalization (142). Murphy and coworkers studied 44 patients presenting to an emergency department with acute asthma (143). Patients received aminophylline or placebo in addition to 125 mg of intravenous methylprednisolone. Measurements of PEFR were made hourly for 5 h. There were no significant differences in PEFR throughout the study period between the two groups. No comments were made on admission rates, although this was commented upon in a similar study by Wrenn and colleagues (144). Although the PEFR did not differ between aminophylline and placebo groups, as in the study by Murphy et al., the authors noted a 6% admission rate in the aminophylline-treated group as compared to 21% in the placebo group ($p = 0.016$). These findings suggest that theophylline may exert other effects that may affect admission and not necessarily the FEV_1. Certainly there are data suggesting that theophylline preparations enhance diaphragmatic function (145,146).

B. Theophylline and Nedocromil/Cromolyn

An earlier study also evaluated the addition of cromolyn and beclomethasone to an asthma treatment regimen in patients whose asthma was not fully controlled by regular β_2-agonists and theophylline (147). Seventeen patients were studied in a double-blind crossover fashion in two 8-week treatment periods. Compared to baseline, both beclomethasone and cromolyn produced similar improvements in morning and evening PEFRs and symptom scores. The beclomethasone arm resulted in further improvements in nocturnal awakenings and morning chest tightness and in reductions in β_2-agonist use.

A second study evaluated the effect of nedocromil 2 mg four times daily in patients who used slow-release theophylline preparations (148). Two hundred patients with moderate asthma (percent predicted FEV_1, 65–67%) were randomized to received nedocromil or placebo. They were initially maintained on theophylline preparations adjusted to a therapeutic level, with inhaled β_2-agonists as needed. After the first 2 weeks of study, the theophylline preparations were withdrawn; after 6 weeks, patients who used oral β_2-agonists (13%) discontinued them. Patients were allowed to use inhaled β_2-agonists and immediate-release theophylline preparations if the inhaled β_2-agonist did not provide relief.

The cumulative daily symptom scores showed statistically significant differences in favor of nedocromil throughout the study ($p \leq 0.02$). The withdrawal of theophylline did not cause an increase in daytime asthma and cough symptoms in the nedocromil-treated group but a leveling off in the previous improvement. Nighttime asthma scores also were in favor of nedocromil and returned to pretheophylline withdrawal levels during weeks 7–14 ($p = 0.006$). FEV_1 also improved in the nedocromil group, from 4.01 $\pm$ 0.17 at baseline to 4.23 $\pm$ 0.15 L. This is in contrast to the placebo group, where the baseline FEV_1 was 3.79 $\pm$ 0.14 L ($p = 0.32$ as compared with the nedocromil group at baseline) and decreased to 3.37 $\pm$ 0.18 ($p < 0.0001$ as compared to nedocromil at week 14). Patients did complain about the taste of nedocromil, but adverse events such as cough, bronchospasm, and headache were reported with equal frequency. Thus, these results indicated that nedocromil provided an additional benefit to adult patients with asthma receiving slow-release theophylline preparations and β_2-agonists.

C. Theophylline and Leukotriene Modifiers

To date, no double-blind, placebo-controlled studies have been performed evaluating the combination of theophylline and any of the leukotriene modifiers without concomitant inhaled corticosteroids. However, they are used in combination clinically, and the leukotriene D4-receptor antagonists have been reported not to affect serum theophylline levels. However, a case report by Katial et al. reveals that this may not be accurate (149). A 15-year-old girl with asthma had been taking theophylline (Slo-bid) 300 mg twice daily, attaining serum levels of approximately 11 μg/mL. After beginning zafirlukast at 20 mg twice daily, her theophylline level increased to 24 μg/mL. Attempts were made to restart theophylline therapy at progressively lower doses to a minimum of 75 mg/day; each attempt was accompanied by an elevated theophylline level of 18–27 µg/mL. The investigators measured serum zafirlukast levels in this patient (not routinely done), and they were in the expected range according to previous pharmacokinetic studies. On resuming 300 mg of theophylline twice daily after stopping zafirlukast, her level again ranged from 10–11 µg/mL. Despite the data provided by the manufacturers, it is prudent to measure serum theophylline levels in patients for whom a leukotriene D4-receptor antagonist is added. In regard to 5-lipoxygenase inhibitors such as zileuton, there is already a known interaction with theophylline; thus the measurement of serum levels in the setting is also recommended.

V. Cromolyn/Nedocromil and Other Agents

Cromolyn and nedocromil without concomitant inhaled corticosteroids have been studied primarily in combination with inhaled β_2-agonists in exercise-induced asthma. The formulation of both nedocromil 4 mg and salbutamol 200 µg in a metered-dose inhaler was compared to salbutamol alone in 12 children with exercise-induced asthma (150). In a randomized, double-blind, placebo-controlled crossover fashion, 12 children aged 7–13 years received either the combination, salbutamol, or placebo alone 20 min before exercise. Both the nedocromil/salbutamol combination and salbutamol alone offered significant protection against a fall in FEV_1 compared to placebo (percent fall in FEV_1: 25.7 ± 18%, 2.2 ± 2.7%, and 3.7 ± 4.4% in placebo, nedocromil/salbutamol, and salbutamol groups, respectively; $p < 0.05$). There were no statistically or clinically significant differences between the nedocromil/salbutamol and salbutamol responses. When individual protection was evaluated, complete protection ($<10\%$ fall in FEV_1) was provided in 100% of children when receiving the nedocromil/salbutamol combination, 92% when receiving the salbutamol alone, and 16% when receiving placebo. The difference between the nedocromil/salbutamol protection and salbutamol protection was not significant. In addition, only two children exhibited a fall $> 10\%$ while on salbutamol, to 12 and 13%. Although the authors concluded that a minority of patients may benefit from the nedocromil/salbutamol combination, a more detailed pharmacoeconomic analysis should be performed before this can be recommended.

Nedocromil in combination with furosemide has been studied in children with exercise-induced asthma (151). Twenty-four children aged 6–16 years with mild asthma were randomized to inhaled furosemide (30 mg), nedocromil (4 mg), the combination of the two drugs, and placebo in a double-blind cross-over design. Both active drugs were more efficacious than placebo, as the mean fall in FEV_1 was $28.5 \pm 13.8\%$ on placebo, $15.4 \pm 8.4\%$ after nedocromil ($p < 0.001$), and $11.4 \pm 9.1\%$ after furosemide ($p < 0.001$). When the drugs were given together, there was a statistically significant additive effect, as the mean fall in FEV_1 was $5.8 \pm 3.6\%$. The proposed mechanism of furosemide's action includes blockade of chloride secretion by furosemide, which has been shown to prevent bronchoconstriction induced by various triggers such as nebulized distilled water, cold air, metabisulfite, allergen and lysine-aspirin, but not methacholine or histamine (151–157).

Cromolyn has been studied in combination with terbutaline for the treatment of exercise-induced asthma and pediatric asthma (158,159). Woolley and colleagues evaluated whether the combination of cromolyn 2 mg and terbutaline 0.5 mg offered a longer duration of action than terbutaline alone, cromolyn alone, or placebo (158). Twelve patients with mild asthma were randomized to treatments in a double-blind fashion using a Latin square design. Of the 12 subjects, 1 patient used beclomethasone, 3 used cromolyn and 2 used theophylline preparations. FEV_1 was measured immediately before and after exercise and at 15 min, 2, 4, and 6 h after the medication.

Compared with placebo, the fall in FEV_1 was significantly reduced by either cromolyn alone or terbutaline alone for up to 2 h. The combination of cromolyn and terbutaline afforded protection (a fall in FEV_1 of $< 10\%$ postexercise) for up to 4 h after inhalation ($p < 0.05$ when the combination was compared to either drug alone and placebo). No difference in protection was seen between the combination and cromolyn or terbutaline alone during the initial 2 h postexercise. Thus, the combination of a β_2-agonist and cromolyn may offer prolonged effective protection from the fall in FEV_1. The authors hypothesized that inhaled β_2-agonist use may increase the surface area of the airways exposed to cromolyn, thus allowing it to exert a greater effect.

In the treatment of pediatric asthma, cromolyn, terbutaline, and the combination have been studied by Shapiro and coworkers (159). Twenty-seven children aged 6–12 years with mild-to-moderate asthma were randomized to cromolyn 20 mg, terbutaline 0.1 mg/kg up to 4 mg, or the combination three times daily in a double-blind crossover fashion. After 24 weeks (8 weeks per treatment period), daily diary scores were generally lower with cromolyn or the combination. Similarly, morning PEFR was higher with the combination ($p < 0.05$), whereas evening PEFRs were higher with either cromolyn or the combination ($p < 0.01$). Methacholine challenge demonstrated less bronchial hyperresponsiveness with the combination or cromolyn alone as compared with terbutaline ($p < 0.02$). In addition, the patients required a total of four prednisone bursts while taking terbutaline alone as compared to one burst while taking cromolyn alone and none while using the combination (statistics not performed). Not surprisingly, the use of an anti-inflammatory agent in the asthma treatment regimen is superior to inhaled β_2-agonist alone.

Cromolyn has also been combined with fenoterol, a short-acting inhaled β_2-agonist used in the study of exercise-induced asthma by Clarke and colleagues (160). Twenty subjects were randomized using a Latin square design to cromolyn alone, fenoterol alone, or the combination. Each of the single treatment arms was accompanied by a placebo. These results revealed that fenoterol alone or in combination with cromolyn increased the FEV_1 by up to 25% before and after exercise. In these patients, cromolyn was of no benefit in eliminating the fall in FEV_1 after exercise. Interestingly, the group exhibited a mean fall in FEV_1 of 43.9% at screening compared with a change of 9.8% while on placebo.

VI. Anticholinergic Medications and Other Agents

Ipratropium bromide (Atrovent) is the first-line choice for the therapy of chronic obstructive pulmonary disease. However, it has also been evaluated in the treatment of acute asthma and in pediatric asthma. The studies described below address the use of the combination of ipratropium and an inhaled β_2-agonist in these settings. The combination has been studied in acute asthma for more than 10 years (161–171). Glycopyrrolate has also been studied in combination with albuterol in acute asthma (172). Lin and coworkers concluded that ipratropium should be combined with albuterol via nebulizer in treatment of asthmatic patients in the emergency department (161). They evaluated 55 adult asthmatics with PEFRs < 200 L/min who were randomly assigned to receive nebulized albuterol alone (2.5 mg followed by two more doses at 20-min intervals) or the same albuterol regimen plus ipratropium (0.5 mg combined with the initial dose of albuterol only). The primary endpoints were changes in PEFR and change in percentage predicted PEFR over time. PEFRs were assessed at baseline and at 20-min intervals for a 1-h period.

The increases in PEFR and percent predicted PEFR over time were both significantly greater in the combined ipratropium/albuterol group as compared to albuterol alone ($p < 0.001$) (Fig. 8). In addition, the proportion of admitted patients was less in the combination group (3 of 27) as compared to the albu-

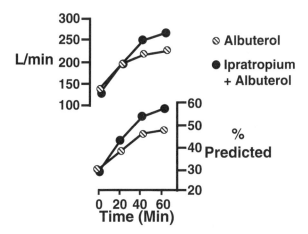

Figure 8 Peak expiratory flow rate (PEFR) responses after albuterol (striped circles) and ipratropium + albuterol (closed circles) expressed as a geometric mean (top graph), and geometric means of percentages of predicted values (bottom graph). Time is expressed in minutes. (Adapted from Ref. 161.)

terol group (10 of 28) (95% Cl: 3–46%, $p = 0.03$). These data suggest that ipratropium should be combined with albuterol for patients with acute asthma, especially those with PEFRs <200 L/min.

In contrast to these results, Karpel and colleagues showed no benefit of adding ipratropium to albuterol for the treatment of acute asthma (163). They randomized 384 patients presenting to the emergency department with acute asthma to either nebulized albuterol 2.5 mg or the combination of albuterol and ipratropium 0.5 mg at entry and at 45 min. These patients differed from those in the Lin study, as approximately 30% used theophylline preparations and 30% used either inhaled and/or oral corticosteroid preparations. In the Lin study, only 13% used inhaled corticosteroids and none used theophylline. In addition, Lin et al. measured PEFR and Karpel et al. measured FEV$_1$. In the Karpel study, the median change in FEV$_1$ was 0.53 L in the ipratropium/ albuterol group and 0.42 L in the albuterol group ($p = 0.35$). There were also no significant differences between the groups in the need for additional therapy or the number requiring hospitalization.

Earlier studies by Summers et al. (165) and Higgins et al. (166) evaluating ipratropium in the treatment of acute asthma concluded that ipratropium did not confer added benefit in one study (165) but did in the other (166). For instance, Higgins et al. randomized 40 patients who presented with acute asthma to either nebulized salbutamol 5 mg or salbutamol mixed with ipratropium 0.5 mg on presentation to the hospital and again 2 h later. The PEFR in both groups increased at 2 h, but there was no statistically significant difference between them. The authors compared their results to those of two other studies (167,173). When the differences in the bronchodilator responses were pooled, the mean percentage improvement in lung function after an inhaled β_2-agonist was 31.5%; after inhaled β_2-agonist plus ipratropium, the percentage improvement was 44%. The improvement in bronchodilation offered by ipratropium was 12.5%, with a 95% Cl of 1.2–23.8%. Therefore, pooled data do appear to confirm a small advantage with combined treatment. Although complications with ipratropium are uncommon, Hall and colleagues report that acute angle-closure glaucoma occurred as a complication of ipratropium in a 66-year-old woman treated for acute asthma in the emergency department (174).

Ipratropium has also been studied in the treatment of asthma in the pediatric population (175–179). Qureshi and colleagues studied 434 children aged 2–18 years. The patients were randomized to either nebulized albuterol, 2.5 or 5 mg per dose depending on body weight, plus placebo every 20 min for three doses or ipratropium 0.5 mg, with the second and third doses of albuterol. Prednisone or prednisolone 2 mg/kg was also given to each subject.

Overall, the hospitalization rate was lower in the ipratropium group than in the control group: 59 of 215 vs. 80 of 219 in the ipratropium and control groups, respectively, $p = 0.05$. When the group was divided according to severity of asthma, hospitalization rates were lower in the ipratropium group with severe asthma (PEFR < 50% predicted) as compared to the severe control group ($p = 0.02$). There was no difference in hospitalization rates in the patients with PEFR 50–70% predicted. As in the adult studies, ipratropium appeared to benefit those patients with more severe asthma.

The benefit of ipratropium in the patients with more severe asthma was again shown in the study of pediatric patients by Schuh and colleagues (176). This study design was slightly different in that these patients exhibited FEV_1 < 50% predicted prior to entry and were randomized to either three doses of ipratropium at 0.25 mg with albuterol within 60 min, one dose of ipratropium with albuterol, or no ipratropium. Pulmonary function measurements were performed every 20 min for up to 120 min.

At 120 min, the mean percentage predicted FEV_1 improved from 33.4–56.7% in the group, who received three doses of ipratropium, 34.2–52.3% in the single-dose ipratropium group, and 35.4–48.3% in the group that received no ipratropium ($p = 0.0001$). Overall, the hospitalization rates were lowest in the group that received three doses of ipratropium, but the differences were not significant. However, in patients with $FEV_1 < 30\%$ predicted, the hospitalization rates were 27% in the group that received three doses of ipratropium, 56% in the group that received the single dose of ipratropium, and 83% in the group that received no ipratropium ($p = 0.027$). No toxic effects were attributable to ipratropium. Again, the group with severe asthma seemed to benefit most from ipratropium.

Several studies have evaluated the combination of atropine and albuterol in children and adults with acute asthma and in nocturnal worsening of asthma (180–182). Instead of ipratropium, adult asthmatics presenting with an exacerbation to the emergency department were randomized to one of three therapies added to three doses of 2.5 mg nebulized albuterol: saline placebo, 2.0 mg atropine added to the second and third albuterol treatments, and 2.0 mg atropine added to the first and third albuterol treatments. There were no significant differences between the three groups in PEFR, hospitalization rates, or adverse events. In this study, atropine did not offer any significant benefit over albuterol alone.

The combination of nebulized atropine and albuterol was studied in nocturnal asthma in 11 patients (182). Patients were randomized to nebulized albuterol with either placebo or atropine methylnitrate in a crossover fashion at 10 P.M. on each of 4 consecutive nights. As these patients used inhaled corticosteroids, they would receive each medication regimen on and off steroids. There were no differences in the overnight fall in FEV_1 between the groups. In another study evaluating nocturnal asthma, 21 patients were randomized to controlled-release terbutaline tablets 10 mg twice daily, ipratropium 0.40 mg four times daily, and the two drugs in combination (183). Although the nocturnal decline in PEFR was lowest with terbutaline and with the combination of the two drugs as compared to treatment with ipratropium alone, these differences were not significant. Therefore, the combination of ipratropium and albuterol does not appear to be efficacious in the treatment of nocturnal asthma.

VII. Leukotriene Modifiers and Other Agents

Most studies evaluating the leukotriene modifiers have studied their effects without other medications, and inhaled β_2-agonists were used as needed. However, one study evaluated the effects of zafirlukast and loratadine on the early- and late-phase responses in asthma (184). Twelve subjects with mild asthma and atopy underwent allergen bronchoprovocation at baseline and after 1 week of treatment with zafirlukast 80 mg twice daily, after 1 week of treatment with the antihistamine loratadine 10 mg twice daily, and after 1 week of therapy with both agents in a double-blind crossover fashion. Zafirlukast alone reduced the fall in lung function occurring during the early and late responses by 62 $\pm$ 11% and 55 $\pm$ 12%, respectively ($p < 0.05$ vs. control). Loratadine alone inhibited the early and late responses by 25 $\pm$ 14% and 40 $\pm$ 16%, respectively ($p < 0.05$ vs. control). The combination of the two agents reduced the early and late responses even further, by 75 $\pm$ 8% and 74 $\pm$ 14%, respectively ($p < 0.05$ vs. control). These findings are intriguing, but further studies are needed in order to recommend this regimen as treatment for chronic asthma.

VIII. Antihistamines and Other Agents

It is known that treatment of sinusitis and allergic rhinitis improves asthma symptoms (185–189). Corren and colleagues conducted a randomized, double-blind, placebo-controlled trial evaluating the efficacy of loratidine 5 mg plus pseudoephedrine 120 mg twice daily in patients with allergic rhinitis and mild asthma (189). After 6 weeks, rhinitis and asthma symptom scores were significantly reduced in patients receiving therapy as compared to those on placebo. PEFR improved 26.2 $\pm$ 4.6 L/min, as compared to 8.5 $\pm$ 3.5 L/min in the control group, $p = 0.002$). In contrast, Ekstrom and colleagues found that loratadine alone at 20 mg twice daily offered no significant benefit over placebo when PEFR, FEV_1, FVC, daily symptoms, and nocturnal symptoms were evaluated (190). The subjects in the study by Ekstrom et al. had more severe disease than those in the study by Corren et al., and not all of them had symptoms of atopy. Last, the Corren study was performed during an allergy season, which was not done in the Ekstrom study. Thus, antihistamines with or without decongestants may have benefit in the asthmatic patient with an allergic component, especially during an allergy season. In addition, antihistamines did not appear to interact with the ability of albuterol to bronchodilate, as shown by Spector and colleagues in their evaluation of cetirizine in mild to moderate asthma (191).

IX. Concluding Remarks

Combination therapy offers the ability to treat several aspects of asthma simultaneously and potentially also to decrease side effects. Fixed-combination regi-

Table 2 Compliance Results[a]

Drug	Method of Analysis	Day-by-Day Use, % of Days			
		Correct Dose	<50% of Dose[+]	All Doses Omitted	Extra Doses Taken
Budesonide	A	30	56	38	5
	B	41	52	31	6
	C	36	48	26	6
	D	30	42	17	7

[a] Percent compliance, 60 ± 37.

mens are also attractive, although they have not necessarily improved compliance, as shown by Bosely et al. (192) and Braunstein et al. (193). Bosley et al. demonstrated that combining budesonide and terbutaline in one inhaler did not improve compliance as compared to the use of separate inhalers of budesonide and terbutaline (192). The average compliance was 60–70%. Treatment was taken as prescribed on only 30–40% of study days. Only 15% of patients took the medications as prescribed on 80% of the study days (Table 2). Braunstein and colleagues studied compliance with a fixed-dose nedocromil/salbutamol combination at two actuations four times daily as compared to nedocromil alone at 2 mg four times daily (193). The mean number of two actuation doses per day was 2.1 ± 1.3 for nedocromil and 2.4 ± 2.1 for the combination. Similar to the Bosley study, 35% of the nedocromil group and 34% of the combination group were compliant (6–10 actuations per day) >60% of days. As always, education in asthma is essential and may ultimately improve compliance. However, fixed-combination regimens do offer convenience for the patient if both medications are to be used with the same frequency. As the ultimate goals in asthma therapy are to reduce airway inflammation, decrease bronchial hyperresponsiveness, and improve quality of life, combination therapy may offer the opportunity to accomplish these goals at the lowest doses of medications possible.

References

1. Barnes PJ, Pedersen S, Busse WW. Efficacy and safety of inhaled corticosteroids: new developments. Am J Respir Crit Care Med 1998; 157:S1–S53.
2. Barnes PJ, Pedersen S. Efficacy and safety of inhaled corticosteroids in asthma:

report of a workshop held in Eze, France, October 1992. Am Rev Respir Dis 1993; 148:S1–S26.

3. Dompeling E, van Schayck CP, van Grunsven PM, van Herwaarden CL, Akkermans R, Molema J, Folgering H, van Weel C. Slowing the deterioration of asthma and chronic obstructive pulmonary disease observed during bronchodilator therapy by adding inhaled corticosteroids. A 4-year prospective study. Ann Intern Med 1993; 118:770–778.

4. Haahtela T, Alanko K, Muittari A, Lahdensuo A, Sahlstrom K, Vilkka V. The superiority of combination beclomethasone and salbutamol over standard dosing of salbutamol in the treatment of chronic asthma. Ann Allergy 1989; 62: 63–66.

5. Turner-Warwick M. Epidemiology of nocturnal asthma. Am J Med 1988; 85: 6–8.

6. McGivern DV, Ward M, MacFarlance JT, Roderick Smith WH. Failure of once daily inhaled corticosteroid treatment to control chronic asthma. Thorax 1984; 39:933–934.

7. Malo JL, Cartier A, Merland N, Ghezzo H, Burek A, Morris J, Jennings BH. Four-times-a-day dosing frequency is better than a twice-a-day regimen in subjects requiring a high-dose inhaled steroid, budesonide, to control moderate to severe asthma. Am Rev Respir Dis 1989; 140:624–628.

8. Toogood JH, Baskerville JC, Jennings B, Lefcoe NM, Johansson SA. Influence of dosing frequency and schedule on the response of chronic asthmatics to the aerosol steroid, budesonide. J Allergy Clin Immunol 1982; 70:288–298.

9. Horn CR, Clark TJH, Cochrane GM. Can the morbidity of asthma be reduced by high dose inhaled therapy? Respir Med 1990; 84:61–66.

10. Horn CR, Clark TJH, Cochrane GM. Inhaled therapy reduces morning dips in asthma. Lancet 1984; 1:1143–1145.

11. Prahl P, Jensen T, Bjorregaard-Anderson H. Adrenocortical function in children on high dose steroid aerosol therapy. Allergy 1987; 42:541–544.

12. Pincus DJ, Szefler SJ, Ackerson LM, Martin RJ. Chronotherapy of asthma with inhaled steroids: the effect of dosage timing on drug efficacy. J Allergy Clin Immunol 1995; 95:1172–1178.

13. Waalkens HJ, Gerritsen J, Koeter GH, Krouwels FH, van Aalderen WM, Knol K. Budesonide and terbutaline or terbutaline alone in children with mild asthma: effects on bronchial hyperresponsiveness and diurnal variation in peak flow. Thorax 1991; 46:499–503.

14. van Essen-Zandvliet EEM, Hughes MD, Waalkens HJ, Duiverman EJ, Kerrebijn KF. Remission of childhood asthma after long-term treatment with an inhaled corticosteroid (budesonide): can it be achieved? Eur Respir J 1994; 7:63–68.

15. Inoue T, Doi S, Takamatsu I, Murayama N, Kameda M, Hayashida M, Nishida M, Toyoshima K. Effects of inhaled beclomethasone on height growth and bone metabolism in children with asthma. Arerugi 1995; 44:678–684.

16. Varsano I, Volovitz B, Malik H, Amir Y. Safety of 1 year of treatment with

budesonide in young children with asthma. J Allergy Clin Immunol 1990; 85: 914–920.

17. Merkus PJ, van Essen-Zandvliet EE, Duiverman EJ, van Houwelingen HC, Kerrebijn KF, Quanjer PH. Long-term effect of inhaled corticosteroids on growth rate in adolescents with asthma. Pediatrics 1993; 91:1121–1126.

18. Konig P, Ford L, Galant S, Lawrence M, Lemanske R, Mendelson L, Pearlman D, Wyatt R, Allen D, Baker K, Hamedani A, Kellerman D. A 1-year comparison of the effects of inhaled fluticasone propionate (FP) and placebo on growth in prepubescent children with asthma. Eur Respir J 1996; 9:294S.

19. Allen DB, Mullen M, Mullen B. A meta-analysis of the effect of oral and inhaled corticosteroids on growth. J Allergy Clin Immunol 1994; 93:967–976.

20. Ganassini A, Rossi A. Short-term regular beta 2-adrenergic agonists treatment is safe in mild asthmatics taking low doses of inhaled steroids. J Asthma 1997; 34:61–66.

21. Tormey VJ, Faul J, Leonard C, Lennon A, Burke CM. A comparison of regular with intermittent bronchodilators in asthma patients on inhaled steroids. Ir J Med Sci 1997; 166:249–252.

22. Laitinen LA, Laitinen A, Haahtela T. A comparative study of the effects of an inhaled corticosteroid, budesonide, and a beta$_2$-agonist, terbutaline, on airway inflammation in newly diagnosed asthma: a randomized, double-blind, parallel-group controlled trial. J Allergy Clin Immunol 1992; 90:32–42.

23. Lundgren R, Soderberg M, Horstedt P, Stenling R. Morphological studies of bronchial mucosal biopsies from asthmatics before and after ten years of treatment with inhaled steroids. Eur Respir J 1988; 1:883–889.

24. Laursen LC, Taudorf E, Borgeskov S, Kobayasi T, Jensen H, Weeke B. Fiberoptic bronchoscopy and bronchial mucosal biopsies in asthmatics undergoing long-term high-dose budesonide aerosol treatment. Allergy 1988; 43:284–288.

25. Laitinen LA, Laitinen A, Heino M, Haahtela T. Eosinophilic airway inflammation during exacerbation of asthma and its treatment with inhaled corticosteroid. Am Rev Respir Dis 1991; 143:423–427.

26. Vathenen AS, Knox AJ, Wisniewski A, Tattersfield AE. Time course of change in bronchial reactivity with an inhaled corticosteroid in asthma. Am Rev Respir Dis 1991; 143:1317–1321.

27. Wempe JB, Tammeling EP, Koeter GH, Hakansson L, Venge P, Postma DS. Blood eosinophil numbers and activity during 24 hours: effects of treatment with budesonide and bambuterol. J All Clin Immunol 1992; 1992:757–765.

28. Adelroth E, Rosenhall L, Johansson SA, Linden M, Venge P. Inflammatory cells and eosinophilic activity in asthmatics investigated by bronchoalveolar lavage: the effects of antiasthmatic treatment with budesonide or terbutaline. Am Rev Respir Dis 1990; 142:91–99.

29. Djukanovic R, Wilson JW, Britten KM, Wilson SJ, Walls AF, Roche WR, Howarth PH, Holgate ST. Effect of an inhaled corticosteroid on airway inflammation and symptoms in asthma. Am Rev Respir Dis 1992; 145:669–674.

30. De Baets FM, Goeteyn M, Kerrebijn KF. The effect of two months of treatment with inhaled budesonide on bronchial responsiveness to histamine and house dust mite antigen in asthmatic children. Am Rev Respir Dis 1990; 142:581–586.

31. Wong CS, Wahedna I, Pavord ID, Tattersfield AE. Effect of regular terbutaline and budesonide on bronchial reactivity to allergen challenge. Am J Respir Crit Care Med 1994; 150:1268–1273.

32. Cockcroft DW, Ruffin RE, Frith PA, Cartier A, Juniper EF, Dolovich J, Hargreave FE. Determinants of allergen-induced asthma: dose of allergen, circulating IgE antibody concentration, and bronchial responsiveness to inhaled histamine. Am Rev Respir Dis 1979; 120:1053–1058.

33. Svedmyr N. Action of corticosteroids on beta-adrenergic receptors: clinical aspects. Am Rev Respir Dis 1990; 141:S31–S38.

34. Adcock IM, Stevens DA, Barnes PJ. Interactions of glucocorticoids and β_2-agonists. Eur Respir J 1996; 9:160–168.

35. Nielson CP, Hadjokas NE. Beta-adrenoceptor agonists block corticosteroid inhibition in eosinophils. Am J Respir Crit Care Med 1998; 157:184–191.

36. Cockcroft DW, Swystun VA, Bhagat R. Interaction of inhaled beta$_2$-agonist and inhaled corticosteroid on airway responsiveness to allergen and methacholine. Am J Respir Crit Care Med 1995; 152:1485–1489.

37. National Heart, Lung, and Blood Institute, National Institutes of Health. International consensus report on diagnosis and treatment of asthma. Eur Respir J 1992; 5:601–641.

38. Guidelines on the management of asthma. Statement by the British Thoracic Society, the British Paediatric Association, the Research Unit of the Royal College of Physicians of London, the King's Fund Center, the National Asthma Campaign, the Royal College of General Practitioners, the General Practitioners in Asthma Group, the British Association of Accident and Emergency Medicine, and the British Paediatric Respiratory Group [published errata appear in Thorax 1994; 49:96 and 49:386]. Thorax 1993; 48:S1–S24.

39. Asthma: a follow-up statement from an international paediatric asthma consensus group. Arch Dis Child 1992; 67:240–248.

40. van der Molen T, Postma DS, Turner MO, Meyboom-de Jong B, Malo JL, Chapman K, Grossman R, de Graaff CS, Riemersma RA, Sears MR. Effects of the long acting β-agonist formoterol on asthma control in asthmatic patients using inhaled corticosteroids. Thorax 1996; 52:535–539.

41. Wilding P, Clark M, Coon JT, Lewis S, Rushton L, Bennett J, Oborne J, Cooper S, Tattersfield AE. Effect of long-term treatment with salmeterol on asthma control: a double blind, randomised crossover study. BMJ 1997; 314:1441–1446.

42. Greening AP, Ind PW, Northfield M, Shaw G. Added salmeterol versus higher-dose corticosteroid in asthma patients with symptoms on existing inhaled corticosteroids. Lancet 1994; 344:219–224.

43. Woolcock A, Lundback B, Ringdal N, Jacques LA. Comparison of addition of salmeterol to inhaled steroids with doubling of the dose of inhaled steroids. Am J Respir Crit Care Med 1996; 153:1481–1488.

44. Sears MR, Taylor DR, Print CG, Lake DC, Herbison GP, Flannery EM. Increased inhaled bronchodilator vs increased inhaled corticosteroid in the control of moderate asthma. Chest 1992; 102:1709–1715.

45. Pauwels RA, Lofdahl CG, Postma DS, Tattersfield AE, O'Byrne P, Barnes PJ, Ullman A. Effect of inhaled formoterol and budesonide on exacerbations of asthma: Formoterol and Corticosteroids Establishing Therapy (FACET) International Study Group [published erratum appears in N Engl J Med 1998; 338: 139]. N Engl J Med 1997; 337:1405–1411.

46. Kalra S, Swystun VA, Bhagat R, Cockcroft DW. Inhaled corticosteroids do not prevent the development of tolerance to the bronchoprotective effect of salmeterol. Chest 1996; 109:953–956.

47. Bhagat R, Kalra S, Swystun VA, Cockcroft DW. Rapid onset of tolerance to the bronchoprotective effect of salmeterol. Chest 1995; 108:1235–1239.

48. Cheung D, Timmers C, Zwinderman AH, Bel EH, Dijkman JH, Sterk PJ. Long-term effects of a long-acting β_2-adrenoceptor agonist, salmeterol, on airway hyperresponsiveness in patients with mild asthma. N Engl J Med 1992; 327:1198–1203.

49. Ramage L, Lipworth BJ, Ingram CG, Cree IA, Dhillon DP. Reduced protection against exercise induced bronchoconstriction after chronic dosing with salmeterol. Respir Med 1994; 88:363–368.

50. Newnham DM, McDevitt DG, Lipworth BJ. Bronchodilator subsensitivity after chronic dosing with eformoeterol in patients with asthma. Am J Med 1994; 97: 29–37.

51. O'Connor BJ, Aikman SL, Barnes PJ. Tolerance to the nonbronchodilator effects of inhaled beta$_2$-agonists in asthma. N Engl J Med 1992; 327:1204–1028.

52. Yates DH, Sussman HS, Shaw MJ, Barnes PJ, Chung KF. Regular formoterol treatment in mild asthma: effect on bronchial responsiveness during and after treatment. Am J Respir Crit Care Med 1995; 152:1170–1174.

53. Fitzpatrick MF, Mackay T, Driver H, Douglas NJ. Salmeterol in nocturnal asthma: a double blind, placebo controlled trial of a long acting inhaled β_2 agonist. BMJ 1990; 301:1365–1368.

54. Dahl R, Earnshaw JS, Palmer JBD. Salmeterol: a four week study of a long-acting beta-adrenoceptor agonist for the treatment of reversible airways disease. Eur Respir J 1991; 4:1178–1184.

55. Dahl R, Pedersen B, Hagglof B. Nocturnal asthma: effect of treatment with oral sustained-release terbutaline, inhaled budesonide, and the two in combination. J Allergy Clin Immunol 1989; 83:811–815.

56. Selby C, Engleman HM, Fitzpatrick MF, Sime PM, Mackay TW, Douglas NJ. Inhaled salmeterol or oral theophylline in nocturnal asthma? Am J Respir Crit Care Med 1997; 155:104–108.

57. Weersink EJ, Douma RR, Postma DS, Koeter GH. Fluticasone propionate, salmeterol xinafoate, and their combination in the treatment of nocturnal asthma. Am J Respir Crit Care Med 1997; 155:1241–1246.

58. Butchers PR, Vardey CJ, Johnson M. Salmeterol: a potent and long-acting inhibitor of inflammatory mediator release from human lung. Br J Pharmacol 1991; 104:672–676.

59. Kraft M, Wenzel SE, Bettinger CM, Martin RJ. The effect of salmeterol on nocturnal symptoms, airway function, and inflammation in asthma. Chest 1997; 111:1249–1254.

60. Williams HL, Lubin A, Goodnow JJ. Impaired performance with acute sleep loss. Psychol Monogr 1959; 73:1–26.

61. Friedman RC, Bigger JT, Kornfield DS. The intern and sleep loss. N Engl J Med 1971; 285:201–203.

62. Fitzpatrick MF, Cheshire K, Whyte KF, Deary IJ, Shapiro CM, Douglas NJ. Sleep quality and daytime cognitive performance in nocturnal asthma (abstr). Thorax 1990; 45:338.

63. Weersink EJ, van Zomeren EH, Koeter GH, Postma DS. Treatment of nocturnal airway obstruction improves daytime cognitive performance in asthmatics. Am J Respir Crit Care Med 1997; 156:1144–1150.

64. Verberne AA, Frost C, Duiverman EJ, Grol MH, Kerrebijn KF. Addition of salmeterol versus doubling the dose of beclomethasone in children with asthma: The Dutch Asthma Study Group. Am J Respir Crit Care Med 1998; 158:213–219.

65. Meijer GG, Postma DS, Mulder PG, van Aalderen WM. Long-term circadian effects of salmeterol in asthmatic children treated with inhaled corticosteroids. Am J Respir Crit Care Med 1995; 152:1887–1892.

66. Simons FE, Gerstner TV, Cheang MS. Tolerance to the bronchoprotective effect of salmeterol in adolescents with exercise-induced asthma using concurrent inhaled glucocorticoid treatment. Pediatrics 1997; 99:655–659.

67. Nelson JA, Strauss L, Skowronski M, Ciufo R, Novak R, McFadden ER Jr. Effect of long-term salmeterol treatment on exercise-induced asthma. N Engl J Med 1998; 339:141–146.

68. Clark CD, Ferguson HD, Siddorn JA. Respiratory arrests in young asthmatics on salmeterol. Respir Med 1993; 87:227–228.

69. Gardiner PV, Ward C, Booth H, Allison A, Hendrick DJ, Walters EH. Effect of eight weeks of treatment with salmeterol on bronchoalveolar lavage inflammatory indices in asthmatics. Am J Respir Crit Care Med 1994; 150:1006–1011.

70. Chung KF. The complementary role of glucocorticosteroids and long-acting β-adrenergic agonists. Allergy 1998; 53:7–13.

70a. Chapman KR, Ringdal N, Backer Vibeke, Palmqvist M, Saarelainen S, Briggs M. Salmeterol and fluticasone proprionate (50/150 μg) administered via combination Diskus inhaler: As effective as when given via separate Diskus inhaler. Can Respir J 1999; 6:46–51.

70b. Bateman ED, Britton M, Carillo T, Almeida J, Wixon C. Salmeterol/fluticasone (50/100 µg) combination inhaler. A new, effective and well tolerated treatment for asthma. Clin Drug Invest 1998; 16:193–201.

71. Evans DJ, Taylor DA, Zetterstrom O, Chung KF, O'Connor BJ, Barnes PJ. A comparison of low-dose inhaled budesonide plus theophylline and high-dose inhaled budesonide for moderate asthma. N Engl J Med 1997; 337:1412–1418.

72. Ukena D, Harnest U, Sakalauskas R, Magyar P, Vetter N, Steffen H, Leichtl S, Rathgeb F, Keller A, Steinijans VW. Comparison of addition of theophylline to inhaled steroid with doubling of the dose of inhaled steroid in asthma. Eur Respir J 1997; 10:2754–2760.

73. Edmunds AT, McKenzie S, Baillie E, Tooley M, Godfrey S. A comparison of oral choline theophyllinate and beclomethasone in severe perennial asthma in children. Br J Dis Chest 1979; 73:149–156.

74. Nassif EG, Weinberger M, Thompson R, Huntley W. The value of maintenance theophylline in steroid-dependent asthma. N Engl J Med 1981; 304:71–75.

75. Youngchaiyud P, Permpikul C, Suthamsmai T, Wong E. A double-blind comparison of inhaled budesonide, long-acting theophylline, and their combination in treatment of nocturnal asthma. Allergy 1995; 50:28–33.

76. Meltzer EO, Orgel HA, Ellis EF, Eigen HN, Hemstreet MP. Long-term comparison of three combinations of albuterol, theophylline, and beclomethasone in children with chronic asthma. J Allergy Clin Immunol 1992; 90:2–11.

77. Rebuck AS, Kesten S, Boulet LP, Cartier A, Cockcroft D, Gruber J, Laberge F, Lee-Chuy E, Keshmiri M, MacDonald GF. A 3-month evaluation of the efficacy of nedocromil sodium in asthma: a randomized, double-blind, placebo-controlled trial of nedocromil sodium conducted by a Canadian multicenter study group. J Allergy Clin Immunol 1990; 85:612–617.

78. O'Hickey SP, Rees PJ. High-dose nedocromil sodium as an addition to inhaled corticosteroids in the treatment of asthma. Respir Med 1994; 88:499–502.

79. Svendsen UG, Jorgensen H. Inhaled nedocromil sodium as additional treatment to high dose inhaled corticosteroids in the management of bronchial asthma. Eur Respir J 1991; 4:992–999.

80. Anderson SD, du Toit JI, Rodwell LT, Jenkins CR. Acute effect of sodium cromoglycate on airway narrowing induced by 4.5 percent saline aerosol: outcome before and during treatment with aerosol corticosteroids in patients with asthma. Chest 1994; 105:673–680.

81. National Asthma Education and Prevention Program, National Institutes of Health. National Heart, Lung and Blood Institute Guidelines for the Diagnosis and Management of Asthma. Expert Panel Report 2. 1997.

82. Manning PJ, Watson RM, Margolskee DJ, Williams VC, Schwartz JI, O'Byrne PM. Inhibition of exercise-induced bronchoconstriction by MK-571, a potent leukotriene D4-receptor antagonist. N Engl J Med 1990; 323:1736–1739.

83. Cloud ML, Enas GC, Kemp J, Platts-Mills T, Altman LC, Townley R, Tinkel-

man D, King T Jr, Middleton E, Sheffer AL. A specific LTD4/LTE4-receptor antagonist improves pulmonary function in patients with mild, chronic asthma. Am Rev Respir Dis 1989; 140:1336–1339.

84. Gaddy JN, Margolskee DJ, Bush RK, Williams VC, Busse WW. Bronchodilation with a potent and selective leukotriene D4 (LTD4) receptor antagonist (MK-571) in patients with asthma. Am Rev Respir Dis 1992; 146:358–363.

85. Impens N, Reiss TF, Teahan JA, Desmet M, Rossing TH, Shingo S, Zhang J, Schandevyl W, Verbesselt R, Dupont AG. Acute bronchodilation with an intravenously administered leukotriene D4 antagonist, MK-679. Am Rev Respir Dis 1993; 147:1442–1446.

86. Hui KP, Bames NC. Lung function improvement in asthma with a cysteinyl-leukotriene receptor antagonist. Lancet 1991; 337:1062–1063.

87. Dahlen B, Nizankowska E, Szczeklik A, Zetterstrom O, Bochenek G, Kumlin M, Mastalerz L, Pinis G, Swanson LJ, Boodhoo TI, Wright S, Dube LM, Dahlen SE. Benefits from adding the 5-lipoxygenase inhibitor zileuton to conventional therapy in aspirin-intolerant asthmatics. Am J Respir Crit Care Med 1998; 157:1187–1194.

88. Stevenson DD, Simon RA. Aspirin sensitivity: respiratory and cutaneous manifestations. In: Middleton JE, Reed CE, Sllis EF, Adkinson NF, Yunginger JW, eds. Allergy. Principles and Practice. St. Louis: Mosby, 1988: 1537–1554.

89. Dahlen B, Kumlin M, Margolskee DJ, Larsson C, Blomqvist H, Williams VC, Zetterstrom O, Dahlen SE. The leukotriene-receptor antagonist MK-0679 blocks airway obstruction induced by inhaled lysine-aspirin in aspirin-sensitive asthmatics. Eur Respir J 1993; 6:1018–1026.

90. Yamamoto H, Nagata M, Kuramitsu K, Table K, Kiuchi H, Sakamoto Y, Yamamoto K, Dohi Y. Inhibition of analgesic-induced asthma by leukotriene receptor antagonist ONO-1078. Am J Respir Crit Care Med 1994; 150:254–257.

91. Israel E, Fischer AR, Rosenberg MA, Lilly CM, Callery JC, Shapiro J, Cohn J, Rubin P, Drazen JM. The pivotal role of 5-lipoxygenase products in the reaction of aspirin-sensitive asthmatics to aspirin. Am Rev Respir Dis 1993; 148: 1447–1451.

92. Nasser SM, Bell GS, Foster S, Spruce KE, MacMillan R, Williams AJ, Lee TH, Arm JP. Effect of the 5-lipoxygenase inhibitor ZD2138 on aspirin-induced asthma. Thorax 1994; 49:749–756.

93. Christie PE, Tagari P, Ford-Hutchinson AW, Charlesson S, Chee P, Arm JP, Lee TH. Urinary leukotriene E4 concentrations increase after aspirin challenge in aspirin-sensitive asthmatic subjects. Am Rev Respir Dis 1991; 143:1025–1029.

94. Reiss TF, Sorkness CA, Stricker W, Botto A, Busse WW, Kundu S, Zhang J. Effects of montelukast (MK-0476): a potent cysteinyl leukotriene receptor antagonist, on bronchodilation in asthmatic subjects treated with and without inhaled corticosteroids. Thorax 1997; 52:45–48.

95. Virchow JC, Hassall SM, Summerton L, Harris A. Improved asthma control

over 6 weeks with Accolate (zafirlukast) in patients on high-dose inhaled corticosteroids (abstr). J Invest Med 1997; 45:286A.

96. Tamaoki J, Kondo M, Sakai N, Nakata J, Takemura H, Nagai A, Takizawa T, Konno K. Leukotriene antagonist prevents exacerbation of asthma during reduction of high-dose inhaled corticosteroid: The Tokyo Joshi-Idai Asthma Research Group. Am J Respir Crit Care Med 1997; 155:1235–1240.

97. Knorr B, Matz J, Bernstein JA, Nguyen H, Seldenberg BC, Reiss TF, Becker A. Montelukast for chronic asthma in 6- to 14-year-old children: a randomized, double-blind trial: Pediatric Montelukast Study Group. JAMA 1998; 279: 1181–1186.

98. Shapiro GG, Sharpe M, DeRouen TA, Pierson WE, Furukawa CT, Virant FS, Bierman CW. Cromolyn versus triamcinolone acetonide for youngsters with moderate asthma. J Allergy Clin Immunol 1991; 88:742–748.

99. Simons FE. A comparison of beclomethasone, salmeterol, and placebo in children with asthma: Canadian Beclomethasone Dipropionate-Salmeterol Xinafoate Study Group. N Engl J Med 1997; 337:1659–1665.

100. van Essen-Zandvliet EE, Hughes MD, Waalkens HJ, Duiverman EJ, Pocock SJ, Kerrebijn KF. Effects of 22 months of treatment with inhaled corticosteroids and/or beta$_2$-agonists on lung function, airway responsiveness, and symptoms in children with asthma: The Dutch Chronic Non-specific Lung Disease Study Group. Am Rev Respir Dis 1992; 146:547–554.

101. Kraemer R, Modelska K, Aebischer CC, Schoni MH. Comparison of different inhalation schedules to control childhood asthma. Agents Actions Suppl 1993; 40:211–221.

102. Guttman A, Afilalo M, Colacone A, Kreisman H, Dankoff J. The effects of combined intravenous and inhaled steroids (beclomethasone dipropionate) for the emergency treatment of acute asthma: The Asthma ED Study Group. Acad Emerg Med 1997; 4:100–106.

103. Rodrigo G, Rodrigo C. Inhaled flunisolide for acute severe asthma. Am J Respir Crit Care Med 1998; 157:698–703.

104. Volovitz B, Bentur L, Finkelstein Y, Mansour Y, Shalitin S, Nussinovitch M, Varsano I. Effectiveness and safety of inhaled corticosteroids in controlling acute asthma attacks in children who were treated in the emergency department: a controlled comparative study with oral prednisolone. J Allergy Clin Immunol 1998; 102:605–609.

105. Nana A, Youngchaiyud P, Charoenratanakul S, Boe J, Lofdahl CG, Selroos O, Stahl E. High-dose inhaled budesonide may substitute for oral therapy after an acute asthma attack. J Asthma 1998; 35:647–655.

106. Levy ML, Stevenson C, Maslen T. Comparison of short courses of oral prednisolone and fluticasone propionate in the treatment of adults with acute exacerbations of asthma in primary care. Thorax 1996; 51:1087–1092.

107. Ono Y, Kondo T, Tanigaki T, Ohta Y. Furosemide given by inhalation ameliorates acute exacerbation of asthma. J Asthma 1997; 34:283–289.

108. Freed AN, Kelly LJ, Menkes HA. Airflow-induced bronchospasm: imbalance between airway cooling and airway drying? Am Rev Respir Dis 1987; 136: 595–599.

109. Saban R, Dick EC, Fishleder RI, Buckner CK. Enhancement by parainfluenza 3 infection of contractile responses to substance P and capsaicin in airway smooth muscle from the guinea pig. Am Rev Respir Dis 1987; 136:586–591.

110. Boulet LP, Cartier A, Cockcroft DW, Gruber JM, Laberge F, MacDonald GF, Malo JL, Mazza JA, Moote WD, Sandham JD. Tolerance to reduction of oral steroid dosage in severely asthmatic patients receiving nedocromil sodium. Respir Med 1990; 84:317–323.

111. Read J, Rebuck AS. Steroid-sparing effect of disodium cromoglycate ("Intal") in chronic asthma. Med J Aust 1969; 1:566–569.

112. Toogood JH, McCourtie DR, Jennings BH, Lefcoe NM, Mullin JK. Changes in corticosteroid usage by chronic asthma patients during a year of cromoglycate treatment. J Allergy Clin Immunol 1973; 52:334–345.

113. Goldin JG, Bateman ED. Does nedocromil sodium have a steroid sparing effect in adult asthmatic patients requiring maintenance oral corticosteroids? Thorax 1988; 43:982–986.

114. Sung L, Osmond MH, Klassen TP. Randomized, controlled trial of inhaled budesonide as an adjunct to oral prednisone in acute asthma. Acad Emerg Med 1998; 5:209–213.

115. Becker AB, Nelson NA, Simons FE. The pulmonary index: assessment of a clinical score for asthma. Am J Dis Child 1984; 138:574–576.

116. Schuckman H, DeJulius DP, Blanda M, Gerson LW, DeJulius AJ, Rajaratnam M. Comparison of intramuscular triamcinolone and oral prednisone in the outpatient treatment of acute asthma: a randomized controlled trial [published erratum appears in Ann Emerg Med 1998; 31:795]. Ann Emerg Med 1998; 31: 333–338.

117. Green SS, Lamb GC, Schmitt S, Kaufman J, et al. Oral versus repository corticosteroid therapy after hospitalization for treatment of asthma. J Allergy Clin Immunol 1995; 95:15–22.

118. Willey RF, Fergusson RJ, Godden DJ, Crompton GK, Grant IW. Comparison of oral prednisolone and intramuscular depot triamcinolone in patients with severe chronic asthma. Thorax 1984; 39:340–344.

119. McLeod DT, Capewell SJ, Law J, MacLaren W, Seaton A. Intramuscular triamcinolone acetonide in chronic severe asthma. Thorax 1985; 40:840–845.

120. Ogirala RG, Aldrich TK, Prezant DJ, Sinnett MJ, Enden JB, Williams MH Jr. High-dose intramuscular triamcinolone in severe, chronic, life-threatening asthma [published erratum appears in N Engl J Med 1991; 324:1380]. N Engl J Med 1991; 324:585–589.

121. Peake MD, Cayton RM, Howard P. Triamcinolone in corticosteroid-resistant asthma. Br J Dis Chest 1979; 73:39–44.

122. Szczeklik A, Nizankowska E, Dworski R, Domagala B, Pinis G. Cyclosporin for steroid-dependent asthma. Allergy 1991; 46:312–315.
123. Alexander AG, Barnes NC, Kay AB. Trial of cyclosporin in corticosteroid-dependent chronic severe asthma. Lancet 1992; 339:324–328.
124. Lock SH, Kay AB, Barnes NC. Double-blind, placebo-controlled study of cyclosporin A as a corticosteroid-sparing agent in corticosteroid-dependent asthma. Am J Respir Crit Care Med 1996; 153:509–514.
125. Mullarkey MF, Blumenstein BA, Andrade WP, Bailey GA, Olason I, Wetzel CE. Methotrexate in the treatment of corticosteroid-dependent asthma: a double-blind crossover study. N Engl J Med 1988; 318:603–607.
126. Dyer PD, Vaughan TR, Weber RW. Methotrexate in the treatment of steroid-dependent asthma. J Allergy Clin Immunol 1991; 88:208–212.
127. Kremer JM, Lee JK. The safety and efficacy of the use of methotrexate in long-term therapy for rheumatoid arthritis. Arthritis Rheum 1986; 29:822–831.
128. Shiner RJ, Nunn AJ, Chung KF, Geddes DM. Randomised, double-blind, placebo-controlled trial of methotrexate in steroid-dependent asthma. Lancet 1990; 336:137–140.
129. Erzurum SC, Leff JA, Cochran JE, Ackerson LM, Szefler SJ, Martin RJ, Cott GR. Lack of benefit of methotrexate in severe, steroid-dependent asthma. A double-blind, placebo-controlled study. Ann Intern Med 1991; 114:353–360.
130. Ogirala RG, Sturm TM, Aldrich TK, Meller FF, Pacia EB, Keane AM, Finkel RI. Single, high-dose intramuscular triamcinolone acetonide versus weekly oral methotrexate in life-threatening asthma: a double-blind study. Am J Respir Crit Care Med 1995; 152:1461–1466.
131. Bernstein IL, Bernstein DI, Dubb JW, Faiferman I, Wallin B. A placebo-controlled multicenter study of auranofin in the treatment of patients with corticosteroid-dependent asthma: Auranofin Multicenter Drug Trial. J Allergy Clin Immunol 1996; 98:317–324.
132. Muranaka M, Miyamoto T, Shida T, Kabe J, Makino S, Okumura H, Takeda K, Suzuki S, Horiuchi Y. Gold salt in the treatment of bronchial asthma—a double-blind study. Ann Allergy 1978; 40:132–137.
133. Bernstein DI, Bernstein IL, Bodenheimer SS, Pietrusko RG. An open study of auranofin in the treatment of steroid-dependent asthma. J Allergy Clin Immunol 1988; 81:6–16.
134. Nierop G, Gijzel WP, Bel EH, Zwinderman AH, Dijkman JH. Auranofin in the treatment of steroid dependent asthma: a double blind study. Thorax 1992; 47:349–354.
135. Nelson HS, Hamilos DL, Corsello PR, Levesque NV, Buchmeier AD, Bucher BL. A double-blind study of troleandomycin and methylprednisolone in asthmatic subjects who require daily corticosteroids. Am Rev Respir Dis 1993; 147:398–404.
136. Siracusa A, Brugnami G, Fiordi T, Areni S, Severini C, Marabini A. Troleando-

mycin in the treatment of difficult asthma. J Allergy Clin Immunol 1993; 92: 677–682.

137.   Wald JA, Friedman BF, Farr RS. An improved protocol for the use of troleando-mycin (TAO) in the treatment of steroid-requiring asthma. J Allergy Clin Immunol 1986; 78:36–43.

138.   Kaplan MA, Goldin M. The use of triacetyloleandomycin in chronic infectious asthma. In: Welch H, Marti-Ibanez F, eds. Antibiotics Annual—1958–1959. New York: Interscience, 1959:273.

139.   Spector SL, Katz FH, Farr RS. Troleandomycin: effectiveness in steroid-dependent asthma and bronchitis. J Allergy Clin Immunol 1974; 54:367–379.

140.   McGivney SA, Ogirala RG. Effect of high-dose intramuscular triamcinolone in older adults with severe, chronic asthma. Lung 1994; 172:73–78.

141.   Huang D, O'Brien RG, Harman E, Aull L, Reents S, Visser J, Shieh G, Hendeles L. Does aminophylline benefit adults admitted to the hospital for an acute exacerbation of asthma? Ann Intern Med 1993; 119:1155–1160.

142.   Self TH, Abou-Shala N, Burns R, Stewart CF, Ellis RF, Tsiu SJ, Kellermann AL. Inhaled albuterol and oral prednisone therapy in hospitalized adult asthmatics: does aminophylline add any benefit? Chest 1990; 98:1317–1321.

143.   Murphy DG, McDermott MF, Rydman RJ, Sloan EP, Zalenski RJ. Aminophylline in the treatment of acute asthma when beta₂-adrenergics and steroids are provided. Arch Intern Med 1993; 153:1784–1788.

144.   Wrenn K, Slovis CM, Murphy F, Greenberg RS. Aminophylline therapy for acute bronchospastic disease in the emergency room. Ann Intern Med 1991; 115:241–247.

145.   Aubier M, De Troyer A, Sampson M, Macklem PT, Roussos C. Aminophylline improves diaphragmatic contractility. N Engl J Med 1981; 305:249–252.

146.   Moxham J. Aminophylline and the respiratory muscles: an alternative view. Clin Chest Med 1988; 9:325–336.

147.   Harper GD, Neill P, Vathenen AS, Cookson JB, Ebden P. A comparison of inhaled beclomethasone dipropionate and nedocromil sodium as additional therapy in asthma. Respir Med 1990; 84:463–469.

148.   North A. A double-blind multicenter group comparative study of the efficacy and safety of nedocromil sodium in the management of asthma. Chest 1990; 97:1299–1306.

149.   Katial RK, Stelzle RC, Bonner MW, Marino M, Cantilena LR, Smith LJ. A drug interaction between zafirlukast and theophylline. Arch Intern Med 1998; 158:1713–1715.

150.   de Benedictis FM, Tuteri G, Pazzelli P, Solinas LF, Niccoli A, Parente C. Combination drug therapy for the prevention of exercise-induced bronchoconstriction in children. Ann Allergy Asthma Immunol 1998; 80:352–356.

151.   Novembre E, Frongia G, Lombardi E, Veneruso G, Vierucci A. The preventive effect of nedocromil or furosemide alone or in combination on exercise-induced asthma in children. J Allergy Clin Immunol 1994; 94:201–206.

152. Moscato G, Dellabianca A, Falagiani P, Mistrello G, Rossi G, Rampulla C. Inhaled furosemide prevents both the bronchoconstriction and the increase in neutrophil chemotactic activity induced by ultrasonic "fog" of distilled water in asthmatics. Am Rev Respir Dis 1991; 143:561–566.

153. Grubbe RE, Hopp R, Dave NK, Brennan B, Bewtra A, Townley R. Effect of inhaled furosemide on the bronchial response to methacholine and cold-air hyperventilation challenges. J Allergy Clin Immunol 1990; 85:881–884.

154. Nichol GM, Alton EW, Nix A, Geddes DM, Chung KF, Barnes PJ. Effect of inhaled furosemide on metabisulfite- and methacholine-induced bronchoconstriction and nasal potential difference in asthmatic subjects. Am Rev Respir Dis 1990; 142:576–580.

155. Bianco S, Pieroni MG, Refini RM, Rottoli L, Sestini P. Protective effect of inhaled furosemide on allergen-induced early and late asthmatic reactions. N Engl J Med 1989; 321:1069–1073.

156. Vargas FS, Croce M, Teixeira LR, Terra-Filho M, Cukier A, Light RW. Effect of inhaled furosemide on the bronchial response to lysine-aspirin inhalation in asthmatic subjects. Chest 1992; 102:408–411.

157. O'Connor BJ, Chen-Worsdell YM, Fuller RW, Chung KF, Barnes PJ. Effect of inhaled furosemide on adenosine 5′-monophosphate and histamine-induced bronchoconstriction in asthmatic subjects (abstr). Thorax 1990; 45:333.

158. Woolley M, Anderson SD, Quigley BM. Duration of protective effect of terbutaline sulfate and cromolyn sodium alone and in combination on exercise-induced asthma. Chest 1990; 97:39–45.

159. Shapiro GG, Furukawa CT, Pierson WE, Sharpe MJ, Menendez R, Bierman CW. Double-blind evaluation of nebulized cromolyn, terbutaline, and the combination for childhood asthma. J Allergy Clin Immunol 1988; 81:449–454.

160. Clarke PS, Ratowsky DA. Effect of fenoterol hydrobromide and sodium cromoglycate individually and in combination on postexercise asthma. Ann Allergy 1990; 64:187–190.

161. Lin RY, Pesola GR, Bakalchuk L, Morgan JP, Heyl GT, Freyberg CW, Cataquet D, Westfal RE. Superiority of ipratropium plus albuterol over albuterol alone in the emergency department management of adult asthma: a randomized clinical trial. Ann Emerg Med 1998; 31:208–213.

162. FitzGerald JM, Grunfeld A, Pare PD, Levy RD, Newhouse MT, Hodder R, Chapman KR. The clinical efficacy of combination nebulized anticholinergic and adrenergic bronchodilators vs nebulized adrenergic bronchodilator alone in acute asthma: Canadian Combivent Study Group. Chest 1997; 111:311–315.

163. Karpel JP, Schacter EN, Fanta C, Levey D, Spiro P, Aldrich T, Menjoge SS, Witek TJ. A comparison of ipratropium and albuterol vs albuterol alone for the treatment of acute asthma. Chest 1996; 110:611–616.

164. Karpel JP, Appel D, Breidbart D, Fusco MJ. A comparison of atropine sulfate and metaproterenol sulfate in the emergency treatment of asthma. Am Rev Respir Dis 1986; 133:727–729.

165. Summers QA, Tarala RA. Nebulized ipratropium in the treatment of acute asthma. Chest 1990; 97:425–429.
166. Higgins RM, Stradling JR, Lane DJ. Should ipratropium bromide be added to beta-agonists in treatment of acute severe asthma? Chest 1988; 94:718–722.
167. Rebuck AS, Chapman KR, Abboud R, Pare PD, Kreisman H, Wolkove N, Vickerson F. Nebulized anticholinergic and sympathomimetic treatment of asthma and chronic obstructive airways disease in the emergency room. Am J Med 1987; 82:59–64.
168. Ward MJ, Fentem PH, Smith WH, Davies D. Ipratropium bromide in acute asthma. BMJ 1981; 282:598–600.
169. Bryant DH. Nebulized ipratropium bromide in the treatment of acute asthma. Chest 1985;88:24–29.
170. Watson WT, Becker AB, Simons FE. Comparison of ipratropium solution, fenoterol solution, and their combination administered by nebulizer and face mask to children with acute asthma. J Allergy Clin Immunol 1988; 82:1012–1018.
171. Leahy BC, Gomm SA, Allen SC. Comparison of nebulized salbutamol with nebulized ipratropium bromide in acute asthma. Br J Dis Chest 1983; 77:159–163.
172. Cydulka RK, Emerman CL. Effects of combined treatment with glycopyrrolate and albuterol in acute exacerbation of asthma. Ann Emerg Med 1994; 23:270–274.
173. Ward MJ, Macfarlane JT, Davies D. A place for ipratropium bromide in the treatment of severe acute asthma. Br J Dis Chest 1985; 79:374–378.
174. Hall SK. Acute angle-closure glaucoma as a complication of combined β-agonist and ipratropium bromide therapy in the emergency department. Ann Emerg Med 1994; 23:884–887.
175. Qureshi F, Pestian J, Davis P, Zaritsky A. Effect of nebulized ipratropium on the hospitalization rates of children with asthma. N Engl J Med 1998; 339:1030–1035.
176. Schuh S, Johnson DW, Callahan S, Canny G, Levison H. Efficacy of frequent nebulized ipratropium bromide added to frequent high-dose albuterol therapy in severe childhood asthma. J Pediatr 1995; 126:639–645.
177. Greenough A, Yuksel B, Everett L, Price JF. Inhaled ipratropium bromide and terbutaline in asthmatic children. Respir Med 1993; 87:111–114.
178. Beck R, Robertson C, Galdes-Sebaldt M, Levison H. Combined salbutamol and ipratropium bromide by inhalation in the treatment of severe acute asthma. J Pediatr 1985; 107:605–608.
179. Storr J, Lenney W. Nebulised ipratropium and salbutamol in asthma. Arch Dis Child 1986; 61:602–603.
180. Vichyanond P, Sladek WA, Sur S, Hill MR, Szefler SJ, Nelson HS. Efficacy of atropine methylnitrate alone and in combination with albuterol in children with asthma. Chest 1990; 98:637–642.
181. Diaz JE, Dubin R, Gaeta TJ, Pelczar P, Bradley K. Efficacy of atropine sulfate

in combination with albuterol in the treatment for acute asthma. Acad Emerg Med 1997; 4:107–113.

182. Sur S, Mohiuddin AA, Vichyanond P, Nelson HS. A random double-blind trial of the combination of nebulized atropine methylnitrate and albuterol in nocturnal asthma. Ann Allergy 1990; 65:384–388.

183. Tammivaara R, Elo J, Mansury L. Terbutaline controlled-release tablets and ipratropium aerosol in nocturnal asthma. Allergy 1993; 48:45–48.

184. Roquet A, Dahlen B, Kumlin M, Ihre E, Anstren G, Binks S, Dahlen SE. Combined antagonism of leukotrienes and histamine produces predominant inhibition of allergen-induced early and late phase airway obstruction in asthmatics. Am J Respir Crit Care Med 1997; 155:1856–1863.

185. Henriksen JM, Wenzel A. Effect of an intranasally administered corticosteroid (budesonide) on nasal obstruction, mouth breathing, and asthma. Am Rev Respir Dis 1984; 130:1014–1018.

186. Welsh PW, Stricker WE, Chu CP, Naessens JM, Reese ME, Reed CE, Marcoux JP. Efficacy of beclomethasone nasal solution, flunisolide, and cromolyn in relieving symptoms of ragweed allergy. Mayo Clin Proc 1987; 62:125–134.

187. Corren J, Adinoff AD, Buchmeier AD, Irvin CG. Nasal beclomethasone prevents the seasonal increase in bronchial responsiveness in patients with allergic rhinitis and asthma. J Allergy Clin Immunol 1992; 90:250–256.

188. Watson WT, Becker AB, Simons FE. Treatment of allergic rhinitis with intranasal corticosteroids in patients with mild asthma: effect on lower airway responsiveness. J Allergy Clin Immunol 1993; 91:97–101.

189. Corren J, Harris AG, Aaronson D, Beaucher W, Berkowitz R, Bronsky E, Chen R, Chervinsky P, Cohen R, Fourre J, Grossman J, Meltzer E, Pedinoff A, Stricker W, Wanderer A. Efficacy and safety of loratadine plus pseudoephedrine in patients with seasonal allergic rhinitis and mild asthma [published erratum appears in J Allergy Clin Immunol 1998; 101:792]. J Allergy Clin Immunol 1997; 100:781–788.

190. Ekstrom T, Osterman K, Zetterstrom O. Lack of effect of loratadine on moderate to severe asthma. Ann Allergy Asthma Immunol 1995; 75:287–289.

191. Spector SL, Nicodemus CF, Corren J, Schanker HM, Rachelefsky GS, Katz RM, Siegel SC. Comparison of the bronchodilatory effects of cetirizine, albuterol, and both together versus placebo in patients with mild-to-moderate asthma. J Allergy Clin Immunol 1995; 96:174–181.

192. Bosley CM, Parry DT, Cochrane GM. Patient compliance with inhaled medication: does combining beta-agonists with corticosteroids improve compliance? Eur Respir J 1994; 7:504–509.

193. Braunstein GL, Trinquet G, Harper AE. Compliance with nedocromil sodium and a nedocromil sodium/salbutamol combination: Compliance Working Group. Eur Respir J 1996; 9:893–898.

8

COPD—Combination Therapy

E. Rand Sutherland and Richard J. Martin

National Jewish Medical and Research Center
Denver, Colorado

I. Introduction

Chronic obstructive pulmonary disease (COPD) comprises a group of pulmonary disorders characterized by expiratory airflow limitation that is difficult to reverse and slowly progressive over months to years of observation (1). Exposure to tobacco smoke is the primary risk factor for COPD. COPD is common, affecting approximately 14 million patients in the United States. The prevalence of COPD is increasing, particularly among women and minorities, and—in contrast to declining mortality rates seen with coronary and cerebral vascular disease—COPD mortality is increasing (2,3).

Several classes of drugs have been utilized for the treatment of COPD. This review briefly discusses therapeutic mechanisms of single agents used for the treatment of COPD (see previous chapters for more detailed descriptions of individual therapeutic agents) and then focuses extensively on the role of combinations of these single agents for the treatment of COPD.

II. Pathophysiology and Clinical Manifestations of COPD

Long-term cigarette dependence and abuse are primary risk factors for the development of COPD. Patients with COPD are described as having emphysema, chronic bronchitis, or a combination of both. Emphysema is "a condition of the lung characterized by abnormal permanent enlargement of airspaces distal to the terminal bronchiole, accompanied by destruction of their walls without obvious fibrosis" (4). Chronic bronchitis is an inflammatory condition of the airways resulting in the excessive production of mucus by the tracheobronchial tree. Specific causes of airways disease such as bronchiectasis and asthma are usually excluded as causes of COPD.

Patients with COPD complain of dyspnea, productive cough, and recurrent respiratory tract infections. Physical examination often reveals expiratory phase prolongation, decreased breath sounds, and evidence of hyperinflation. Wheezing occasionally occurs in COPD. Chest radiography may be helpful in confirming the diagnosis of COPD by demonstrating hyperinflation, bullous disease, and hyperlucency. The spirometric finding of an obstructive ventilatory defect [i.e., decreased forced expiratory volume in 1 s (FEV_1) or FEV_1/ forced vital capacity (FVC) %], along with increased lung volumes and a low diffusing capacity, are the typical physiological manifestations of COPD (5).

III. Natural History and Prognosis of COPD

The clinical course of COPD is marked by a progressive decline in FEV_1 at a rate greater than that of nonsmoking controls, with frequent episodes of acute worsening of airflow limitation ("exacerbations") and recurrent pulmonary infections. The rate of decrease in FEV_1 increases with both patient age and intensity of cigarette smoking. Following smoking cessation, some lung function may or may not be regained, but the rate of decline in lung function will decrease to almost match that of never-smoking controls (6,7).

Mortality in COPD is high; in patients with $FEV_1 < 0.75$ L, mortality rates of 30% at 1 year and 95% at 10 years have been reported (8). Advancing age, severity of airflow limitation (as measured by FEV_1), and abnormalities of gas exchange (hypoxemia and/or hypercapnia) are important predictors of mortality in patients with COPD. Death in COPD usually occurs as a result of an acute complication of the disease itself, such as pneumonia, pneumothorax, pulmonary embolism, dysrhythmia, or acute hypoventilatory respiratory failure (1).

IV. Goals of Therapy in COPD

In COPD, the goals of therapy are improving symptoms of airflow limitation, increasing quality of life, and reducing overall mortality. These goals may be achieved by treating the airway inflammation and bronchoconstriction responsible for airflow limitation. The prevention and treatment of secondary complications of COPD such as hypoxemia and recurrent respiratory infection can result in fewer episodes of emergency care or hospitalization, with an overall reduction in associated health care costs. Other therapeutic goals include improving exercise tolerance, reducing the number of acute exacerbations of COPD, modifying disease progression by slowing deterioration of lung function, and improving overall health status and sense of well-being. It should be noted that there is no good evidence that pharmacotherapy has any salutary effects on disease progression or mortality in COPD (9); it may, however, significantly improve quality of life and even slow the rate of decline in FEV_1 (10).

V. Individual Agents for Pharmacological Therapy of COPD

Many COPD patients suffer from persistent and only mildly reversible symptoms of airflow limitation. Pharmacotherapy in COPD is utilized to facilitate bronchodilation, a reduction in airways inflammation, and an increase the clearance of secretions from the airways. Several different classes of medications are routinely employed to effect these goals. Individual agents may provide relief of symptoms in many patients with COPD, but multiple agents are often required for greater control of symptoms.

A. Bronchodilators

Ipratropium Bromide

Ipratropium bromide is an inhaled quaternary anticholinergic agent that produces at least comparable if not superior bronchodilation in patients with COPD to that seen with β-agonist use. Ipratropium bromide inhibits the action of acetylcholine on airway smooth muscle muscarinic receptors, indirectly leading to bronchodilation via inhibition of smooth muscle contraction. Ipratropium's bronchodilatory effect is maintained over years of use and is seen with drug delivered by both metered-dose inhaler (MDI) and nebulizer routes.

This agent lasts approximately 4 h; thus patients may feel the need to use it more frequently than prescribed. In patients with moderate to severe COPD, ipratropium bromide should be dosed as three to four actuations (21 μg per actuation) four times per day.

The sensitivity of cholinergic receptors, unlike adrenergic receptors, does not diminish with age. For this reason, the anticholinergic effects of ipratropium may result in significant bronchodilation over years of use (11), whereas β_2-adrenergic receptor agonists may become less valuable over time because of receptor desensitization. There is also evidence that adding ipratropium to standard-dose albuterol improves spirometric variables and results in a more prolonged bronchodilator effect than does albuterol alone (12).

β_2-Adrenergic Receptor Agonists

β_2-adrenergic receptor agonist aerosols are often utilized for their bronchodilating properties in the treatment COPD. β-agonists produce significantly less bronchodilation in COPD than in asthma, although most patients with COPD will still demonstrate a measurable improvement in FEV_1 following inhalation of β-agonists (13). Agents such as albuterol are available as both metered-dose inhalers (MDIs) and solutions for nebulized delivery. β-agonists initiate an enzymatic pathway that ultimately leads to an increase in intracellular cyclic adenosine monophosphate (cAMP), which results in bronchodilation. β-agonists may also stimulate clearance of the airways via the mucociliary elevator mechanism (14) and by improving airflow and cough effectiveness (15). Patients often note a subjective improvement in symptoms of airflow limitation with β-agonists as well as objective improvements in spirometry.

Albuterol and other intermittent-acting agents last only 3–4 h; thus patients commonly feel the need to use these medications more than four times per day. Salmeterol is a long-acting (12-h) β_2-adrenergic agonist that has been shown to result in effective bronchodilation in patients with COPD (16). Although the onset of action is slower than that of albuterol (30–40 min vs. 5–10 min), its extended duration of action provides longer bronchodilation; when dosed twice a day, this lasts throughout the day and night and reduces the incidence of "breakthrough" symptoms and the need for "as needed" albuterol. The typical dose of salmeterol is two inhalations (25 μg per actuation) delivered twice a day.

Theophylline

Theophylline is an orally administered methylxanthine usually employed as a bronchodilator in patients with COPD. Theophylline's mode of action is by inhibition of phosphodiesterase, resulting in increased levels of intracellular cAMP, causing bronchodilation. However, theophylline also improves respiratory muscle strength and endurance, which can aid COPD patients (17). This study of 60 patients with severe, but stable, COPD (FEV_1 31.5 ± 13% predicted; associated with hypoxia, Pa_{O_2} 62 ± 11 mmHg; and hypercarbia Pa_{CO_2} 48 ± 8 mmHg) demonstrated that theophylline improved respiratory function and dyspnea, which were probably due to better respiratory muscle performance. On theophylline compared to placebo, there was an increased generation of maximal inspiratory force. This effect improved the respiratory muscle reserve by about 29% in these patients. Associated with this was a significant improvement in gas exchange (Pa_{O_2} improved by 5 mmHg and Pa_{CO_2} fell by 5 mmHg) and lung function in regard to the FEV_1 and FVC. Dyspnea additionally improved by approximately 25%.

Mahler and colleagues used very precise measures of dyspnea to evaluate the effect of theophylline in regard to dyspnea in COPD patients (18). They determined that sustained-released theophylline significantly decreased the components of functional impairment ($p = 0.02$) and magnitude of task ($p = 0.02$) relating to dyspnea as well as the overall dyspnea rating ($p = 0.01$).

Of interest, the classic measures of improved lung function (i.e., FEV_1 and FVC) may not be the appropriate index in COPD. Chrystyn et al. demonstrated that spirometric measurement showed only a minimal dose response to theophylline (19). However, the measure of trapped gas volume (the difference between the lung volume measured by body plethysmography and helium dilution) showed a linear dose-dependent fall, with increased theophylline doses producing serum theophylline levels between 5 and 10, 10 and 15, and 15 and 20 µg/mL. Associated with this dose-dependent fall in trapped gas volume was a progressive increase in the 6-min walking distance.

Other effects of theophylline that can be beneficial for COPD patients include improvements in mucociliary clearance (20), cardiac function (21), respiratory drive (17), and nocturnal lung function (22). The most common complaint among patients with COPD is related to poor sleep. In one study by Martin and Pak, the overnight fall in lung function at baseline was 20%. Using a long-acting once-daily theophylline preparation dosed at 6–7 P.M., these patients maintained their overnight lung function (22). Further studies need to be performed to determine whether improvement in overnight lung function translates into improved symptoms related to sleep in general.

Theophylline can be a very helpful agent in patients with COPD. A blood level in the range of 10–15 µg/mL is appropriate. If a once-daily preparation is used, the peak level occurs about 10–12 h postdose. If the drug is dosed for nocturnal control, a 5–7 P.M. dosing schedule should be used. The 7–8 A.M. blood level can then be used to gauge the effects of therapy.

B. Anti-Inflammatory Therapy

Although inflammation of the airways is a prominent part of the pathophysiology of asthma, its role in the pathogenesis of COPD has not been fully established. Only a small number of patients with COPD benefit from courses of corticosteroids (inhaled or systemic), and no clinical or physiological indicators have been identified indicating which patients with COPD will respond to corticosteroid therapy (23). Thus, they are generally considered inadequate as monotherapy for COPD. A meta-analysis of the role of corticosteroids in patients with stable airflow limitation suggested that only about 10% of patients will benefit from such therapy (24). This benefit is most substantial when steroids are given in high systemic doses (25). By contrast, in acute exacerbations of COPD, a far greater percentage of patients will derive benefit from a course of systemic corticosteroids (26).

Theophylline has been shown to have important anti-inflammatory effects in asthma (27–29), but this same benefit has yet to be established in COPD. Leukotriene pathway modifiers, commonly used in asthma to interrupt inflammatory pathways (30), may have an important role in reducing sputum production in COPD, although this benefit remains to be established.

C. Other Agents

The major precipitant of acute exacerbations of COPD is respiratory tract infection (31), both viral and bacterial. The airways' inflammatory response caused by acute infection leads to increased production of mucus and limitation of airflow. Antibiotics may be employed in COPD exacerbations to speed symptomatic recovery (32). Pharmacological measures to improve the clearance of mucus—such as attempting to decrease sputum viscosity with mucolytics and rehydration or the addition of an expectorant medication—are largely ineffective and provide little added improvement in respiratory symptoms or function.

VI. Pharmacological Combinations in the Treatment of COPD

A stepwise approach to the management of COPD (Table 1) has been advocated by many authors. Combinations of pharmacological agents with differ-

Table 1 Stepwise Approach to Combination Therapy in COPD

Symptoms	Step I	Step II	Step III	Step IV
		Drug Therapy		
Intermittent symptoms	Intermediate-acting β-agonist (albuterol) 2 actuations qid prn			
Mild persistent symptoms	Ipratropium bromide[a] 2 actuations tid–qid	Intermediate-acting β-agonist (albuterol) (2 actuations qid) prn		
Moderate persistent symptoms	Ipratropium bromide[a] 2–4 actuations qid	Long-acting β-agonist (salmeterol) (2 actuations bid) with albuterol prn for breakthrough symptoms	• Theophylline once- or twice-daily preparations (STC 10–15 μg/mL) • Albuterol prn for breakthrough symptoms	
Severe persistent symptoms	Ipratropium bromide[a] 4 actuations qid	Long-acting β-agonist (salmeterol) (2 actuations bid) with albuterol prn for breakthrough symptoms	• Theophylline once- or twice-daily preparations (STC 10–15 μg/mL) • Albuterol prn for breakthrough symptoms	
Exacerbation	Ipratropium bromide[a] 4 actuations qid	Intermediate-acting β-agonists (albuterol) are used for "rescue" due to rapid onset of action	• Theophylline once- or twice-daily preparations (STC 10–15 μg/mL)	Oral corticosteroid Antibiotic[b] trial

Abbreviations: qid = four times daily; tid = three times daily; bid = twice daily; prn = as needed; STC+ = serum theophylline concentration. Once-daily preparation, blood should be drawn about 12 h postdose. Once-daily dosing time should be between 5–7 P.M. to help improve the overnight decrement in lung function. For twice-daily preparation, blood should be drawn about 8 h postdose.

[a] A combined preparation of ipratropium and albuterol (Combivent) may be efficacious and is more convenient.

[b] The most common bacterium found in COPD exacerbations is *Haemophilus influenzae*.

ent modes of action are often recommended for patients who do not obtain relief of symptoms with ipratropium bromide or β-agonist therapy alone. Combination pharmacotherapy in the treatment of COPD provides several potential benefits: adherence to a regimen of inhaled medications may be improved by simplifying it (e.g., by the use of a single MDI containing two different agents), costs of therapy may be lessened, and additive effects may be obtained from therapies with different mechanisms of action.

A. Anticholinergic/β-Agonist Combinations

Airway smooth muscle tone is maintained by a balance of activity between the sympathetic (adrenergic) and parasympathetic (cholinergic) autonomic nervous systems. Bronchodilation may be obtained either by stimulating adrenergic receptors with β-agonists (e.g., albuterol, fenoterol, salbutamol, salmeterol) or by inhibiting the action of acetylcholine at muscarinic receptors with agents such as ipratropium bromide.

Beginning in the mid-1970s, investigators began conducting trials to evaluate the utility of combining inhaled bronchodilators to alleviate symptoms of chronic airflow limitation. A 1975 report by Petrie and Palmer stimulated interest in combination therapy when it revealed that that both salbutamol and ipratropium bromide led to significant bronchodilation in eight patients with chronic bronchitis, but that the combination of the two produced a slightly greater and more prolonged effect than did either agent alone (33). Following this report, a number of trials were published evaluating different β-agonists— such as fenoterol, metaproterenol, and salbutamol (albuterol)—in combination with ipratropium bromide.

Ipratropium/Fenoterol Combinations

In 1979, Marlin et al. reported an additive bronchodilator effect when fenoterol and ipratropium bromide were administered together to patients with chronic, partially reversible airways obstruction (34). In 20 patients with chronic airflow limitation and $\geq 15\%$ response in FEV_1 to β-agonist bronchodilators, Duovent (a proprietary combination MDI preparation of fenoterol, 100 μg per actuation, and ipratropium bromide, 40 μg per actuation, which is not available in the United States) was shown to produce near maximal bronchodilation in this patient population with two inhaled actuations. Higher doses of either fenoterol or ipratropium (up to eight actuations) yielded only minimal additional bronchodilation at the expense of greater systemic side effects (35).

A benefit of combination bronchodilator therapy was also seen in patients who did not demonstrate significant reversibility on physiological testing. In 1982, Jenkins et al. demonstrated that the combination of nebulized ipratropium bromide and fenoterol administered simultaneously produced greater improvement in FEV_1 than when only one of the two agents was administered to eight patients with obstructive airways disease (36). Ulmer reported a series of 92 patients treated with a metered-dose aerosolized fenoterol/ipratropium bromide combination, demonstrating that patients could safely be treated with this combination for up to 160 months and that when the two agents were administered simultaneously, a 50% reduction in the dose of fenoterol was possible (37). When it was studied in nonasthmatic subjects (i.e., patients without clinically significant reversible airflow limitation), Duovent produced greater bronchodilation than did salbutamol (38) or terbutaline (39) alone. Published commentary on Duovent noted that these preparations safely combined two widely prescribed agents with complementary actions, allowed for a 50% reduction in the β-agonist dose, were more convenient than using two separate MDIs, and were associated with fewer side effects (40). The safety and efficacy of this preparation were further documented in COPD patients by Cecere (41) in 1986 and Stewart (42) in 1987. Additional small studies further reinforced that the combination of fenoterol and ipratropium was safe (43) and more effective in facilitating bronchodilation than either agent alone. This effect was seen with drug delivered either as nebulized solution or aerosol (44).

A double-blind crossover trial of ipratropium bromide 40 µg (two puffs) and fenoterol hydrobromide 200 µg (two puffs) alone and in combination in patients with COPD (FEV_1 < 70% of predicted) was published by Wesseling et al. in 1992 (45). In this trial both ipratropium bromide and fenoterol alone, delivered as two doses separated by 1 h, were shown to result in a significant improvement in FEV_1 and airways resistance when compared with placebo. A slightly greater bronchodilator effect was seen, however, with the combination of the two agents. Twenty minutes after dosing, an increase in FEV_1 of $17.7 \pm 9.6\%$ was noted with ipratropium bromide; with fenoterol, a $34 \pm 14.2\%$ increase was seen; with the combination of the two drugs, an improvement of $38 \pm 17.7\%$ in the FEV_1 was noted. The clinical importance of this small extra improvement with regard to symptoms is questionable.

Ipratropium/Metaproterenol Combinations

In a study published in 1996, Tashkin et al. evaluated the effect of adding nebulized ipratropium bromide to bronchodilator therapy with nebulized metaproterenol sulfate (46). This study enrolled 213 patients with symptomatic, stable COPD (age ≥ 40 years, $FEV_1 < 65\%$ of predicted, $FEV_1/FVC < 70\%$, smoking history >10 pack/years) and randomized them to treatment with nebulized metaproterenol (15 mg) plus placebo or nebulized metaproterenol (15 mg) plus ipratropium bromide (500 μg) dosed three times daily. Patients were allowed to continue other medications during the trial, including theophylline, oral or inhaled corticosteroids, and other forms (MDI, oral, subcutaneous) of β-agonist. More than 85% of patients in both groups were taking other respiratory medications concurrently.

Throughout the 85-day follow-up period, the combination of ipratropium bromide and metaproterenol consistently produced significantly greater bronchodilation, as measured by FEV_1, than did metaproterenol alone ($p < 0.0004$). The response in FVC was comparable. In addition, the duration of effect seen with the combination of bronchodilators was greater than that seen with metaproterenol. These effects persisted throughout the course of the trial. Mean morning and evening peak expiratory flow rates (PEFR) did not change in either group, and patients reported no differences in symptoms of wheezing, dyspnea, or cough. Approximately 25% of patients in each group added or increased the use of systemic corticosteroids during the trial.

Small Trials of Salbutamol (Albuterol)/Ipratropium Combinations

A 1978 study by Leitch et al. evaluated 24 patients meeting the Medical Research Council's criteria for chronic bronchitis and demonstrated that the combination of aerosol ipratropium and salbutamol resulted in small increases in FEV_1, FVC, and exercise tolerance as compared with therapy with either drug alone (47). This additive effect was also reported by Douglas et al. in 1979, when they reported that administration of ipratropium followed by salbutamol led to greater bronchodilation than did the use of either agent alone (48). In a crossover trial in a mixed population of 21 patients with both asthma and chronic bronchitis, Lightbody et al. showed that the combination of aerosolized salbutamol (200 μg, or two puffs, qid) and ipratropium (40 μg, or two puffs, qid) led to greater bronchodilation than did monotherapy with either agent (49). This additive effect has also been demonstrated with drugs administered as nebulized solutions. A placebo-controlled study of 20 patients with COPD and FEV_1 of approximately 33% of predicted showed that the combination of nebulized ipratropium (0.5-mg nebulized solution) and salbutamol (5-mg nebulized solution) produced a bronchodilator response of greater magnitude than that seen with either agent alone. It should be noted that some patients in this study were taking theophylline preparations, although no added effect from theophylline was measured in these patients (50).

Two studies were published in the mid-1980s that called the role of combination therapy with ipratropium bromide and albuterol into question. Easton et al. performed a study in patients with stable COPD in which a maximum dose of either albuterol or ipratropium was administered by aerosol (the first drug was chosen at random), followed by a maximum dose of the other agent (51). They could not demonstrate any additive effect of the second agent to the bronchodilation produced by the first drug. They additionally noted that the bronchodilator effects produced by both ipratropium bromide and albuterol were similar, and that there was no significant difference between the two drugs. They concluded that the two drugs were equipotent and that the combination of the two had no additive effect when maximum doses were given. A study by Lloberes et al. of 13 patients with COPD exacerbation, in which salbutamol, ipratropium, and aminophylline were administered in random sequence, did not demonstrate a greater effect with combination therapy than that attained with the first agent alone (52).

Large Trials of Salbutamol (Albuterol)/Ipratropium Combinations

Although the weight of evidence appeared to support the conclusion that combinations of a β-agonist and ipratropium bromide produced superior bronchodilation than either agent alone, that conclusion was based on numerous small, often statistically underpowered studies of heterogeneous populations. In addition, the endpoints of these trials were almost exclusively spirometric data, not symptom scores, quality of life, or other outcomes relevant to patients. Perhaps because of this paucity of compelling data, combination bronchodilator therapy had never been recommended in the United States, despite its availability in other parts of world. In the early 1990s, the first in a pair of large multicenter, prospective, randomized studies was conducted in the United States to investigate the utility of combination albuterol and ipratropium bromide delivered together as one metered-dose inhalation or as a combined nebulized solution for the management of COPD.

The first study randomized 534 patients with stable COPD [defined as $FEV_1 \leq 65\%$ of predicted and FEV_1/FVC (%) $\leq 70\%$ of predicted, a smoking history, and the requirement of at least two drugs for chronic disease management] to one of three treatment arms: albuterol MDI (two puffs qid at 100 μg per actuation), ipratropium bromide MDI (two puffs qid at 21 μg per actuation), or a Combivent MDI (two puffs qid of aerosol containing 120 μg of albuterol and 21 μg of ipratropium bromide in each actuation). The patients were then followed for 85 days. All drugs were administered four times per

Sutherland and Martin

day. Eighty percent of patients in each group were taking theophylline preparations before randomization and were allowed to continue them during the trial. Of note, patients in this trial were not evaluated for reversibility of airflow limitation prior to randomization.

The results of this trial were as follows (Table 2): first, all three treatment arms produced a clinically significant (i.e., ≥15% above baseline) improvement in the FEV_1. Albuterol alone produced a 24–27% improvement in peak FEV_1, ipratropium alone produced a 24–25% improvement, and the albuterol-ipratropium combination produced increases of between 31 and 33% over baseline FEV_1. The magnitude of this superior ipratropium-albuterol response was statistically significant. A significant improvement was also seen in FVC when combination therapy was compared with bronchodilator monotherapy: albuterol alone yielded an improvement of 24–29%, ipratropium alone a 25–28% improvement, and the combination a 30–40% improvement in FVC. Fewer patients using the bronchodilator combination required rescue therapy with systemic corticosteroids. COPD symptom scores and PEFR did not differ among the treatment arms. The therapeutic effect persisted at 81-day follow up, and no safety issues or important side effects were noted during the trial. This study clearly demonstrated a short-term (85-day) improvement in spirometry with the albuterol/ipratropium combination that was superior to that seen with either agent alone.

Table 2 Results of a Trial ($n = 534$) of Combination Bronchodilator Therapy Delivered via Metered-Dose Inhaler

	Improvement in FEV_1 (L)[a]	Improvement in FVC (%)[b]	Symptom Score	Steroid Rescue (%)[c]
Albuterol MDI	0.29 ($p < 0.001$)	24–29	No significant difference	10.4
Ipratropium MDI	0.30 ($p < 0.001$)	25–28	No significant difference	6.1
Albuterol/ ipratropium MDI	0.37	30–40	No significant difference	3.8

[a] Reported values are from end-of-trial testing, data from other test dates are also significantly different; p values represent comparison with combination therapy.
[b] Reported values are from test dates throughout trial; combination therapy is significantly better than individual therapy.
[c] p-Values not reported.
Source: Ref. 95.

A second study of 652 patients with stable COPD (inclusion criteria identical to those of the previous study) was published by the same group using the combination of albuterol and ipratropium bromide delivered via thrice-daily nebulized solution. Patients were randomized to either albuterol (3 mg nebulized solution in 2.5 mL), ipratropium bromide (0.5 mg nebulized solution in 2.5 mL), or the combination delivered by small-volume nebulizer. Although the medication was prescribed for use three times per day, patients were allowed two extra doses per day on an as-needed basis. Patients were allowed to continue any additional medications that they might have been using prior to the study, including theophylline and oral or inhaled corticosteroids.

In this trial a significant improvement in FEV_1 was noted in all treatment arms, and combination therapy was again shown to be most effective in improving spirometry (Table 3). Improvements in FVC similar to those in FEV_1 were also noted. Evening PEFR measurements in the combination therapy group were significantly higher than those in the albuterol group. Quality-of-life scores were similar in all treatment groups. Therapy was well tolerated by all patients despite the use of higher drug doses in a nebulized form.

Pharmacoeconomic Evaluation—Ipratropium/Albuterol

In a post hoc pharmacoeconomic evaluation of two double-blind trials with a total of 1067 patients with COPD, ipratropium alone or in combination with

Table 3 Results of a Trial ($n = 652$) of Combination Bronchodilator Therapy Delivered via Small-Volume Nebulizer

	Improvement in FEV_1 (L)[a]	Symptom Score	Steroid Rescue
Albuterol	0.29 ($p = 0.001$)	No significant difference	No significant difference
Ipratropium	0.27 ($p < 0.001$)	No significant difference	No significant difference
Albuterol/ Ipratropium	0.34	No significant difference	No significant difference

[a] Reported values are from end-of-trial testing, data from other test dates are also significantly different; p values represent comparison with combination therapy.
Source: Ref. 96.

albuterol was the most cost-effective therapy (53). Ipratropium was used at two actuations (42 µg) four times a day, albuterol was dosed at two actuations (240 µg) four times a day; the combination came from a single MDI. The combination therapy was superior to either agent alone in improving FEV_1. Compared with albuterol, the combination therapy and ipratropium groups experienced significantly fewer exacerbations and patient-days of exacerbations. Also, in the albuterol-alone group, a significant increase in the number of hospital days and antibiotic and corticosteroid use was associated with the exacerbations. The total cost of treatment in this study was significantly less for the ipratropium group ($156 per patient) and for the ipratropium-plus-albuterol group ($197 per patient) than for albuterol group ($269 per patient).

B. β-Agonist/Theophylline Combinations

As noted above, β-adrenergic agonists and theophylline preparations have distinct mechanisms of bronchodilation. Given that β-agonists work to increase the intracellular production of cAMP and that theophyllines work to inhibit cAMP breakdown by phosphodiesterase, in theory a synergistic effect could be obtained by using these two agents in combination.

Many of the studies evaluating the use of theophylline with inhaled bronchodilators are small, crossover-design trials that have shown some degree of therapeutic benefit with this combination of agents. A 1982 study by Lamont and colleagues utilized a crossover design to treat 11 patients with serial regimens of microcrystalline theophylline (375 mg orally), terbutaline (5 mg orally), the combination of both agents, and placebo (54). The authors concluded that the combination of the two drugs led to greater bronchodilation than either drug given alone. In 1985, Taylor and colleagues published a crossover trial of 25 patients with COPD, a mean FEV_1 of approximately 39% of predicted, and varying degrees of reversibility in which patients received serial courses of sustained-release theophylline, inhaled salbutamol (200 µg by MDI qid), the combination of both agents, and placebo in random order over 3-week intervals (55). In this study both theophylline alone and the combination of both agents led to fewer treatment failures (as defined by a deterioration in clinical condition) than did monotherapy with salbutamol, although combination therapy led to the fewest number of treatment failures and higher mean daily peak flow rates. Improvements in FEV_1 and FVC were also seen with combination therapy as compared with placebo. In a similar crossover trial, Tandon and Kailis studied a population of 30 patients with COPD and reversible airflow limitation and showed that a combination of terbutaline (1 mg qid) and theophylline was superior to monotherapy with either agent and placebo in reducing treatment failures and improving mean daily peak flows. In this study, by contrast, inhaled terbutaline was found to be better than monotherapy with theophylline (56).

In 1993, McKay et al. published a trial of escalating theophylline doses in 20 COPD patients who were already being treated with corticosteroids and inhaled bronchodilators. During three separate 6-week-long treatment periods, patients randomly received placebo, theophylline doses to achieve a serum concentration of 10 µg/mL, and theophylline doses to achieve a serum concentration of 17 µg/mL (57). A less impressive effect of theophylline on symptoms was noted by Nishimura and colleagues when they added oral theophylline (400 mg p.o. qd for 2 weeks followed by 600 mg p.o. qd for 2 weeks) to the regimen of patients already treated with salbutamol (200 µg by MDI qid) and ipratropium bromide (40 µg by MDI qid). Although the addition of theophylline significantly improved FEV_1 and daily peak flows, patients noted no significant improvement in symptoms of airflow limitation (58).

C. Inhaled Bronchodilator/Corticosteroid Combinations

Although systemic and/or inhaled corticosteroids are routinely utilized in the long-term control of symptoms of airflow limitation in asthma, the role of corticosteroids in the treatment of stable COPD remains controversial. Despite this controversy, the use of inhaled corticosteroids appears to be increasing among patients with COPD (59). Although there is no clinical evidence (see below) demonstrating a benefit to patients who take inhaled corticosteroids in combination with inhaled bronchodilators, there is some evidence for a theoretical role for the use of corticosteroids in COPD. In in vitro models, corticosteroids increase the number of β-adrenergic receptors (60), increase the pharmacological effect of β-agonists (61), and may even reduce desensitization of β-receptors to β-agonist bronchodilators (62).

These theoretical benefits are not borne out in clinical trials, however. A crossover trial of 10 patients with COPD demonstrated that treatment with inhaled budesonide (1.6 mg/day for 3 weeks) or oral prednisone (40 mg p.o. qd for 8 days) did not significantly improve response to inhaled ipratropium bromide, salbutamol, or the combination of both bronchodilators (63). A crossover trial by Watson et al. of 14 subjects with mild airways obstruction compared the effects of 3 months of treatment with an inhaled budesonide (600 µg bid) with placebo on responses to inhaled bronchodilators (salbutamol 5 mg and ipratropium bromide 0.5 mg) (64). No significant changes in FEV_1, vital capacity, or bronchodilator responsiveness were noted at the end of 3 months. Following the 3-month crossover trial, six subjects were maintained on budesonide for 9 months, and the results were compared with those of six subjects who received no treatment for the subsequent nine months. No improvements in baseline spirometry, home peak flow measurements, or bronchoconstrictor/bronchodilator responsiveness were observed after a total of 12 months of budesonide treatment. In 1998 crossover trial, Corden and Rees investigated 20 patients with COPD who were already being treated with various combinations and doses of inhaled β-agonists, inhaled anticholinergic agents, and inhaled corticosteroids (65). The subjects received in sequence placebo or prednisolone, 30 mg p.o. qd, for 3 weeks and then were crossed over to the other agent. Although there was a trend toward improvement of baseline spirometry after treatment with prednisolone, this study failed to demonstrate a clinically significant increase in bronchodilator response to β-agonists or anticholinergics after treatment with corticosteroids.

Two recent studies of inhaled corticosteroids provide conflicting data as to their effect in patients with stable COPD. The first study, by Bourbeau and colleagues, was designed to evaluate the role of high-dose inhaled corticosteroids for the management of stable COPD in patients who did show spirometric improvement after a course of oral corticosteroids (66). The first phase of the study identified patients who did not respond to oral corticosteroids, and—consistent with previously published data (24)—approximately 90% (in this study, 86.5%) of subjects with COPD did not improve their spirometry after a 2-week course of prednisone, 40 mg p.o. qd. Nonresponders were then randomized to treatment with inhaled budesonide, 400 μg by inhaler bid for 6 months or to placebo. At the end of the study period there were no differences in FEV_1, exercise capacity, quality of life, or symptom scores between the two groups. All patients were treated with at least one bronchodilating agent throughout the course of the study.

The second study, by Paggiaro et al., did not stratify patients by corticosteroid responsiveness prior to their entry into the trial (67). The study included subjects with a diagnosis of COPD who did not have evidence of significant reversibility on spirometry after treatment with salbutamol. Patients were randomly assigned to either placebo or two puffs (250 μg) of fluticasone dipropionate bid for 6 months. Patients were allowed to continue short-acting β-agonists (e.g., salbutamol), anticholinergics (e.g., ipratropium bromide), and xanthine derivatives (e.g., theophylline) as desired throughout the study. Daily cough scores were reduced in patients treated with fluticasone, as was daily sputum volume. There were no significant differences in the use of additional bronchodilator medications or in symptoms of breathlessness. During the trial periods, there was a significant increase in peak expiratory flow rates as well as in FEV_1. Statistically significant increases in both FEV_1 (9.4% or 0.15 L) and FVC (5.6% or 0.33 L) were noted at the end of the study. However, these improvements, though statistically significant, do not meet spirometric criteria for clinically relevant improvements in airflow limitation.

A 1999 meta-analysis of three long-term prospective, randomized, placebo-controlled clinical trials of inhaled corticosteroids (68–70) was designed to evaluate the effect of inhaled corticosteroids on decline in lung function in COPD as measured by FEV_1 (71). Many of the patients in the original studies demonstrated a high level of bronchodilator response and were therefore not felt to adequately represent patients with COPD. The authors of this meta-analysis used original clinical data from each trial, including only patients who met strict diagnostic criteria for COPD as defined by a constellation of symptoms, advanced age, smoking history, reduced FEV_1, and the absence of significant response in FEV_1 to β-agonist bronchodilators. In patients treated with inhaled corticosteroids (varied medications and doses) along with concomitant use of bronchodilators—including β-agonists, anticholinergics, and theophylline—an annual increase in prebronchodilator FEV_1 of 0.034 L/year and postbronchodilator FEV_1 of 0.039L/year were noted. This stands in contrast to the typical decrease in FEV_1 of approximately 0.06 L/year described in population studies of patients with COPD. No significant difference in the number of COPD exacerbations was noted.

VII. COPD Exacerbations

A. Combination Bronchodilator Therapy in Exacerbations of COPD

It remains questionable whether combination bronchodilator therapy improves outcomes in acute exacerbations of COPD. In a study of patients admitted to a large urban emergency department, Shrestha et al. demonstrated that the addition of nebulized ipratropium bromide (36 and 54 µg as two or three puffs) to isoetharine (at 5 mg as 0.5 mL of 1% solution) caused a more rapid subjective improvement and allowed patients to be discharged more rapidly from the emergency department (72). All subjects were treated with theophylline preparations as well. No significant differences in FEV_1 or FVC were seen in patients who received combination therapy as compared with patients receiving only isoetharine.

Other studies show no benefit to combinations of inhaled bronchodilators in COPD exacerbations. A study of 51 patients with acute exacerbations of COPD by Rebuck et al. showed that treatment with regimens of ipratropium bromide (0.5 mg of nebulized solution), fenoterol (1.25 mg of nebulized solution), or both all resulted in similar improvements in FEV_1 after 45–90 min of emergency department observation (73). A smaller crossover study of ipratropium bromide and metaproterenol in which patients with COPD exacerbation first received either ipratropium bromide MDI (54 µg in three puffs) or metaproterenol MDI (1.95 mg) alone, followed 90 min later by the other agent, confirmed that the agents did not produce any added effect when administered serially (74). In a 1995 study of 70 patients admitted with COPD exacerbation and randomized to nebulized salbutamol (5 mg) or nebulized salbutamol (5 mg) plus nebulized ipratropium bromide (500 µg), there were no differences in length of stay, symptoms, or spirometric measurements between the two groups (75). Thus, although there are minimal data to support the routine use of combination therapy in COPD exacerbations, some authors recommend employing combination therapy when patients fail to respond adequately to therapy with a single inhaled bronchodilator (76).

B. Antibiotic Therapy in Exacerbations of COPD

Bacterial respiratory tract infections play an important role in the pathogenesis of COPD exacerbations. *Haemophilus influenzae* is the bacterium most commonly isolated from sputum in patients with COPD exacerbation, although other organisms, including *Streptococcus pneumoniae*, may be isolated (77). A meta-analysis of nine randomized trials of antibiotics in COPD exacerbations demonstrated a small overall benefit to the use of antibiotics as measured by a summary estimate combining the diverse endpoints of the included trials. In addition, a small improvement in PEFR of 10.75 L/min was noted in patients receiving antibiotics (32). A recent qualitative review of antibiotic use in COPD notes that appropriate antibiotic therapy in exacerbations of COPD may prevent respiratory failure and hospitalization, thereby improving clinical outcomes and resulting in lower overall health care expenditures (78).

VIII. Nonpharmacological Therapy of COPD

Although many pharmacological measures are available for the treatment of COPD, additional nonpharmacological modalities have proved to be important

Table 4 Important Adjuncts to Pharmacotherapy of COPD

Patient education
Smoking cessation
Long-term oxygen therapy (if hypoxemia or cor pulmonale is
  present)
Exercise and pulmonary rehabilitation
Vaccination for pneumococci and influenza

additions to the management of COPD (Table 4). Smoking cessation is recommended for all patients with COPD, and supplemental oxygen therapy has a clearly defined role in reducing mortality in those patients with COPD who are hypoxemic. Preventive care by means of routine immunizations and exercise may also help improve quality of life in patients with COPD.

A. Smoking Cessation

Smoking cessation is associated with a significant reduction in the rate of decline in FEV_1. Rates of smoking cessation as high as 30% after 1 year as well as improvements in FEV_1, have been reported in patients receiving care from specialty smoking cessation programs (79). Patients who stop smoking can reduce their rate of decline in FEV_1 to match that of never-smokers, thus slowing disease progression. For this reason, every effort should be made to encourage abstinence from tobacco in patients with COPD. A successful regimen for smoking cessation is dependent on multiple interventions, including clinician support, a strong social support network, and pharmacological intervention to reduce nicotine withdrawal symptoms (80). Effective pharmacological interventions for smoking cessation are reviewed elsewhere (81) and include nicotine replacement (by transdermal route or polacrilex chewing gum) and sustained-release oral bupropion.

B. Long-Term Oxygen Therapy

Supplemental oxygen therapy has been shown to reduce mortality in certain subsets of patients with COPD. Other benefits of long-term oxygen therapy include improved exercise tolerance, correction of erythrocytosis, and prevention/regression of cor pulmonale and pulmonary hypertension. Two separate controlled studies—the Medical Research Council (MRC) study (82), which compared oxygen therapy for 15 h/day with no oxygen, and the Nocturnal Oxygen Therapy Trial (NOTT) (83), which compared continuous oxygen with nocturnal oxygen—demonstrated that long-term oxygen therapy improved survival in hypoxemic COPD patients. This reduction in mortality is likely due to a reduction in secondary pulmonary hypertension due to chronic alveolar hypoxia.

Secondary pulmonary hypertension is a common and progressive complication of advanced COPD. Patients treated with oxygen in the MRC study (82) showed no significant increase in pulmonary arterial pressure after approximately 2 years when compared with controls; in the NOTT (83), patients treated with continuous oxygen demonstrated a reduction in pulmonary arterial pressure at 6 months, whereas patients receiving nocturnal oxygen had stable pulmonary artery pressures. Longer-term follow-up studies have supported the shorter-term results seen in these studies. In one prospective series in which patients were followed for 6 years, long-term oxygen therapy for 14 to 15 h/day resulted in a reduction in pulmonary artery pressures over the first 2 years. After the first 2 years of the study, pulmonary artery pressures returned to their initial levels but stabilized. This effect on pulmonary hypertension occurred despite progression of arterial hypoxemia and expiratory airflow limitation (84).

Patients who are not hypoxemic at rest may demonstrate oxygen desaturation during exercise or during sleep, with resultant pulmonary hypertension. Oxygen therapy during sleep may militate against the development of pulmonary hypertension, and supplemental oxygen during exercise relieves exertional dyspnea and improves exercise tolerance (85); it can also prevent transient increases in pulmonary vascular resistance and pulmonary artery pressure (86). Supplemental oxygen also reduces the work and oxygen cost of breathing, improves neuropsychological performance, and reduces arousals during sleep. It should be noted that anecdotal concerns about oxygen therapy causing suppression of respiratory drive are overemphasized; the therapeutic benefit of correcting tissue hypoxia and pulmonary hypertension far outweigh the small risk of carbon dioxide retention (87).

The decision to initiate long-term oxygen therapy is based on arterial blood gas analysis or oxygen saturation while breathing room air. Current recommendations state that long-term oxygen therapy should be considered in COPD patients with a resting $Pa_{O_2} \leq$ mmHg or an oxygen saturation $(Sp_{O_2}) \leq 89\%$ (Table 5). These guidelines are utilized by Medicare and insurance companies for reimbursement. After the initiation of therapy, pulse oximetry may be used to titrate flow rates at rest, with exertion, and during sleep to a goal of $Sp_{O_2} \geq 90\%$. Patients who must travel by airline should increase the oxygen flow rate by 1–2 L/min during flight (88).

Table 5 Indications for Long-Term Oxygen Therapy

Continuous supplemental oxygen
  Resting $Pa_{O_2} \leq 55$ mmHg
  Resting $Sp_{O_2} \leq 89\%$
  Pa_{O_2} 55–59 mmHg or $Sp_{O_2} \geq 89\%$ in the presence of cor pulmonale or
    congestive heart failure
Intermittent supplemental oxygen
  $Pa_{O_2} \leq 55$ mmHg or $Sp_{O_2} \leq 89\%$ with exercise (low-level)
  $Pa_{O_2} \leq 55$ mmHg or $Sp_{O_2} \leq 89\%$ during sleep not corrected by CPAP/BiPAP

Abbreviations: CPAP = continuous positive airway pressure; BiPAP = bilevel positive airway pressure.

C. Pulmonary Rehabilitation

Referral for pulmonary rehabilitation should be considered in patients with moderate to severe COPD. An effective pulmonary rehabilitation program comprises rehabilitation techniques aimed at improving quality of life and overall health status. Components of a typical pulmonary rehabilitation program include exercise training, breathing retraining to increase respiratory muscle strength and function, home care (when needed), and psychosocial support (89).

Although pulmonary rehabilitation programs have not been shown to improve survival and do not routinely improve airflow limitation, several studies support the role of pulmonary rehabilitation in improving quality of life in patients with COPD. Compared with education alone, a comprehensive pulmonary rehabilitation program results in improvements in maximal exercise tolerance and oxygen uptake, exercise endurance, and symptoms of perceived breathlessness and muscle fatigue (90). Most outpatient rehabilitation programs are hospital-based, but participation in a home-based program (now more common, given increased pressures to reduce both the number and duration of hospitalizations) also significantly improves quality-of-life measures (91). In addition to improving quality of life, pulmonary rehabilitation programs have been shown to reduce the utilization of health care resources by patients with COPD. Two studies of patients who had undergone pulmonary rehabilitation demonstrated a subsequent reduction in the total number of days spent in the hospital for pulmonary disease (92,93).

D. Health Care Maintenance

Health care maintenance in COPD should consist of routine preventive care, with special attention to reducing the risk of respiratory tract infections. As such, it is recommended that all patients with COPD be immunized against influenza on a yearly basis and receive a pneumococcal vaccine once every 5 years. A large number of COPD patients are chronically malnourished, so careful attention should also be paid to maintaining nutritional balance and ideal body weight (94).

IX. Summary

Therapeutic interventions in COPD must be approached by both pharmacological (Table 1) and nonpharmacological (Tables 4–5) strategies to effect the best outcome for the patient. Patient education, no matter what the disease, is paramount, as this will lead to a better understanding of what the caregiver is trying to accomplish and thus better compliance with the entire program. Smoking cessation is one of the most important aspects of the program, as well as supplemental oxygen if needed. Health maintenance—with vaccination and rehabilitation programs—adds to the beneficial outcomes.

Although COPD is commonly associated with ''nonreversibility'' of airflow obstruction, patients do respond to bronchodilation therapy. Table 1 gives a general algorithm that can be altered to best suit the individual patient. In the patients with more moderate to severe COPD, a common mistake is to underdose ipratropium bromide. Overall, combination therapy is superior to a single agent in COPD. The most commonly used combination therapy is ipratropium and a β_2-agonist. However, individual patients may respond very well to the addition of theophylline. As we learn more about the phenotype of the COPD patient who is helped by inhaled steroids, this form of additive therapy will be better directed.

References

1. American Thoracic Society. Standards for the diagnosis and care of patients with chronic obstructive pulmonary disease: definitions, epidemiology, pathophysiology, diagnosis, and staging. Am Rev Respir Dis 1995; 152:S78–S83.
2. Higgins MW, Thom T. Incidence, prevalence and mortality: intra- and inter-county differences. In: Hensley MD, Saunders NA, eds. Clinical Epidemiology of Chronic Obstructive Pulmonary Disease. New York: Marcel Dekker, 1990: 23–43.
3. Feinleib M, Rosenberg HM, Collins JG, Delozier JE, Pokras R, Chevarley FM. Trends in COPD morbidity and mortality in the United States. Am Rev Respir Dis 1989; 140:S9–S18.

4. NHLBI. The definition of emphysema. Report of a National Heart, Lung, and Blood Institute Division of Lung Diseases workshop. Am Rev Respir Dis 1985; 132:182–185.
5. American Thoracic Society. Lung function testing: selection of reference values and interpretative strategies. Am Rev Respir Dis 1991; 144:1202–1218.
6. Anthonisen NR, Connett JE, Kiley JP, Altose MD, Bailey WC, Buist AS, Conway WAJ, Enright PL, Kanner RE, O'Hara P, Owens GR, Scanlon PO, Tashkin DP, Wise RA. Effects of smoking intervention and the use of an inhaled anticholinergic bronchodilator on the rate of decline of FEV_1. The Lung Health Study. JAMA 1994; 272:1497–1505.
7. Camilli AE, Burrows B, Knudson RJ, Lyle SK, Lebowitz MD. Longitudinal changes in forced expiratory volume in one second in adults: effects of smoking and smoking cessation. Am Rev Respir Dis 1987; 135:794–799.
8. Hodgkin JE. Prognosis in chronic obstructive pulmonary disease. Clin Chest Med 1990; 11:555–569.
9. Celli BR. Standards for the optimal management of COPD: a summary. Chest 1998; 113:283S–287S.
10. Vollmer WM, Johnson LR, Buist AS. Relationship of response to a bronchodilator and decline in forced expiratory volume in one second in population studies. Am Rev Respir Dis 1985; 132:1186–1193.
11. Gross NJ. Ipratropium bromide. N Engl J Med 1988; 319:486–494.
12. Levin DC, Little KS, Laughlin KR, Galbraith JM, Gustman PM, Murphy D, Kram JA, Mardie G, Reuter C, Ostransky D, McFarland K, Petty TL, Silvers W, Rennard SI, Mueller M, Repsmer LM, Zuwallack RL, Vale R. Addition of anticholinergic solution prolongs bronchodilator effect of $beta_2$ agonists in patients with chronic obstructive pulmonary disease. Am J Med 1996; 100:40S–48S.
13. Anthonisen NR, Wright EC. Bronchodilator response in chronic obstructive pulmonary disease. Am Rev Respir Dis 1986; 133:814–819.
14. Wanner A, Salathe M, O'Riordan TG. Mucociliary clearance in the airways. Am J Respir Crit Care Med 1996; 154:1868–1902.
15. Madison JM, Irwin RS. Chronic obstructive pulmonary disease. Lancet 1998; 352:467–473.
16. Boyd G, Morice AH, Pounsford JC, Siebert M, Peslis N, Crawford C. An evaluation of salmeterol in the treatment of chronic obstructive pulmonary disease (COPD). Eur Respir J 1997; 10:815–821.
17. Murciano D, Auclair MH, Pariente R, Aubier M. A randomized, controlled trial of theophylline in patients with severe chronic obstructive pulmonary disease. N Engl J Med 1989; 320:1521–1525.
18. Mahler DA, Matthay RA, Snyder PE, Wells CK, Loke J. Sustained-release theophylline reduces dyspnea in nonreversible obstructive airway disease. Am Rev Respir Dis 1985; 131:22–25.
19. Chrystyn H, Mulley BA, Peake MD. Dose response relation to oral theophylline in severe chronic obstructive airways disease. BMJ 1988; 297:1506–1510.

20. Ziment I. Theophylline and mucociliary clearance. Chest 1987; 92:38S–43S.
21. Matthay RA, Berger HJ, Davies R, Loke J, Gottschalk A, Zaret BL. Improvement in cardiac performance by oral long-acting theophylline in chronic obstructive pulmonary disease. Am Heart J 1982; 104:1022–1026.
22. Martin RJ, Pak J. Overnight theophylline concentrations and effects on sleep and lung function in chronic obstructive pulmonary disease. Am Rev Respir Dis 1992; 145:540–544.
23. Chapman KR. Therapeutic approaches to chronic obstructive pulmonary disease: an emerging consensus. Am J Med 1996; 100:5S–10S.
24. Callahan CM, Dittus RS, Katz BP. Oral corticosteroid therapy for patients with stable chronic obstructive pulmonary disease: a meta-analysis. Ann Intern Med 1991; 114:216–223.
25. Wedzicha JA. Inhaled corticosteroids in COPD: awaiting controlled trials. Thorax 1993; 48:305–307.
26. Thompson WH, Nielson CP, Carvalho P, Charan NB, Crowley JJ. Controlled trial of oral prednisone in outpatients with acute COPD exacerbation. Am J Respir Crit Care Med 1996; 154:407–412.
27. Sullivan P, Bekir S, Jaffar Z, Page C, Jeffery P, Costello J. Anti-inflammatory effects of low-dose oral theophylline in atopic asthma (published erratum appears in Lancet 1994; 343:1512). Lancet 1994; 343:1006–1008.
28. Kidney J, Dominguez M, Taylor PM, Rose M, Chung KF, Barnes PJ. Immunomodulation by theophylline in asthma: demonstration by withdrawal of therapy. Am J Respir Crit Care Med 1995; 151:1907–1914.
29. Finnerty JP, Lee C, Wilson S, Madden J, Djukanovic R, Holgate ST. Effects of theophylline on inflammatory cells and cytokines in asthmatic subjects: a placebo-controlled parallel group study. Eur Respir J 1996; 9:1672–1677.
30. Rodgers IW. Leukotrienes, asthma, and the preclinical science of montelukast. Eur Respir Rev 1998; 8:358–360.
31. Wilson R. The role of infection in COPD. Chest 1998; 113:242S–248S.
32. Saint S, Bent S, Vittinghoff E, Grady D. Antibiotics in chronic obstructive pulmonary disease exacerbations: a meta-analysis. JAMA 1995; 273:957–960.
33. Petrie GR, Palmer KN. Comparison of aerosol ipratropium bromide and salbutamol in chronic bronchitis and asthma. BMJ 1975; 1:430–432.
34. Marlin GE, Berend N, Harrison AC. Combined cholinergic antagonist and beta$_2$-adrenoceptor agonist bronchodilator therapy by inhalation. Aust NZ J Med 1979; 9:511–514.
35. Packe GE, Archer PS, Cayton RM. A dose-response and duration of action assessment of a combined preparation of fenoterol and ipratropium bromide (Duovent). Postgrad Med J 1984; 60:18–22.
36. Jenkins CR, Chow CM, Fisher BL, Marlin GE. Ipratropium bromide and fenoterol by aerosolized solution. Br J Clin Pharmacol 1982; 14:113–115.
37. Ulmer WT. Treatment of obstructive disease with fenoterol-ipratropiumbromid

dosage aerosol (IK 6): short and long-terms results. Med Klin 1979; 74:1548–1552.

38. Marangio E, Pesci A, Mori A, Marchioni M, Bertorelli G. Clinical physiological data on the bronchodilator effect of Duovent versus salbutamol in chronic obstructive lung disease. Respiration 1986; 50:165–168.

39. Longhini E, Bozzoni M, Mastropasqua B, Marazzini L. Evaluation of the intensity and duration of the bronchodilatory action of fenoterol-ipratropium bromide in combination compared with terbutaline and placebo in patients with chronic obstructive lung disease. Respiration 1986; 50:169–172.

40. Phillips VJ. The background to Duovent. Postgrad Med J 1984; 60:13–17.

41. Cecere L, Funaro G, De Cataldis G, Carnicelli P, Pinto R. Long-term treatment with "Duovent" in elderly patients affected by chronic obstructive lung disease. Respiration 1986; 50:245–248.

42. Stewart DE, Gillies AJ. A dose response study comparing Duovent vs salbutamol. NZ Med J 1987; 100:742–744.

43. Serra C, Giacopelli A. Controlled clinical study of a long-term treatment of chronic obstructive lung disease using a combination of fenoterol and ipratropium bromide in aerosol form. Respiration 1986; 50:249–253.

44. Marlin GE. Studies of ipratropium bromide and fenoterol administered by metered-dose inhaler and aerosolized solution. Respiration 1986; 50:290–293.

45. Wesseling G, Mostert R, Wouters EF. A comparison of the effects of anticholinergic and beta$_2$-agonist and combination therapy on respiratory impedance in COPD. Chest 1992; 101:166–173.

46. Tashkin DP, Bleecker E, Braun S, Campbell S, DeGraff AC Jr, Hudgel DW, Boyars MC, Sahn S. Results of a multicenter study of nebulized inhalant bronchodilator solutions. Am J Med 1996; 100:62S–69S.

47. Leitch AG, Hopkin JM, Ellis DA, Merchant S, McHardy GJ. The effect of aerosol ipratropium bromide and salbutamol on exercise tolerance in chronic bronchitis. Thorax 1978; 33:711–713.

48. Douglas NJ, Davidson I, Sudlow MF, Flenley DC. Bronchodilatation and the site of airway resistance in severe chronic bronchitis. Thorax 1979; 34:51–56.

49. Lightbody IM, Ingram CG, Legge JS, Johnston RN. Ipratropium bromide, salbutamol and prednisolone in bronchial asthma and chronic bronchitis. Br J Dis Chest 1978; 72:181–186.

50. Chan CS, Brown IG, Kelly CA, Dent AG, Zimmerman PV. Bronchodilator responses to nebulised ipratropium and salbutamol singly and in combination in chronic bronchitis. Br J Clin Pharmacol 1984; 17:103–105.

51. Easton PA, Jadue C, Dhingra S, Anthonisen NR. A comparison of the bronchodilating effects of a beta-2 adrenergic agent (albuterol) and an anticholinergic agent (ipratropium bromide), given by aerosol alone or in sequence. N Engl J Med 1986; 315:735–739.

52. Lloberes P, Ramis L, Montserrat JM, Serra J, Campistol J, Picado C, Agusti-

Vidal A. Effect of three different bronchodilators during an exacerbation of chronic obstructive pulmonary disease. Eur Respir J 1988; 1:536–539.

53. Friedman M, Serby CW, Menjoge SS, Wilson JD, Hilleman DE, Witek TJ Jr. Pharmacoeconomic evaluation of a combination of ipratropium plus albuterol compared with ipratropium alone and albuterol alone in COPD. Chest 1999; 115: 635–641.

54. Lamont H, van der Straeten M, Pauwels R, Moerman E, Bogaert M. The combined effect of theophylline and terbutaline in patients with chronic obstructive airway diseases. Eur J Respir Dis 1982; 63:13–22.

55. Taylor DR, Buick B, Kinney C, Lowry RC, McDevitt DG. The efficacy of orally administered theophylline, inhaled salbutamol, and a combination of the two as chronic therapy in the management of chronic bronchitis with reversible air-flow obstruction. Am Rev Respir Dis 1985; 131:747–751.

56. Tandon MK, Kailis SG. Bronchodilator treatment for partially reversible chronic obstructive airways disease. Thorax 1991; 46:248–251.

57. McKay SE, Howie CA, Thomson AH, Whiting B, Addis GJ. Value of theophylline treatment in patients handicapped by chronic obstructive lung disease. Thorax 1993; 48:227–232.

58. Nishimura K, Koyama H, Ikeda A, Izumi T. Is oral theophylline effective in combination with both inhaled anticholinergic agent and inhaled beta$_2$-agonist in the treatment of stable COPD? Chest 1993; 104:179–184.

59. Van Andel AE, Reisner C, Menjoge SS, Witek TJ. Analysis of inhaled corticosteroids and oral theophylline use among COPD patients from 1987 to 1996. Am J Respir Crit Care Med 1997; 155:A279.

60. Fraser CM, Venter JC. The synthesis of beta-adrenergic receptors in cultured human lung cells: induction by glucocorticoids. Biochem Biophys Res Commun 1980; 94:390–397.

61. Geddes BA, Jones TR, Dvorsky RJ, Lefcoe NM. Interaction of glucocorticoids and bronchodilators on isolated guinea pig tracheal and human bronchial smooth muscle. Am Rev Respir Dis 1974; 110:420–427.

62. Hui KK, Conolly ME, Tashkin DP. Reversal of human lymphocyte beta-adrenoceptor desensitization by glucocorticoids. Clin Pharmacol Ther 1982; 32:566–571.

63. Wempe JB, Postma DS, Breederveld N, Kort E, van der Mark TW, Koeter GH. Effects of corticosteroids on bronchodilator action in chronic obstructive lung disease. Thorax 1992; 47:616–621.

64. Watson A, Lim TK, Joyce H, Pride NB. Failure of inhaled corticosteroids to modify bronchoconstrictor or bronchodilator responsiveness in middle-aged smokers with mild airflow obstruction. Chest 1992; 101:350–355.

65. Corden Z, Rees PJ. The effect of oral corticosteroids on bronchodilator responses in COPD. Respir Med 1998; 92:279–282.

66. Bourbeau J, Rouleau MY, Boucher S. Randomised controlled trial of inhaled corticosteroids in patients with chronic obstructive pulmonary disease. Thorax 1998; 53:477–482.

67. Paggiaro PL, Dahle R, Bakran I, Frith L, Hollingworth K, Efthimiou J. Multicentre randomised placebo-controlled trial of inhaled fluticasone propionate in patients with chronic obstructive pulmonary disease: International COPD Study Group. Lancet 1998; 351:773–780.

68. Renkema TE, Schouten JP, Koeter GH, Postma DS. Effects of long-term treatment with corticosteroids in COPD. Chest 1996; 109:1156–1162.

69. Kerstjens HA, Brand PL, Hughes MD, Robinson NJ, Postma DS, Sluiter HJ, Bleeker ER, Dekmuijzen PN, De Jong PM, Mengelers MJ, Overbeek SE, Schoonbrood DFME. A comparison of bronchodilator therapy with or without inhaled corticosteroid therapy for obstructive airways disease: Dutch Chronic Non-Specific Lung Disease Study Group. N Engl J Med 1992; 327:1413–1419.

70. Derenne JP. Effects of high dose inhaled beclomethasone in the rate of decline in FEV_1 in patients with chronic obstructive pulmonary disease: results of a two-year prospective multicenter study. Am J Respir Crit Care Med 1995; 151:A463.

71. Fletcher C, Peto R, Tinker C, Speizer FE. The Natural History of Chronic Bronchitis and Emphysema: An Eight-Year Study of Early Chronic Obstructive Lung Disease in Working Men in London. Oxford, UK: Oxford University Press, 1976.

72. Shrestha M, O'Brien T, Haddox R, Gourlay HS, Reed G. Decreased duration of emergency department treatment of chronic obstructive pulmonary disease exacerbations with the addition of ipratropium bromide to beta-agonist therapy. Ann Emerg Med 1991; 20:1206–1209.

73. Rebuck AS, Chapman KR, Abboud R, Pare PD, Kreisman H, Wolkove N, et al. Nebulized anticholinergic and sympathomimetic treatment of asthma and chronic obstructive airways disease in the emergency room. Am J Med 1987; 82:59–64.

74. Karpel JP, Pesin J, Greenberg D, Gentry E. A comparison of the effects of ipratropium bromide and metaproterenol sulfate in acute exacerbations of COPD. Chest 1990; 98:835–839.

75. Moayyedi P, Congleton J, Page RL, Pearson SB, Muers MF. Comparison of nebulised salbutamol and ipratropium bromide with salbutamol alone in the treatment of chronic obstructive pulmonary disease. Thorax 1995; 50:834–837.

76. Ikeda A, Nishimura K, Izumi T. Pharmacological treatment in acute exacerbations of chronic obstructive pulmonary disease. Drugs Aging 1998; 12:129–137.

77. Chodosh S. Acute bacterial exacerbations in bronchitis and asthma. Am J Med 1987; 82:154–163.

78. Grossman RF. The value of antibiotics and the outcomes of antibiotic therapy in exacerbations of COPD. Chest 1998; 113:249S–255S.

79. Pederson LL, Williams JI, Lefcoe NM. Smoking cessation among pulmonary patients as related to type of respiratory disease and demographic variables. Can J Public Health 1980; 71:191–194.

80. Kottke TE, Battista RN, DeFriese GH, Brekke ML. Attributes of successful smoking cessation interventions in medical practice: a meta-analysis of 39 controlled trials. JAMA 1988; 259:2883–2889.

81. Jorenby DE, Leischow SJ, Nides MA, Rennard SI, Johnston JA, Hughes AR, Smith SS, Muramoto ML, Daughton D, Doan K, Fiore MC, Baker TB. A controlled trial of sustained-release bupropion, a nicotine patch, or both for smoking cessation. N Engl J Med 1999; 340:685–691.

82. Medical Research Council. Long term domiciliary oxygen therapy in chronic hypoxic cor pulmonale complicating chronic bronchitis and emphysema. Lancet 1981; 1:681–686.

83. Timms RM, Khaja FU, Williams GW. Hemodynamic response to oxygen therapy in chronic obstructive pulmonary disease. Ann Intern Med 1985; 102:29–36.

84. Zielinski J, Tobiasz M, Hawrylkiewicz I, Sliwinski P, Palasiewicz G. Effects of long-term oxygen therapy on pulmonary hemodynamics in COPD patients: a 6-year prospective study. Chest 1998; 113:65–70.

85. Liker ES, Karnick A, Lerner L. Portable oxygen in chronic obstructive lung disease with hypoxemia and cor pulmonale: a controlled double-blind crossover study. Chest 1975; 68:236–241.

86. Dempsey JA, Vidruk EH, Mastenbrook SM. Pulmonary control systems in exercise. Fed Proc 1980; 39:1498–1505.

87. Tarpy SP, Celli BR. Long-term oxygen therapy. N Engl J Med 1995; 333:710–714.

88. Gong H Jr. Air travel and oxygen therapy in cardiopulmonary patients. Chest 1992; 101:1104–1113.

89. ACCP/AACVPR. Pulmonary rehabilitation: joint ACCP/AACVPR evidence-based guidelines. Chest 1997; 112:1363–1396.

90. Ries AL, Kaplan RM, Limberg TM, Prewitt LM. Effects of pulmonary rehabilitation on physiologic and psychosocial outcomes in patients with chronic obstructive pulmonary disease. Ann Intern Med 1995; 122:823–832.

91. Reina-Rosenbaum R, Bach JR, Penek J. The cost/benefits of outpatient-based pulmonary rehabilitation. Arch Phys Med Rehabil 1997; 78:240–244.

92. Lertzman MM, Cherniack RM. Rehabilitation of patients with chronic obstructive pulmonary disease. Am Rev Respir Dis 1976; 114:1145–1165.

93. Hudson LD, Tyler ML, Petty TL. Hospitalization needs during an outpatient rehabilitation program for severe chronic airway obstruction. Chest 1976; 70:606–610.

94. American Thoracic Society. Standards for the diagnosis and care of patients with chronic obstructive pulmonary disease: additional considerations. Am Rev Respir Dis 1995; 152:S111–S113.

95. Combivent Inhalation Aerosol Study Group. In chronic obstructive pulmonary disease, a combination of ipratropium and albuterol is more effective than either agent alone: an 85-day multicenter trial. Chest 1994; 105:1411–1419.

96. Combivent Inhalation Aerosol Study Group. Routine nebulized ipratropium and albuterol together are better than either alone in COPD. Chest 1997; 112:1514–1521.

AUTHOR INDEX

U

SUBJECT INDEX